T0257090

AS THE WORLD AGES

As the World Ages

RETHINKING A DEMOGRAPHIC CRISIS

Kavita
Sivaramakrishnan

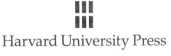

Harvard University Press

Cambridge, Massachusetts
London, England
2018

Copyright © 2018 by the President and Fellows of Harvard College

ALL RIGHTS RESERVED

Printed in the United States of America

First printing

Library of Congress Cataloging-in-Publication Data

Names: Sivaramakrishnan, Kavita, author.
Title: As the world ages : rethinking a demographic crisis / Kavita Sivaramakrishnan.
Description: Cambridge, Massachusetts : Harvard University Press, 2018. | Includes
bibliographical references and index.
Identifiers: LCCN 2017046944 | ISBN 9780674504639 (alk. paper)
Subjects: LCSH: Social gerontology—Developing countries. | Social gerontology—Africa. |
Social gerontology—South Asia. | Aging—Developing countries. | Social planning—
Developing countries. | Africa—Social policy. | South Asia—Social policy.
Classification: LCC HN980 .S567 2018 | DDC 305.2609172/4—dc23
LC record available at https://lccn.loc.gov/2017046944

To Appa and Amma, for their love and inspiration
in the past, present, and future

Contents

Introduction: Coming of Age   1

1   Old Age in Young Nations   22

2   Growing Old in the Time of Chronic Disease   59

3   The Emergence of the International Gerontologist   86

4   New Frontiers: Aging Experts in Asia and Africa   110

5   The Birth of Global Aging and Its Local Afterlives   131

6   International NGOs and the Aged in the
Developing World   169

   Epilogue: From Decolonization to Globalization   196

ABBREVIATIONS   219

NOTES   221

ACKNOWLEDGMENTS   297

INDEX   305

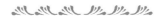

AS THE WORLD AGES

Coming of Age

IN DECEMBER 1984, experts at the first African gerontological conference, held in Dakar, confronted a new problem: the challenge of Africa's aging populations. A report on the conference observed that

> This week, the aging of Africa truly began and with it, the recording of its historic start right here in Dakar. . . . For the first time representatives from all of Africa have met to exchange ideas and find ways and means of maintaining the graceful and dignified aging which has been the heritage of Africa and which is likely to tumble under the rapid social, economic and cultural changes that appear to be the lot of Africa in this century and beyond. . . . Immediately after political independence, African societies abandoned agriculture in favor of industrialization which seemed to them their only way to achieve economic autonomy and assure their development. The technological choices made, however, have contributed to the marginalization of aged persons.[1]

The observation that the moment was uniquely historical is particularly striking. Far from being simple encomium, it highlighted a history that needed to be reset: it underscored a crucial and disruptive aspect of the problem of aging as a sociopolitical issue that required recasting. Aging had so far been approached as an issue that grew out of industrialization and development. The issue defined industrialized Western societies and populations and their present, and, in the same form, represented the remote future of the as-yet undeveloped world. These assumptions colored the approach to what was really a world problem but was still not informed by experiences from other parts of the world. In this report, the writers put their finger on the pulse of the issue: the problems of aging across the world were interwoven with issues and historicities of a recent past in Africa: an uneven process of industrialization, technology shifts, development, and rapid social, economic, and cultural changes. These events and processes needed to be reconciled and integrated into the conceptual apparatus of aging, and the "problems" associated with old age needed to acquire new explanatory sensibilities informed by aging in Africa.

In the 1980s, in Dakar as elsewhere in the global South, aging as a moral and developmental issue was beginning to engage the imaginations of experts and activists. Apart from local politicians, the conference also attracted an impressive number of social experts from across the continent who were advocating for the needs of aging persons. In particular, the meeting drew and shaped a first generation of African gerontological experts and activists interested in the study and field of aging in Africa, who claimed that they could guide the process of mitigating these shifts and renewing African society.[2] Speakers at the conference narrated a story, told and retold since the 1940s, of modernization's and development's ills and the dependence of older persons. The delegates observed that societal choices about development had produced the social and economic predicaments associated with aging populations in Africa. The narratives of aging in developing nations were thereby tied to the aspirations of decolonization in Africa and associated with attempts by various nations to forge ahead on a path of unfettered industrial modernization. This flawed vision led to untold losses in just a few decades: instead of lifting all boats, it diminished certain populations, such as the aged, who lost the support of their families and communities. The aged became the face of unfettered development's failures and challenges.

Changing Demographics, Changing Perspectives

More recently, aging populations have found renewed relevance. For some experts, aging has heralded the promise of dividends over dependence. These experts link the aging with Africa's future and promise rather than its past errors; they project that aging populations can enable equitable change and the harmonious development of African societies. As experts from across the continent lay out their development agenda for the future, aging populations are no longer viewed as neglected, needy, and primarily representing poverty and destitution.[3] For example, at recent meetings of the Organization of African Unity, in which representatives were asked to imagine the "Africa we want" to see by the year 2063, older persons were imagined as having a role in issues relating to youth and women through intergenerational dialogue and pictured as a buffer to future social change. These visions, however, have not necessarily led to real support on the ground.

The swift changes in perspectives about aging among international experts have been partly shaped by demographic patterns, or the speed at which aging is occurring in parts of Asia and Africa. Nations in Europe, such as France and Germany, took over 150 years to register a decline in death rates, followed by falls in fertility.[4] However, over the past fifty years or so, there have been steep improvements in longevity and declines in fertility in China, India, and other parts of the world.[5] This has led to concerns that the absolute number of older persons in the global South will soon rapidly outpace their numbers in the West. Over the coming decades, Africa will experience a faster growth in the number of older people in the population than will other regions of the world. The number of people aged sixty and over in Africa is projected to increase from the 2007 figures of 50.5 million to 64.5 million in 2015 and reach 205 million by 2050.[6] Experts are concerned not simply with the increase in the proportion of the older population but with the speed and accelerated growth of those aged over sixty years in the world.[7]

Historiographic and Critical Approach

While keeping these futures in mind, this book explores the recent past and history of aging as a sociopolitical global health concern by tracing it through the lens and lexicon of international health and development concerns since the Second World War. The making and remaking of aging populations merits this attention because these populations have been reconfigured by broader historical debates and concerns. These include late colonial welfare policies and inquiries into social change in the colonies, scientific and political engagements during the Cold War years, the politics of decolonization and international development, and the changing role and perspectives of neoliberal ideas and global health. These critical bends in the river or historical conjunctures, when knowledge about aging in the international and later global arena was being created, structure this book's historiographical work.

This book also takes a critical approach to the issues of global aging, examining how aging became a site of comparison, intervention, evasion, and engagement in the international arena. How did older populations emerge as definitive classes, and how did social scientists, colonial actors, scientific researchers, international bureaucrats, and social activists "discover" them and view them in particular ways? What discourses and practices, in terms of historical surveys, anthropological and ethnographic accounts, and scientific studies, campaigns, and mobilizations in international policy debates and programs, have defined older populations and their vulnerability since the 1940s?

At the heart of the critical inquiries in this book lies a larger concern: the politics of knowledge about aging populations. The norms and paradigms that constituted modern gerontological knowledge, as well as the developmental agenda for aging from the 1940s until the present, were largely shaped by a "dominant" narrative drawn from the experiences, categories, and concerns of West European and American societies.[8] These norms and paradigms reflected critical historical assumptions about how and when non-Western societies age, how their populations would grapple with sudden transformations, and the characteristics of aging populations as "traditional" societies experienced rapid change. A historical analysis of these concepts and their agenda subverts these standards and normative assumptions about age, diseases, and societies.

Aging has been linked with the modernization of societies and with demographic challenges, economic adjustments, and social futures that are more or less shared across the globe. But these notions of global aging and its future often overlook continuing contextual inequalities and historical legacies of differences and variability between societies. Even though the easiest and most obvious way to make a case for the interests and needs of older persons in decolonized societies was often appealing to a loss of culture and "tradition," scientific and social experts as well as NGO leaders were acutely conscious that these debates and engagements were occurring in an intellectually, economically, and politically unequal world. Aging has been suspended as a global agenda between a belief in the distinct societal interests and rights of the old, which has deepened since the 1980s, as well as its historical nodes, when aging-related debates gained global momentum and resources at times of economic or humanitarian crises, and when negative "imaginaries" of the dependence and perils of aging drew attention to older people.

At the same time, aging's "coming of age" as a global agenda has involved more than simply recognizing aging and older persons alone. It has consisted of the gradual recognition that aging and youth need to be tackled as interdependent issues, as are chronic diseases that present risks across the lifespan rather than in later life alone. In the same vein, this book traces debates that demonstrate that there are no "normal" or predictable places where older persons are found and are at risk—such as the aging peasant left behind by the young who were lured by wages and capital in the cities—since many older persons lead precarious lives in urban slums, and many workers return to villages. This book transcends these persistent values and assumptions about aging based on local contexts, and it outlines emerging models and assumptions about aging in postcolonial Asian and African societies.

Critical Backgrounds: Aging in the Postcolonial World

To further explicate the core approach in this book, it may be useful to recapitulate the ideas voiced at the Conference on Gerontology held at Dakar (1984). From the perspective of several UN representatives, the blueprint for international debates on aging was the plan and strategy proposed by the first UN-sponsored World Assembly on Aging (WAA), held in Vienna two years before the meeting at Dakar. At the WAA held in 1982, approximately 120 representatives from developed and developing nations drafted a plan of action to address the challenges posed by world aging. African nations were expected to adapt and implement the vision of this World Assembly. In Vienna, aging was declared a world problem, and the world's attention had been drawn "to the social, economic, political and scientific questions raised by the phenomenon of aging on a massive scale."[9] The WAA declared that the demographic processes causing population aging were at work across the world, not simply in the developed world.[10] These claims were reiterated in Dakar.

Even as experts in Vienna extolled the gradual, unified unfolding of population aging across the world, local experts at regional meetings recognized that behind the, pervasive, worldwide demographic shifts lay a world of inequalities and diversity. Demographers had been increasingly using population aging, as the United Nations termed it—fixing the threshold of old age at sixty years—as a statistical category and temporal reference point since the late-nineteenth century.[11] Historians have since argued that relying on this so-called global indicator and threshold fails to tell a complete story. It means that experts neglected to consider changing social roles and life expectancy or to acknowledge the uneven value and pace of aging. Setting sixty years as a proxy for aging also associated old age with the welfare- and retirement-centered preoccupations of industrialized societies.

At the Dakar Conference, local social workers and development experts reflected on these tensions. They felt that aging in Africa was not merely a demographic fact or pervasive historic process; rather it was a unique post-colonial condition and dilemma stemming from rapid social change and unstable modernization. According to them, the marginalization of older persons resulted from the politics and inequities of technology and re-sources, in particular the bankruptcy of international aid and develop-ment projects. The aging of Africa comprised two periods: a past, when its population aged "gracefully," and a present, when attempts to modernize gave rise to society-wide changes in attitudes to aging populations.[12] This made Africa part of "world aging," but also distinct from it.

During the discussions in Dakar, many pointed out that Africa's unique, complex pathology of climate, communicable diseases, malnutrition, and poverty, which affect and even accelerate the aging process, was also rede-fining population aging, making it distinct from population aging in other societies. As a result, the pathway to address these gerontological chal-lenges, some delegates noted, was through health, education, and training "that should be rooted in African traditions" rather than in an "undigested imitation of European and American models." This view that aging was diverse rather than unitary was not new. In 1982, two years prior to the Dakar Conference, this view was voiced in conversations at a conference supported by the United Nations Population Fund (UNFPA) in Delhi. At the conference, urban sociologists, demographers, and social activists from across South Asia asserted that most aging populations in Third World countries were acutely marginalized; only a few of the "privileged aged," mostly in urban areas in India, Bangladesh, and Nepal, could access better resources.[13] An urban sociologist and activist involved in slum develop-ment in Delhi observed that a majority of families with elders in South

Asia had few means of economic survival available to them, unlike elders in the West, where citizens were eligible for universal social security, pensions, and other welfare support. For countries in the developing world, the major challenge, therefore, was not reintegrating the retired into political and cultural life. Nor did these particular aging populations need rescuing from their social and psychological isolation, as in Europe and the United States. Rather, the majority of the aged were most adversely affected by the urbanization and migration that compounded the problems of poverty and deepened their vulnerability.[14]

Taken together, the Dakar and Delhi conferences give us a glimpse of the remaking of world agendas and the transactions occurring in sites across Africa and Asia. They also provide evidence of a deep-seated critique of international development in general, particularly the inequities of development and its difficulties in developing nations. More obliquely, many of these development experts and activists were skeptical that "world aging" could be addressed through rounds of high-sounding international conferences followed by a few development projects and assistance funded from abroad. For instance, at the Delhi meeting, it was observed that the long-standing imbalance caused by a "neocolonial world order" that subjected developing countries to inequitable economic and aid policies only compounded the problems of marginalization the old faced in these nations.[15]

The meetings in Dakar and Delhi are useful places to begin a book that explores how universalizing "global" agendas focused on aging populations emerged in the West and were then received and remade—or "provincialized," as the historian Dipesh Chakrabarty has termed it—in "developing countries" as experts in these countries made this knowledge their own by recasting aging in light of the social, economic, and moral imperatives of their societies.[16]

An Interdisciplinary Debate

Aging populations across the world have been the subject of growing policy interest based on demographic, economic, and social forecasts. Their rapid rise in numbers, proportions, and needs across the globe have engendered predictions about the cataclysmic onset of a gray wave, a "second population explosion," or a global "tsunami."[17] These predictions have not merely been the preserve of demographers; security analysts too have predicted that a rapidly aging world will be characterized by developed nations facing a loss of dynamism and world power and a challenge to European pre-eminence.[18] Nations in the global South will rapidly follow the West as they face the challenges and "burdens" posed by aging, even as they are still coming to terms with increasing life expectancy, containing infectious diseases, and continuing malnutrition.

UN reports and global demographic studies have expressed more measured and optimistic views.[19] They have summed up the challenge of population aging, or the rise in the population above sixty years of age around the globe, as unprecedented, profound, and pervasive.[20] According to a 2001 UN report, the global population of older persons was growing at a rate of 2.6 percent annually, with the developing world being likely to reach the same stage in the aging process that the developed world currently occupies by 2050.[21] Many see this juncture in human history as unprecedented because it represents the powerful successes of longevity, such as innovations in health, nutrition, and education; declining birth rates and family size; and the ability to control fertility. Together, these trends and shifts in the structure of populations have created historically unique and long-term challenges.

For historians, however, population changes and their deep-seated influence and impact on politics and society have a precedent in the debates and mobilization around the global population control and family planning programs that intensified across the world in the decades after the Second World War. Rapid changes in population growth were understood to have world-changing implications. However, just as debates about population explosion, as Alison Bashford argues, were initially justified as being an issue of "space" and migration rather than of "sex," debates about population aging have similarly been legitimized as an international agenda under various guises, and the concerns about it have varied over time.[22]

Even though historical demography has put aging on various policy agendas, in terms of institutional regulation and interventions, as Foucault noted, only in the modern era—in the context of industrial capitalism—did the state deploy public-health and population policies to regulate the experience of aging.[23] In the West, older populations emerged as definitive classes in the nineteenth and twentieth centuries, with the social sciences and natural sciences playing a significant role in this by "seeing" them in specific ways.[24] By the mid-twentieth century, social movements led by pensioners and others in Europe and the United States began challenging certain generalizations made by state policies and programs about aging—generalizations related to issues such as retirement, leisure, and social interactions, for example.[25]

The emergence of studies around aging populations worldwide has attracted little interest among historians of global health. Global health histories, with significant exceptions, have focused on colonial medicine and health interventions based on local and regional studies. Historians have also studied large-scale disease or immunization programs and global population control interventions and their politics, as traced through international institutions and philanthropies. Further, they have explored the emergence of global health through its association with public-private partnerships, new disease threats such as HIV, and the neoliberal turn in health priorities.[26] This has created an emphasis on the most "visible" and documented burdens of infectious diseases, epidemic diseases, and public health challenges, which have historically been associated with the environments and populations of Asia and Africa and have taken a devastating toll in these societies. So far, historical scholarship has approached these diseases and health interventions through certain fixed temporal lenses and approaches. For instance, international health and decolonization have mostly been examined through histories of international institutions and international disease programs rather than through a comparative or regional focus. Some historians have pointed out that these perspectives have often created implicit silos and have not sufficiently explored, for instance, the links between colonial medicine and post–Second World War international health and development projects.[27] These perspectives also hold deeper intellectual consequences, because they overlook histories of health conditions, human experiences, diseases at the "borders," and intersectionalities. For instance, chronic diseases and comorbidities, cognitive decline and disabilities, and regional histories of medicine from within the global South are rarely traced; and mobilization and meetings that lie on the edges or margins of large UN institutions or Cold War networks and assistance are also less visible.

Aging populations as a worldwide agenda and its historical roots offer a productive engagement for global health historians. They present a less "predictable" and well-known cast of international social actors as well as less orthodox networks and mobilization. This cast's activities and engagements have often occurred at the margins of influential international institutions; "global" aging circumvents power centers and structures, such as the colonial metropolises or Cold War capitals, and offers insights into alternate pathways and scales of mobilization.[28]

Of all the modern agendas that have emerged over the past decades, aging has reflected a complex and unequal world of global health and development. It has presented uneasy political relationships in a seemingly egalitarian world of demographic predictions and promise, and it has lacked confident "cures" and interventions that can be suggested globally. Experts have argued that health becomes a global issue when it transcends boundaries and needs to be addressed by "cooperative actions," but aging demonstrates that stating historical concerns and asserting an agenda that unites vulnerable populations across borders are not necessarily followed by resources and globally coordinated interventions. Thus aging retains strong moorings in local and regional contexts and approaches.[29] This also makes it vital to understand the plural historical genealogies of aging in societies where disease and demographic transformations are ongoing. These changes need to be understood on their own terms, and they require reflection on how experts have historically framed knowledge about aging and its social implications.

Normative Models of Aging and the Politics of Knowledge

At the start of this book, I trace ideas concerning chronological age and aging in Africa and Asia, and I argue that discourses about aging and modernization were still in the making from the 1940s to the early 1950s. Surveys and studies by colonial officials, Christian missionaries, sociologists, and anthropologists at the Rhodes-Livingston Institute, Zambia and in India displayed an urge to compare and contrast notions of chronological age and to understand the role played by gerontological authority and elders in securing social stability. Soon after this, gerontological, sociological, and demographic writings began representing aging as a classical, normative model characteristic of modern Western societies that reflected these societies' successes in industrialization and modernization.[30] In the decades following the Second World War, the growth of aging populations was widely associated with a historical trajectory of modernization emblematic of "civilized" nations.[31] In fact, this stage of development was held out as a model to be envied and emulated.

In the 1950s, a group of American scientific experts toured research centers and institutional care facilities in Western Europe. They declared that the latter was an "unintended laboratory" to study the social aspects of aging. In the same breath, they also emphasized that America had joined the ranks of other civilized nations in addressing these concerns and problems—the rise in old age dependence, retirement, claims on social security and medical care for the chronic "diseases of aging"—associated with the shared demographic changes in life expectancy and fertility.[32]

American social gerontologists and scientists were referring not simply to the experience of aging but to a stage of industrial, advanced development emblematic of the West; it is significant to note that they characterized population aging as a social condition that liberal, welfare regimes in Western Europe and the United States had in common. The power of the Western gerontological imagination, shaped by research on the so-called diseases of old age, demography, and social policy, was influential. It was premised on an unwavering sense of primacy—of having aged and matured "first"—and it derived from a specific set of circumstances and characteristics of technological changes and the organization of production and labor in the West. A certainty that the changes and experiences of aging in Western societies impacted and shaped changes elsewhere underpinned these claims, and this ideological self-confidence, articulated in the 1950 and 1960s, when American social gerontologists began to deepen their studies of aging, has persisted. Writing in 1960, for instance, American gerontologists Clark Tibbitts and Wilma Donahue opined: "Never in human history has a society set such a rapid pace of change in the manner and means of living as our American society today. In turn, we have set in motion processes that are resulting in accelerated change in the rest of the world, from the USSR to the most primitive areas of Africa and South-East Asia."[33]

Gerontological frameworks and their assumptions that emerged in the West have in turn been supported by ideas and enduring models about disease and demographic change. In the 1940 and 1950s, international health projects, deepened by UN leadership and often led by philanthropies and resources now centered in the United States, recast older colonial stereotypes about disease and demography. Developing nations on the path to industrialization that had not yet modernized were regarded as "young societies," both in developmental and demographic terms, and were associated overwhelmingly with the burden of infectious diseases.[34] Public health programs, including campaigns relating to infectious diseases, high fertility, and maternal and child health, addressed the need for a productive labor force on the one hand and, on the other, were premised on racialized demographic anxieties that ignored the relationship between infections, environmental risks, and chronic diseases such as cancers.[35]

These linear demographic and epidemiological transition models that hold the promise of modernization—as societies progress to conquer infections, influence life expectancy and lower fertility—have significant implications for this book's narrative. By the 1970s, the accepted progress of an epidemiological transition was a linear model with "stages" of progress modeled on industrialization and shifts in life expectancy in Western countries. Non-Western nations, it was predicted, were bound merely to play "catch-up" with this linear model.[36] Public health scholars such as Julio Frenk (1989) have challenged this model, and nuanced anthropological studies of the fluid boundaries between "acute" and "chronic" diseases have emerged. But there has been a lack of historically informed reflection on how these debates played out in the 1940s and 1950s, when the dichotomies between young and old nations, their distinct geographies or environment, and their burdens of acute and chronic diseases were first inscribed and challenged; nor do these binaries allow spaces for alternative narratives.[37]

In this book I trace the emergence of these linear and evolutionist ideas about aging and development in the international arena, and I examine how these ideas and models were questioned, adapted locally, and became more inclusive of alternate perspectives. I argue that political and intellectual possibilities existed to mediate and shape ideas and policies regarding age, aging, and their place in society. In non-Western settings, there was the possibility for experts and activists to engage with these ideas about aging and insert other ways of viewing aging in society, in particular by including discourses regarding families, intergenerational ties, and dependence. Analysis of these normative models is critically important, as it can promote thinking about aging from a historical and contextual perspective and in a way that, rather than simply "exporting" Western experiences to other parts of the globe, identifies commonalities.

Efforts to challenge these notions, or to "provincialize Europe" are crucial not simply as an intellectual agenda that aims to limit, decenter, and localize these ideas but also to inform the field of aging and its policies.[38]

The latter needs to be informed by diverse development approaches and policies that will address aging in the global South on its own terms, without viewing these transformations as deviant or deficient from "standard" norms of age and aging.[39]

Thematic Frames and Historical Intersections
(circa 1940–2000)

This book structures its historical exploration of aging through several broadly chronological thematic frames. They are not mutually exclusive, nor are they confined only to certain decades; rather, they reflect historical intersections or convergences when certain actors or agencies that shared international visions of aging were at a crossroads, engaged in debates, or faced a crisis.

The first encounters I trace were in the late colonial period and the early years of decolonization in Asia and Africa. The encounters were characterized by efforts to "know" and map these "traditional" societies. They are a crucial beginning to our story, and that is why I consciously start this narrative from what were believed to be the edges or margins—the colonies— rather than the Western metropolis. Demographers, epidemiologists, anthropologists, missionaries, colonial officials, and others were the "experts" involved in efforts to measure and manage colonial subjects when colonial policy was veering toward introducing developmental reform in these societies. Their observations about chronological age, elders, and the aged in local communities marked an effort to understand aging in Asia and Africa as being the "opposite" of that in the West. They also demonstrated flexibility in interpreting old age in multiple ways, such as social aging; some social anthropologists, in an effort to address the problems of the "maladjusted" old in America, even characterized traditional societies as models in the adaptability of the old. Investigations of old age and aging in the colonies and in traditional pasts were efforts at controlling local power structures. They demonstrated competing visions, but they were also useful in eventually formulating typologies of aging in "traditional" and "modern" societies.

These views, however, did not immediately shape the agenda of the early international gerontological networks. In the 1940s and 1950s, groups of scientists in Europe and the United States projected aging as primarily a biological and medical challenge. These perspectives coincided with the founding of the first international gerontological associations. Their discourses and partnerships focused on research on "diseases of old age," and some scientists initiated comparative studies of chronic diseases and aging in Asia and Africa in that period. Early gerontological visions focused primarily on Europe and North America, although indirectly these normative claims about aging and chronic diseases, as well as their association with modern societies and lifestyles, were already being challenged in Asia and Africa. Historically, in India and South Africa for instance, this research and its science were being shaped by the politics of decolonization and its aspirations. They showed that these societies faced different and often divergent challenges and that aging and chronic diseases were not necessarily associated with a longer life expectancy and Western lifestyles. In turn, these framings of aging populations have wider implications. They remind us that these stigmatized assumptions regarding chronic disease and modernity have had implications for poor and racially marginalized sections of society not only in formerly colonized worlds but in the developed world as well.

In the following decades, with anxieties about aging and retirement deepening in the West, social scientists became influential in shaping a perspective of aging as a "problem" rooted in social psychological issues of maladjustment, mostly of middle-aged white male populations. In the United States, concerns about employment and labor productivity led to an increasing interest in exploring societies in Europe that had aged earlier. These forays demonstrated that the making of Western gerontology involved facing the challenges of an uneven, contingent terrain. Experts who tried to forge a common international vision of and platform on the social problems of aging found it challenging to do so even between Europe and the United States. The politics of the Cold War in particular shaped notions of aging and civilization, and American demographers tried to center these gerontological collaborations between Western European researchers and American social scientists rather than extend them to Eastern Europe.

As networks of international development and aid deepened and links grew with developing nations after the Second World War, social scientists and social workers became interested in the "old" in developing nations due to concerns that modernization projects and urbanization were leading to changing family ties, creating instability, and making older persons vulnerable and visible in Asia and Africa. However, pensions, welfare, and the age of retirement were not necessarily central issues in their development reports. In many social surveys, the "decline" of family life and the migration of youth attracted interest, and older persons began to be viewed as a socially vulnerable group—poor, needy, and victims of changes in family life and migration.

In the 1970s and 1980s, the promise of development soon took a more pessimistic turn in the international arena with a world economic downturn and recession. With growing pressure from aging experts in the United States and Europe, leadership within the UN summoned a World Assembly to reflect on the "problems" of aging worldwide, and a developmental vision of aging began to take shape. Aging had begun to be associated with dependence and welfare costs in some settings; in other places in the global South, urban sociologists and social workers focused on old age and poverty as a deepening crisis due to the failures of the promise of social development and industrialization. As worries about international or "world" aging began to crystallize, experts stressed the priorities of productivity and development. In the short term, the need to plan measures of mitigation and address the issues of aging populations' vulnerability and marginalization were agreed on.

Finally, by the 1990s and thereafter, international meetings made progress in developing an international agenda that often spurred national initiatives in aging. However, the balance between aging policies and the aspirations of development remained a central concern at all levels. Because these meetings did not yield large-scale resources needed for aging programs as anticipated, some international NGOs began undertaking more visible and aggressive international campaigns in support of the aged in sites of humanitarian crisis in developing countries. Their views about aging were colored by humanitarian empathy, and they attempted to build local networks and diverse international partnerships that aligned with older persons' interests based on local needs.

At the turn of the twenty-first century, gerontological experts and social activists stressed the need for social justice and rights for the aged. They have forged partnerships in the global South, and these campaigns shaped the agenda of a Second World Assembly (2002) held in Madrid. International discourse on aging also increasingly emphasizes individual responsibility, coping strategies, and "success" in controlling and delaying aging (including delaying cognitive decline and disease); this implies that both at the national and international levels, more care-giving responsibilities have devolved on individuals and families. This neoliberal approach leaves those who are the old and vulnerable, such as the oldest of old, older women, aging informal workers, and those who are aged and in poor health due to a lifetime of poverty, poor nutrition, and poor immunity excluded or recognized only symbolically, with very few actual resources committed to them.

The Role of Experts

By the 1980s, aging had increasingly begun to capture the imagination of political and bureaucratic elites as well as enterprising experts in developing countries. On an international scale, groups of well-traveled American gerontologists and a few UN experts were a predictable presence at aging discussions from Dakar to Delhi. These experts—ranging from UN officials, researchers in gerontology, and social scientists to international- and national-level NGO activists and social workers—tried to identify the needs and interests of "aging populations." This book maps how these experts and individuals from various disciplines and fields, including colonial bureaucrats and missionaries in the 1940s, began to collect evidence and articulate agendas around aging in various guises—for instance, in terms of migration, chronic diseases, or as a humanitarian question. Although they seldom considered themselves lifelong flagbearers in support of the agenda of aging populations in the international arena, these experts often moved between the realms of domestic and international politics.

The emergence of global expertise on aging is not a grand narrative that originates primarily from the ranks of the UN bureaucracy or from experts in large international philanthropies based in the United States, such as the Rockefeller Foundation. The concerns relating to aging populations did not receive consistent support from large U.S.-based foundations engaged in international development work, such as those focused on infectious diseases. Nor was there a dedicated international cadre of trained gerontological workers and researchers, as had been the case with population research that created the intellectual climate for the local dissemination of population control programs.[40] More often than not, in the earlier decades the vision and politics of aging were incubated outside of or on the peripheries of UN agencies.

Several scholars have explored the specialized knowledge promoted by development experts, who were engaged in planning and monitoring development projects (such as population control, agricultural development, immunization, disease eradication, and community development projects) or in offering social science expertise in the education sector. Through their ideas and services, these experts framed development projects as a means for decolonized societies to undertake a pathway to social change and economic progress.[41] This book draws from historical scholarship on the politics of development and discussions on the tensions and, often, the skepticism that international health experts encountered locally in Asia and Africa. It draws especially from research that focuses on the more ambiguous place of nonelite experts, such as Peace Corps volunteers and social workers.[42] My research demonstrates that, in the absence of well-funded, transnational programs, the interactions between international gerontological experts, officers from international aging NGOs, and local experts were not based on claims to authority drawn from Western techno-science alone. Indeed, these interactions were only marginally influenced by the power and legitimacy that flowed through UN officials and from a supportive national political elite. Instead, the exercise of authority and initiative was based on day-to-day transactions in relief programs and a shared mind-set to advance gerontological education that was promoted by exchanges at conferences. A paucity of aid funds and human resources created more spaces for experts at various levels to bargain conceptually and administratively regarding teaching, training, and welfare or relief programs for older persons.

Aging was a latecomer to the UN's mission for social development in Asia and Africa. Old age as an issue was raised by individual countries such as Argentina through efforts that attempted to safeguard the rights of older persons, but these sporadic attempts remained early, isolated instances.[43] Only in the mid-1970s did the UN General Assembly give repeated consideration to "the question of the elderly" at a worldwide level, publishing its first report on aging policies a few years later, with data and sources that were mainly drawn from industrialized nations.[44] Until then, the Economic and Social Council (ECOSOC) had gathered information on old-age pension schemes and standards of living among the aged, but most of its seminars and expertise had focused on Europe, on countries where "the socioeconomic conditions of the aged are marked."[45] At a consultation held in 1980 before the First World Assembly on Aging in Vienna, the WHO representative for its Global Program on Aging observed, "WHO's general activities in the field of aging have been limited, except in Europe where they have been very active. *In fact, in 1976 the Director General decided that it would be better to transfer the global responsibility of our aging program to the European office in Copenhagen. He felt that European expertise could help us stimulate interest on a worldwide basis and help countries in other regions to develop their programs.*"[46] What seemed to be a broader worldview or unified coming of age was still overwhelmingly informed by Eurocentric perspectives and backed only by limited funding. The ECOSOC secretariat and its social development department remained the main votaries of the world aging agenda in the 1980s, and in the following years various UN agencies pursued certain dimensions of the aging agenda—in terms of health, labor, family policies, and refugee relief— based on the flows of resources, leadership, and intersections with other coinciding programs.

Western experts, primarily American social scientists, cultivated ties with UN agencies and tried to shape its agenda of "world" aging. They recast their domestic experiences of population aging into a universal narrative and model of how societies and families would modernize. The trajectory of aging in the developing world was projected as either conforming to or being a distortion of the events and ideas about aging populations in the West. As a new field, there was something akin to a missionary enterprise involved in the efforts of many of these experts, as many believed that they were offering moral solutions and righting the wrongs of development. Through their writings, gerontological congresses, and training programs, they aimed to suggest means to rebuild family solidarities and heal societies that had taken a downturn from filial piety to abandonment in the course of their industrialization. Migration remained a consistent and escalating concern for these experts. Over time, as social workers and others joined these concerns and founded international NGOs, there was also an effort to engineer dramatic rescues of the aged during the many political and economic crises that deepened worldwide in the 1980s.

Many international and national experts worried that, unlike in the past, families would be unable to support the old, thus assuming all "traditional" societies shared a common past when the old were looked after due to their social and moral authority. Aging-related issues in developing countries invariably stressed the "failures" of family support, with local leaders being urged to repopulate rural areas with young people to support the old and vulnerable who had been left behind in villages. As early as the 1950s, experts in South Asia had observed that improvements in public health were causing life expectancy to rise, leading to a growing number of old persons even though fertility was not really in decline.[47] They were of the view that there was also a discomfiting visibility of the old in public life. The numbers of the old were rising, but more significant, they were increasingly "seen" in places where earlier they had not been present. They "were out of place" or were simply living longer, even in villages. Older persons had always been present in the countryside, within extended families or on their own, and they had suffered, languished, and died of what has been termed the "poverty of age."[48] They were now manifesting alternate forms of deprivation and dependence that were compounded by growing urban poverty, migration, and economic instabilities in cities that were rapidly expanding all over the developing world.[49] In the words of a long-time activist, the priority was for the state to mitigate the effects of rural decline and to extend support to the elderly in urban slums and shanty towns whose families had left them to the care of state welfare services due to the pressures of urban life in developing countries.[50] The increasing lack of family support for the aged was seen as likely to create pressures that could destabilize the development goals the countries envisaged.

Writing about "Global" Aging

The primary focus of much of this book's narrative is anchored in events, ideas, and voices from South Africa (and later developments in West and North Africa), South Asia, and China. I have used the "global" as an approach to write an intellectual history of the politics of aging by tracing key transformative moments, comparisons, and divergences, rather than attempting or even contemplating a worldwide survey of aging.[51] This approach means that I have concentrated on certain defining moments, historical conjunctures, and representative sites that were formative in aging's emergence as a global concern and were critical to the debates relating to decolonization, development, and modernization. The aim underlying this transnational narrative is to draw attention to the critical intersections when certain turns in international debates and meaningful regional responses were articulated. Many nations that provide fascinating examples of the political inequities around debates on social security and pensions at a national level are mentioned but not discussed in detail. In the accounts of specific events, such as the discussion of age and aging in the context of civil war, genocide, and authoritarian rule in and around Zimbabwe (which

I explore in Chapter 5), there is a focus on local actors and NGOs, leaving a dense set of archival and oral accounts. Given the constraints of space, I have not discussed areas with similar challenges and tensions, in particular Southeast Asia.

There were significant national and regional debates about aging and dependence, and also pioneering concerns relating to social security in Latin America; in particular some of the earliest debates on the identity and social claims of aged persons took place in Argentina.[52] Later, in Brazil, Chile, Colombia, and Mexico, there were efforts to establish links with gerontological researchers in the United States and to build education programs that included gerontological training. Experts in these countries were influential in debates on urbanization and aging and in stressing the intergenerational aspects of aging.[53]

I have chosen to focus on Asia and Africa because they are linked subjects in the developmental arena through cross-regional, historical comparisons and shared intellectual and scientific networks in the period I examine. The purpose here is not to leave any nations out or replace one asymmetry with another, but rather to foreground key historical moments in international debates and scientific controversies when aging populations emerged as an analytical category and identity.

In order to avoid constructing cultural monoliths and binaries about the West and non-West, I have spotlighted social distinctions in the West in relation to views and debates on gerontological research agendas. These include differences between white and African American medical subjects in the United States relating to "diseases of aging" (for example, cancers) in the 1950s; tensions between American and European medical researchers, including between American and Soviet researchers, that, however, did not escalate deeper into Cold War rivalries that marked other spheres of health and development. I have also discussed an emerging strain of critical social gerontology that questioned the paternalist and productivity-centered assumptions of gerontological ideas. Many social gerontologists resisted a chronological, age-based focus on the "problems" of old age in the 1980s, offering instead a perspective based on lifespan and wider social and structural factors affecting old age and aging. What is stressed here are the ideas and expositions projected through UN institutions and mediated by their global agenda. The critical perspective and agenda of this book has remained centered on tracing how aging and its concerns became transnational and how aging and debates on aging came to engage with the lives of "others" in the global South.

What I have aimed to present in this book is a history of the present or a genealogical inquiry of the multiple, overlapping strands of ideas and challenges that represent the diverse nature of global population aging. I have traced its emergence as a collective "worldview" at various points when care and dependence, rather than food, space, and resources (which were characteristic of anxieties about population growth and control in earlier decades) seem to become foregrounded.

In exploring the interconnected lineages of aging, I have dwelled in particular on concerns about the aging scenarios in Asia and Africa, where the norms of chronological age and disease as well as notions of dependence have been recast. At an ideological level, debates on aging have underscored a central tension in international and global affairs, namely the imbalance of an international economic order and a global development process that was viewed as reflecting persistent historical inequalities. Despite long-standing critiques, modernization is still seen as a linear process with an optimal pathway, which is based on Western models. Thus it is assumed that "developing" nations will inevitably confront the problems associated with aging at a particular and predicted time in the process. Asia's transition to aging is seen in contemporary reports as being distorted. China, experts argue, will have to confront aging as a challenge (and implicitly a burden) before "growing rich," when welfare and social security resources to support a needy population of elderly people would be sufficient, based on a Western model. It is this teleology of development and its discourses that are an important focus of my inquiry.

1

Old Age in Young Nations

IN SURVEYS AND assessments initiated between the 1930s and the 1950s, old age was either invisible, because of a focus on younger age groups that might offer labor or affect fertility, or understood as evidence that rapid social and economic changes associated with modernization were disrupting "traditional" networks and ties in these societies. Several social actors, including an influential group of late colonial experts, wanted to map and interpret the "instability" and fast-paced changes associated with modernization and migration in the colonies. In diverse and often contradictory ways, their work and paternalistic plans rendered age and aging more "visible." In this chapter, I trace the narratives of four groups: metropolitan demographers and colonial officials involved in comparative surveys and demographic operations; local demographic experts conducting census surveys in India; a new generation of anthropologists in South Africa and India studying social changes; and "amateur" social experts such as missionaries in Africa, who were also conducting local surveys and analyzing emerging social connections and hierarchies. Transdisciplinary approaches and scientific research in the colonies were powerful, with great potential to shape the creation of further institutional support and influence colonial administrators.

Old Age in Young Nations

In 1939, Robert René Kuczynski observed that "Telling the population of a country is like telling the age of a person."[1] The Colonial Office had charged Kuczynski, a reputable demographer, with consolidating a survey of population statistics in the colonies and mandated areas in Africa. Estimating a person's chronological age either involved "guesswork" or was based on knowledge about personal and public events related to their life. Large-scale population surveys were similar, he concluded, in that they could be either rash estimates or genuine, all-inclusive enumerations. Kuczynski's observations reflected a growing interest in the 1940s and later among experts in the British metropolis in mapping population structures and other vital statistics by opening them up to modern methods, and his contemporaries further elaborated on the problems of deepening demographic and epidemiological knowledge in the colonies. One expert from the London School of Hygiene, a training ground for new epidemiological methods and the collection of medical statistics in the tropics, wrote: "One of the greatest difficulties facing organizers of any census operation among native races occurs when attempts are made to record the ages of people. A combination of reasons, prejudices, and beliefs may lie at the root of the problem. . . . At the higher age-groups difficulties of age determination will probably become more acute. The majority of the primitive peoples have no idea of their ages; unlike their Occidental brothers and sisters, they are not anxious to appear younger than their ages would make them—*they simply do not know.*"[2]

Kuczynski's disparaging allusion to "guesswork," which reflects the politics and preconceptions that colored the enterprise of inscribing age in the colonies, also offers us an entry point into a larger set of questions and assumptions at the intersection of local and international experts: How did experts interpret age and aging in the colonies? What interests shaped the meanings ascribed to aging? How did experts and administrators attempt to learn and impute age among populations who "did not know"?

Interestingly, colonial officials, demographers, anthropologists, and missionaries were all invested, in multiple ways, in the rhetoric and plans of modernization unfolding in these years, but they understood the implications of these social changes, their challenges, and suggested mitigations to them in different ways. Although the "guesswork" of chronological age worried Kuczynski, other experts showed that older persons represented an extended life-course of roles and relationships. These plural identities consisted of people functionally identified as elders and, more rarely, people defined as chronologically old for the purposes of social benefits.

Age and specifically old age were invariably tied up with anxieties and speculation about youth and intergenerational networks. For some, the conditions experienced by older persons were typical of the challenges "static" societies faced in coping with sudden changes such as urbanization, especially since some of these societies were viewed as making a transition from being subordinated gerontocracies.[3] For other experts, aging represented the contingent nature of human migration, and it needed to be situated in ties of interdependence being made and remade in these years between young and old and between villages and cities.

Another significant theme later in this chapter traces how and why some American sociologists were interested in understanding aging and adaptation in "primitive societies." Their anxieties about aging stemmed from concerns about another kind of migration—not of elders left behind by young migrants with the growth of capitalist networks as in the global South, but of the potential disruptive movement of aging African Americans from the rural American South to Northern cities. When examined historically, aging and the modernization project was fundamentally a debate about questions of place and mobility. In the case of the United States, it raised issues of racial inequalities and questions about labor within industrialized societies.

Why trace a narrative of flux and uncertainty, a story that often reinforces the invisibility of chronological age and aging among these experts? I start here because this narrative offers us insights into emerging ideas about poverty and marginality associated with the socially or functionally old, ideas that were already emerging indigenously in developmental debates in Asia and Africa. They were genealogically distinct and independent from the demographic forecasts of aging, falling fertility, and dependency that experts in the West were discussing in these decades; yet the networks between colony and metropolis played a significant role in initiating some of these social and demographic inquiries. We therefore need to begin this story by turning to the worries about population decline preoccupying some experts in these years, a widening "imbalance" between old, civilized societies and youthful colonies, and their futures.

Population Anxieties in the Metropolis

We begin this narrative in England in the 1930s, where a growing, paralyzing anxiety about declining fertility and aging was ironically beginning to broaden the professional possibilities and prospects for demographic experts.[4] In 1936, the Population Investigation Committee (PIC) was set up as an autonomous body to survey the trends of population in Great Britain. Its members urged the government to refine the questions and methods used in the census in Britain and Wales. New demographic techniques, such as the measurement of reproductive rates by leading demographers (e.g., Kuczynski), made it easier to measure and predict fertility shifts. The Victorian population rise had been replaced by a longer life expectancy and a fall in death rates, while the birth rate had stabilized, with fewer children being born. Deepening anxieties about a "stationary" population and fears that the British nation would face severe problems, such as a decline in capital accumulation that would unleash the "devil" of unemployment, were voiced. In these interwar years, population fears were focused on fertility and family size rather than on aging populations and longevity. Works such as *The Struggle for Population* by British sociologist D. V. Glass and other studies on fertility in various developed countries highlighted the decline in the birth rate. C. P. Blacker, the secretary of the Eugenics Society and a member of the PIC, commented: "It is difficult to see how Western powers could maintain their present state of civilization if present trends continue to the year 2000. Let us then not be too complacent. . . . Let us recognize clearly what lies before us . . . if the birth rate continues to fall."[5]

Well-known demographers at the PIC shared the view that the population problems of Great Britain merited "serious scientific investigation." Some PIC members understood the population shift in Great Britain as indicating a similar situation in Europe.[6] To many of these experts, such developments could have dire implications for colonial power and its hold on its colonies.[7] The PIC chairman, Carr Saunders, noted that "cessation in growth" was a larger trend across Europe and held implications for the contest over colonies: colonizing nations could no longer make claims for colonies based on the expanding needs of their population, as they would "look ridiculous."[8] A decline in fertility posed a demographic challenge with social and economic consequences at home; it also created the conditions to deploy the same demographic tools and methods in the colonies.[9]

This partly stemmed from concerns about the imbalance between what were perceived as young, populated lands (which were also witnessing rising discontent and nationalist movements) and a metropolis threatened by a loss of markets, a loss of social enterprise, and national decline.[10] The interest in colonial demographics was also related to efforts to introduce developmental and welfare reforms in the colonies, partially as a response to labor unrest and strikes.[11] Colonial authority (in this case the British) was centered on trying to understand the availability of a young workforce and, later, to control migrations to cities.[12]

In the interwar years in particular, the professional and academic fields of ethnological and demographic expertise proliferated in both Britain and France. A range of actors with ties to both the colonies and the metropolis—demographers, anthropologists, and missionaries, who were keen observers of social change—tried to assess and explain these concerns as well as found new disciplines, with varying degrees of success and diverse interests.[13] Demographic surveys and assessments were social tools to re-evaluate the colonizer's role in the colonies. These surveys and assessments also show a marked recognition of the growing need to understand and better address the social changes and transitions occurring in colonial populations alongside the rise of industries, migration, and urbanization. Outside Britain, for instance, experts such as Pierre Gourou were mapping detailed ethnographies, fertility patterns, and geographies of rural populations in colonial Indochina.[14] In the British colonial metropolis, however, the chronologically old were often overlooked in these colonial administrators' surveys and studies, and the measure of age was a low and marginal priority in census operations.

In 1937, participants at the International Demographic Congress in Paris demonstrated increasing ambition to understand fertility and demographic trends in the colonies. In the same year, experts associated with the PIC in London began expanding their inquiries to the wider reaches of the British Empire and its colonial populations.[15] In this ambitious undertaking, they turned to patrons at home and abroad for support, approaching the Carnegie Corporation in the United States to help finance Robert Kuczynski, the architect of several studies in the colonies and their leading demographer, to begin a survey.[16] In 1937, Kuczynski reviewed the inadequacies in colonial census data and vital statistics in *Colonial Populations*, in a bid to suggest improvements in the Imperial Census operations that were to be undertaken in 1941 but were later abandoned. Kuczynski's was not the first commentary and critique on the colonial censuses; their unevenness and lack of statistical reliability, even between and among the colonies, had struck observers earlier.[17]

In its proposal to the Carnegie Corporation, the PIC announced its intention to expand inquiries to examine the population problems of the British Empire, claiming that the Colonial Office in London was willing to cooperate by offering access to its records. The primary aims were to summarize the situation across the colonies, buried in numerous population records; to examine the details and accuracy of population surveys; to understand the means or mechanism of census taking and the demographic conditions "in a large portion of the area of the world"; and to prepare an account that would advance knowledge about population history in these areas.[18]

This initiative was only one of many points of departure in the 1930s that led to revisiting social, economic, and demographic questions relating to the colonies. Scholars have examined this debate as an interwar "depopulation discourse" that reinforced the geopolitical and territory-based anxieties regarding declining fertility.[19] In the case of the African colonies, pressure and interest already existed in Britain, the United States, and South Africa to deepen research on social problems. This led to demands to establish a center for African studies at the University of Oxford and, later, demands for support from the Rockefeller Foundation to found the International African Institute (originally the International Institute of African Languages and Cultures) in London. In the same years in India, growing nationalist agitation and demands for self-rule provided the background for investigations into welfare, population policies, and health.

Kuczynski and his mentors at the PIC and at the Colonial Office rested on significant precedents, such as the African Survey of 1938 (initiated by the PIC in 1931), that had reinforced the need to collect data about Africa systematically.[20] The African Survey marked efforts for studies and approaches that were not cloistered in geographical compartments. The Survey was led by Lord Malcolm Hailey, a retired governor from the North-Western Provinces in India who, despite his failing health in the latter parts of the survey, was viewed as a servant of India who did a great service for Africa, "by making Europe to understand Africa and for Africa to understand itself."[21] Studies such as the African Survey already showed the power of transdisciplinary approaches and scientific research in the colonies, and their potential to shape the creation of further institutional support and to influence colonial administrators.

Knowing Local Society

In 1935, Malcolm Hailey turned to Kuczynski and his colleagues at the London School of Economics to conduct a survey of the existing data on population in Africa, in particular "sub-Saharan Africa."[22] Kuczynski began this work with a study of the West African mandates, and turned to write a voluminous monograph that reviewed the demography of the Cameroon and Togoland, chosen partly because of the relative denseness of their records as compared to other African states. Subsequently, with the PIC's support, Kuczynski undertook an even more extensive project, *The Demographic Survey of the British Colonial Empire.*[23]

Studies to understand society and economic conditions in Africa were not uncommon in the 1930s, as noted by Shula Marks.[24] The 1940s and 1950s marked a turning point as interest in interpreting and categorizing local society deepened with the growing belief that traditional and "backward" societies needed to be brought into the fold of social and economic modernization. Various Colonial Development and Welfare Acts provided resources from the metropolis for development programs in the colonies, though as historians have noted, a blueprint for reforming existing colonial institutions did not always accompany them.[25] Many of these studies shared the objective of providing a continent-wide overview—on African labor, science, and capital—or consisted of financial and economic histories to inform these new developmental imperatives.[26]

These years marked a moment of change, rethinking, and some uncertainty for the colonial administration. They also served as the backdrop for a growing self-confidence among social experts in their ability to penetrate local society. These experts were concerned with more than merely enumerating and fixing the identities of community, caste, or tribe, as earlier census operations had been; they were also keen to probe, through surveys, further into what lay within homes and to gauge the capacity for labor, productivity, and fertility within households.

Developmental projects and demographic forays were closely aligned, and both were led by colonial bureaucrats and metropolitan experts whose careers often spanned across colonies. In their rhetoric, colonial administrators urged standardization in categories and questions. Some colonies were viewed as more adaptable to this progress and scientific accuracy than others, which languished in a "static" state. Lord Hailey, in line with other late colonial administrators and experts, believed that Africa needed solutions beyond the routine of administration and maintenance of order for its special social development needs. Demographic knowledge was key, since population figures were unreliable: figures of population movement, depopulation, and the total amount of ill-health were still based solely on estimates. Hailey, quoting the instance of successful adoption of Indian models of surveys in settings such as Nyasaland, also believed that the colonies could gradually improve population enumeration and vital statistics.[27]

Kuczynski relied on data collected by the League of Nations in his work, but he also admitted that these country estimates for various colonies and territories were unreliable since they were based on faulty national estimates. In 1934, for instance, of the total world population of 2,080 million, 270 million, or 13 percent, was estimated as living in the colonies or mandated areas, with 55 percent and 42 percent living in Asia and Africa, respectively. Yet for many areas, such as Somaliland, Belgian Congo, and Mozambique, the population had not been enumerated. In other areas, such as Kenya, the census officials themselves declared that no accurate census of the native population had yet been made.[28] A similar state prevailed with birth- and death-related medical statistics. Some returns gave the impression of an unending rise and ebb of infectious diseases year after year rather than yielding precise numbers regarding disease conditions and affected populations. Even in large cities such as Lagos, the birth and death returns were so imprecise that it was impossible to report if mortality caused by diseases had diminished by the 1920s.

In British India, too, where the census set-up was reputedly better, information on births, deaths, and diseases left much to be desired. Although surveys of the army's health were systematically undertaken in British India, even in the 1940s, consistency regarding disease categories was lacking. Deaths by plague and cholera were shown to have dropped as their epidemics had waned, though high rates of other infections, such as tuberculosis, sandfly fevers, dysentery, and fevers were reported. New categories, such as rheumatic diseases, heart disease, and cancers appeared, but their reporting and recording was inconsistent. Even in old colonial hubs with well-trained municipal personnel, like Bombay, these vital returns of births and deaths were deemed erratic. The figures associated with the countryside were far more dire and unreliable. In 1942, for instance, the Indian births and deaths were registered as being the lowest since 1935, but there were no specific explanations for the fluctuations—instead, they were usually attributed "to the defective registration of vital statistics, especially of births in rural as well as in urban areas."[29] Some of the changes were attributed to the threat of war in India in 1941–42 possibly disturbing family life.

To effect improvements in census taking, it was vital to get data on age, fertility, and migration, even though traditionally, the only estimates and collections that existed were classifications by sex, civil condition, and tribe. Lord Hailey described the process by which age classes were introduced in a census planned for Kenya, Uganda, and Tanganyika (but ultimately held only in Uganda) to plot the first age-frequency curve of natives in Africa based on five age-classes (under 1 year, 1–7 years, 7–18 years, poll-tax payers, and aged persons). He noted that, "It would seem, however, that the demand for those details placed too great a strain on the resources of native enumerators, and the returns contained many inaccuracies."[30]

Hailey's induction of Kuczynski into these efforts promised a break from these past practices. Reviewing and consolidating census returns, birth and death reports, special surveys and other statistical records, Kuczynski noted "unacceptable" levels of error, neglect, and ignorance of rudimentary statistical analyses in the demographic reports in Africa. In his *Demographic Survey of the British Colonial Empire*, he noted that the census material in the colonies was based on "reasoned guesses" rather than verifiable evidence.[31] He also complained of a great deal of unevenness in this process among colonies. While information on birth and death registration had been collected in some parts of Africa, such as Sierra Leone in the 1800s, in townships in Nigeria this was done much later, in the 1920s.

Predictably, Kuczynski's efforts to persuade colonial administrators to collect more accurate data by using more refined methodologies and setting up permanent colonial centers for regular data collection were not always well received. Medical administrators and epidemiologists, whose views Percy Granville Edge, an expert on vital statistics in the tropics at the London School of Hygiene, summed up, argued for the need to understand the local context in the colonies—the challenges posed by the tropics—rather than to seek solutions in demographic methods and accurate data alone. Edge and his colleagues spoke of the necessity to carefully negotiate rumors, customs, and habits in census taking and to train native census agents who could overcome these barriers. According to him, "to attempt an enumeration of primitive and illiterate peoples after the highly organized systems followed in the civilized states would be to invite failure and worse at the outset, yet the numbers of such peoples must be known, even if only approximately."[32] However, it was clear that the quest for refining census operations, and even the introduction of "universal" demographic categories and aggregates, was a difficult proposition not only due to local challenges but also because there were seldom enough resources available to translate these visions into action.

What was happening in those years was not simply a struggle between those (like Granville Edge) with local field knowledge of the colonies, working with a raw, untrained rank of enumerators and other limitations, and a new generation of demographers (like Kuczynski) who sought to press new tools, personnel, and categories of analysis "from above" on the census operations. As historians have pointed out, these debates pointed toward a shift in the colonial administration's focus. Colonial censuses in the late-nineteenth and early-twentieth centuries had concentrated on recording ethnological data for enumerative and "civilizational" ends. Now, the census surveys were moving toward welfare- and productivity-centered concerns.[33] In India, for instance, census operations in the early twentieth century represented an effort to collect mostly social and physical data.

Imputing Age

Even as experts conducting demographic surveys tried to identify distinct age groups and distinguish between young and old populations in Asia and Africa, they also often commented on the absence of "identities" based on chronological age. Local officials were aware of the social and ritual definitions of elder status, gerontocratic maturity, and gerontocratic values and had engaged with these hierarchies in colonial administration.[34] However, the censuses and social survey records were rarely reflexive in exploring alternate constructions of the life cycle or how and why age norms developed. They reported that chronological age and aging was difficult to compute because its indicators were only vaguely understood in local societies. Later, by the mid-twentieth century, the developmental paradigm rationalizing these surveys narrowed the focus of their interests even further.

In the early twentieth-century censuses in India, for instance, officials complained that accuracy in measuring chronological age and knowledge of the changing proportions of certain age groups in the population were elusive, remarking that the extent to which age returns were "vitiated by misstatements" was extremely unsatisfactory.[35] The implication here was clear: in "premodern" cultures such as those in many colonies, orality prevailed over written, formal traditions, and this affected how a personal and collective past was both understood and put forward.[36] As a result, there were inexact and competing notions of age, and this required the demographic expert to intervene and suggest uniform and singular events that could capture the age structure in a population.

In a lengthy review of age-related information, census officials in India observed that while misstatements of age in the West were due partly to ignorance, carelessness, or deliberate misinformation, in India they were frequently associated with ignorance. The challenges posed in obtaining accurate information about age, they asserted, were not restricted to the census alone; they were also obvious in rarefied environments, such as the British Indian law courts. "The common people have so little idea of their real age and give such absurd replies when questioned regarding it that Magistrates seldom trouble to ask persons appearing before them what their age is, preferring to guess it for themselves. In the same way, at the census, the age of respondents [was] usually guessed by the enumerators who were taught to estimate age. The latter was not satisfactory either," a census official wrote. "If the latter had been educated persons, the result might not have been unsatisfactory; but ordinarily they were not so, and their guesses often have been very wide of the mark."[37] Sometimes intentional misstatements occurred, including "in the case of unmarried girls who had attained the age of puberty, and in the case of very old people who were prone to exaggerate their age, and of young wives with children, who also are nearly always entered as older than they are."[38]

Officials observed that age was often prompted or inscribed by external authorities, to avoid misstatements given by individuals. It was noted that when figures of authority and power ascribed age, errors were different from the erratic disclosures made by individual natives and could be smoothed over to be statistically satisfactory.

Census officials in British India observed that age-related statistics served a twofold purpose. The first was demographic and epidemiological, for the calculation of death and birth rates and "the probable duration of life at

Table 1   Proportions Calculated on the Unadjusted Ages

Province and number of persons per mille aged	0–15	15–50	50+
India	384	503	113
Bengal	406	497	97
Bombay	372	521	107
Burma	378	502	120
Madras	381	493	126
Punjab	384	494	122

Source: Gait, "Age," *Census of India, 1911,* 149.

different ages."[39] The second purpose, significant in the everyday life of courts, was to help govern social practices "such as early marriage and enforced widowhood, or the liability to certain infirmities at various periods of life."[40] Work on the census in India, and the significance of age and its social control, demonstrated the tensions of trying to regulate local customs such as child marriage that frequently stirred controversies between English and Indian feminists.[41]

These early priorities and focus have an important implication for our narrative. As Table 1 shows, those in the older age brackets tended to be grouped together, while all others were divided into quinquennial periods. The most variable age periods were "0–15" and "15 and over," where the population was growing; the group 15–50 contained the largest section of the population. Officials noted that in the case of India, however, this grouping of the population needed to be between "15 and 40," because "old age comes in quicker in India" and also because this corresponded to the reproductive ages of the population.[42]

While census surveys in India offered some figures relating to populations by age, population experts such as Kuczynski commented that, by contrast, few age-related details were available in British dependencies in Africa. Sierra Leone was an exception, as age-based data was available from censuses conducted from 1891 to 1931. Even in its literate areas, however, there seemed to be a tendency to misstate age. A census report in 1931 observed that, "there seems to be, among the older ones, a certain amount of disinterestedness; they are hazy about their ages and do not appear to think it a matter of any importance and, in many cases, give their ages as 'about' a certain age, instead of exactly." Although younger ages were still easy to ascertain, assessing age "after the age of 20 is mostly a matter of guess-work." But, as Kuczynski observed in his analysis of the census in

Lagos, where early twentieth-century vital statistics were seen as being "untrustworthy" in the age group five to nine years and of infants below one year, even the early age groups were often poorly documented. For instance, according to the census officer, infant mortality was high because most deaths were registered, though probably not all births were.[43]

This aspect attracted medical administrators interested in understanding childhood infections, mortality, and remediable deaths at a younger stage. Most "tropical people," an expert remarked, were carriers of up to two or three infections, and it was hard to separate the onset and end of diseases in adults. In the absence of more exact data on age, some medical experts investigating childhood diseases of the spleen in the Yoruba nation in West Africa chose other "empirical" methods to measure age. They used empirical age scales that compared anthropometric measurements of "Negro" children "who had been extensively weighed and measured" with native people who the researcher noted rarely knew their age due to their superstitions.[44]

What were the underlying assumptions in these efforts to impute age? A statistically deduced and time-dependent "age" associated with these populations not only indexed the course of life; it also served as a principle of social organization for societies that needed to be modernizing.[45] Some experts believed that age would be accurately established in the long run when civilized techniques and tools penetrated more deeply, and its accuracy held the promise of modernity. Meanwhile, others were devising means to collect age data across populations—in this case, by comparing and fixing supposedly racial characteristics and comparing the marginalized colonial subject with the more civilized and modern African American body that had been measured and pathologized in a more scientific manner.[46]

These official demographic accounts rarely referred to the intersections of class and local status except in passing, but it was clear from some private sources that in urban areas, groups of subjects could more easily be classified by age. For a fraction of the population in these colonies, data was better recorded and life expectancy had improved. Actuarial estimates regarding pensions and deaths among white officers had already been addressed in the late nineteenth century through data about pension funds and by means of improved vital statistics of British officers, who were now less prone to premature deaths in the colonies due to better hygiene and public health. Even though actuaries trained in Britain were often disappointed when asked to examine data in India and complained about its "primitive" nature, the educated and wealthy class of Indians who enjoyed the same life conditions as Europeans were now being afforded the same life insurance by private companies.[47]

Defining old age according to chronological thresholds remained a somewhat neglected exercise, but not only because of natives' "ignorance": colonial officials often chose to keep these categories contingent and open-ended. Even in the 1940s, nineteenth-century notions of the constraints of racial difference and torrid climates lingered in administrative discussions, but now they were filtered through the scientific vocabulary of differences in survival, measures of life expectancy, and welfare.[48] Old age as a recognizable stage was given a local and contextual derivation, based on the Indian environment and constitutions, that hastened dependency and functional aging in ways distinct from the pathologies of aging in industrialized societies.

Often, officials grappled not so much with the "precise" age of young and old persons but with what constituted old age and dependence, frequently resorting to criteria based on functional age and dependence to decide who was old. Administrators give us some glimpses into the reasons why they preserved flexibility and discretion in defining old age, in, for example, the fascinating case for pensions titled the "Fixing of 'Old Age' in India." In this case, colonial officials were discussing the award of dependents' pensions to the parents of Emergency Commissioned Officers. Their correspondence demonstrated their interest was not in "proof" of chronological age or in determining its exactness, but to understand when functional "incapacity" or conditions of dependence started in India. The "state of old age" in India, it was noted, could not be related to that in the UK, since the latter was fixed by examination of sickness rates and sickness insurance.

Old age was by definition a state of dependence "when a state of incapacity preceded death by a varying period," but in India this state was reached earlier partly because "age limits" or life expectancy were lower. Colonial officials thus decided to award pensions to "old" parents at an earlier age (fifty-five and sixty for women and men, respectively, rather than sixty and sixty-five) since the "beginning of incapacity" was earlier and since, "Because of climate, race, medical facilities, standards of hygiene and living . . . mortality rates are appreciably heavier than in the United Kingdom."[49] The question of who had the power to set chronological thresholds of age, based on social needs and institutional priorities, was indirectly raised here in this correspondence between the India Office and the Government of India; in some cases the state relented, citing "difference" in Indian bodies and their aging or weathering. The same notions of difference and plurality in defining aging, as we shall see in the next chapter, would be inverted and also be used by less powerful actors— Indian and South African scientists—to make a case for the prevalence of cancer and aging in the developing world.

From Ethnographic Knowledge to National Development

Though Kuczynski and others voiced pronouncements regarding the gaps in demographic knowledge in the colonies from the metropolis, thinking among local officials regarding the scope of census operations was shifting as well. Even as fixing chronological age continued to be elusive, new concerns, such as the collection of vital statistics, emerged in the census and other operations. In the 1940s, when the office of the Indian census commissioner was planning the last census before the colonial transfer of power (1947), census officials continued to express interest in questions of race, caste, and language, but a newer interest in collecting data on work, dependence, and diseases and conditions affecting labor and productivity was also evident.[50] The purpose of these newer questions was to understand the extent of employment and productivity. In departmental files, officials debated at length about how populations in various provinces would respond to these newer questions and whether the enumerators themselves would grasp the questions being posed. The earlier interest in "ethnological" knowledge and social facts was declining among census officials not only in India, but also in countries such as Nigeria.[51] The latter's first, comprehensive census in 1951 showed an interest in economic and developmental questions, with an emphasis on fertility, migration, and occupations.

By the 1940s–1950s, not only colonial administrators but also Indian experts were commandeering the census in the context of decolonization. The latter sometimes inserted a new political slant to the collection of demographic and vital statistics that underscored a nationalist over an imperial agenda. They offered a critique of the collection of data used for imperialist propaganda and against the Indian people. Instead, they advocated building a wider "civic consciousness" to support these surveys and their ends—to build a more substantial foundation of facts "about ourselves" on which to base sound national policies and development.[52]

A year after Indian independence, in 1948, an influential population expert and health policymaker in independent India, Sripati Chandrasekar, wrote a tract on census and statistics in India explaining both the drawbacks and the promise of census data in India. Unlike in the West, he argued, the chain to collect census data was through the local administration and village watchmen, or *chowkidars*, who reported and recorded vital statistics. The census was entrusted to the village administration, and these agencies saw these surveys as one of their many cumbersome and competing responsibilities. The census was therefore termed "a by-product of administration activities" and viewed as a comet appearing in the statistical firmament once in ten years, "attracting much information in its culmination, but passing away eventually unnoticed."[53] Urban middle-class experts such as Chandrasekhar continued to use many of the same stereotypes employed by colonial administrators regarding the collection of population figures and vital statistics, terming India "unchanging" and "slow-moving," and writing reprovingly of the "superstition" and "suspicion" of Indians living in villages.

Chandrasekhar's work is interesting in that he attributed past errors in the census to the prior political conditions in India, such as the nationalist agitation and civil disobedience movements that disrupted census operations in 1921 and 1931.[54] But old challenges such as measuring age, or "the embarrassing problem of deciding the age of the individual," remained. Echoing Kuczynski, Chandrasekhar noted that age was "merely the result of guesswork," with "the degree of error depending on the intelligence of the guess and shrewdness of the census enumerator. So the age hunt of the individual during each census is almost amusing, if it were not so tragic."

Chandrasekhar's remarks about the challenges of mapping chronological age were accompanied by some shifts in approaches, as the need to ascribe and know the age of each citizen, old and young, had become marked. To go beyond relying on the quick-wittedness of the village enumerator, census officials devised other means to fix age among the population. They made use of a calendar of events going back about eighty years, with important landmarks in "public memory," which included well-known incidents of national and local importance, "like the first World War, the death of Queen Victoria, the famine of 1880 . . . the Moplah Rebellion, Mahatma

Gandhi's Salt March in 1932," and other earthquakes, famines and political upheavals.[55] Local- and state-level administrators asked the popu-
lace to provide their age relative to such events, which were likely to linger
in the memory of each person. Disasters especially were perceived as familiar to illiterate peasants of every age, in particular older ones who were
least likely to have records.[56]

Indian census officials in this case were making an initial and tentative
effort to shape national memories and a sense of the past. But for those
who were old in the 1950s, this consisted partly of milestones from a colonial and nationalist past of political events dating to the early twentieth
century and partly of "landmarks" rooted in a symbolic memory of nature
and environmental calamities as shared experiences. Historians have explored the implications for defining old age through memories, including
the "Big Wind" in Ireland (1839), which was used to verify an eligibility
age of seventy years and above for the Old Age Pensions Act (1908). In this
case, the efforts in India through the census were intended primarily to
more accurately order identities based on age, rather than to address old-
age poverty.[57]

Anthropologists, Elders, and a Changing Society

The deepening state-led demographic surveys and developmental visions
coincided with the fieldwork and research of other experts: anthropologists. While anthropological research focused on "elders" and studied
aging in "traditional, hierarchical cultures," it also cultivated a greater interest in generational ties and relations in societies experiencing rapid
changes. For instance, the authority elders wielded in African societies had
been associated with the subordinate and traditional nature of power structures and social relations. Anthropological studies conducted in these
years increasingly focused on the transformation of these relations.[58] In
India in the 1950s, anthropologists' focus shifted away from an interest in
"pre-literate" communities dating back to colonial anthropological surveys
and toward ethnographies of changing social relationships in villages—
caste relationships in particular. Sociological and anthropological village
studies began to focusing on generational ties, and changes to those ties,
in rural areas.[59]

In the 1930s through the 1940s, however, preceding these studies of social change, anthropologists focused on studying remote, primitive cul-

tures in Africa. Such studies included Evans Pritchard's classic exploration of age-sets among the Nuers, a Nilotic ethnic group primarily living in Sudan whose "age-sets" performed an integrated role through their membership in the group, and research on the age grades of primitive tribes such as the Masai, who associated significant privileges to each stage from infancy to old age.[60] A focus on "primitive" societies that were defined by nomadic life, and kinship- or descent-based ties and age-based solidarities that cut across family loyalties characterized these studies. The "old" in these accounts were portrayed as leaders of well-entrenched and carefully ordered patriarchal and territorial networks, and elders and youth were divided by rigid and entrenched differences that determined social conduct and interaction as well as roles in warfare and political power. Although anthropologists often emphasized the role of elders as separate from the role of youthful warriors, it was not clear if the "elders" were always old; the focus was on their shifting power in internal matters.[61]

Alfred Hollis noted in his study that the male Masai had a well-developed system of age grades starting from initiation and circumcision and that the elders had normative control over the warriors, who were responsible for military operations or raids. They were defined by a status and function that was rooted in raids and warfare, but once they stopped being warriors, an unproductive life of "dependence" was ascribed to them. Hollis elaborated, "In olden days a Masai did not become an elder and marry until he had been on several raids and reached the age of 27 or 30; but in these more peaceful times the tendency is to quit the ranks of warriors earlier for their life, though not without its pleasures, is subject to various restrictions. An elder on the other hand may eat and drink what he likes, get drunk and smoke, and generally take his ease."[62] However, though unproductive and dependent on the young, a "gerontocracy" of elders was termed as controlling the young and exercising authority over both entrenched customs and the tribe's resources, and these ideas were further extended in colonial critiques of "subordination" to gerontocracies in African societies.[63]

Old persons, in particular old men, formed a focus of interest for many anthropologists and colonial administrators. British Indirect Rule was in place since the 1920s in large swathes of British Africa, and the changing roles of "tribal" elders frequently appeared in contemporary debates relating to it. Colonial policies began aiming at consolidating "native authority" or acting through the mediating political role of headmen and elders, though colonial administrators sought to use or abuse this "collaboration" based on local exigencies.[64]

Explaining Rapid and Unstable Social Changes

Anthropological research to this point had been characterized by ethnological studies of local cultures and behavior in Africa, but by the 1950s, many anthropological studies also reflected a growing concern in Asia and Africa about a rapid, unstable social transition to modernization. Colonial subjects were moving swiftly "forward" to industrialization and urbanization, but in complex and maladjusted terms.[65] The experience of modernization in contemporary anthropological analysis was colored by the lingering weight of traditional societies and unequal colonial structures. Both the old and young were regarded as unfit to cope smoothly with these changes. Violence, disorder, and instability were always perceived as lurking beneath the surface. These narratives captured the tension and interplay of generational relations in Africa—between the young, migrant workers who moved across the region to join the booming copper industry in Central Africa's Copperbelt and those who were left behind in rural areas.

How did these anthropological studies understand and interpret aging in societies in which fundamental economic and technological transitions in the use of labor and capital were leading to the migration of youth to towns and industry? Ideas and concerns about youth, and even a critique of rapid urbanization and the social tensions associated with migration and mobility, featured in the anthropological quest to understand how primitive societies modernized, but these writings largely neglected the changing lives of older persons. Many of these anthropological accounts described aging with little or no reference to changes in the status and functions of the "aged" over time, and they largely overlooked how deep social forces were profoundly reshaping these roles. These studies mostly reconstructed the family life of the old, as characterized by dependence and filial responsibility. The social ties of old people in some of these narratives rarely captured the diverse range of roles they played in mediating between families and communities. The tasks that marked the old as productive may also have been "hard tasks," and once they became unable to carry out those tasks, these accounts were quick to dub certain groups old and inactive or dependent, rather than considering their contributions to household labor and childcare. The old were described as part of a lifecycle of age and aging marked by "age-sets," and old age within the family was described in terms of decrepit dependence or as a characteristic of traditional societies and rewarded by filial care.

In an account of the social institutions of the Dorobo tribe, the author observed that "most Dorobo are fond of their parents, and treat them in old age with much kindness and consideration. . . . The more helpless the parent, the greater the trouble taken to make them comfortable. The old father of Pilo . . . was such a one. . . . He had to be helped in and out, and fed and looked after like a child; but it was all done cheerfully by Coimim and his wife, in whose hut the old man lived, and if they could not attend to him, Pilo and his wife did."[66] In a description of religion and morality among the Ibo in Nigeria, the boundaries between dependence and idleness are seen as quite permeable; the researcher noted "that while there is little intoxication [among the Ibo], older men sometimes drink because 'They have little else to do.'"[67] The last remark is interesting, and invites the question of whether the anthropologist's own observation was being attributed to local discourse.

Anthropological narratives of the time also tended to identify the old with a primordial and paternalist ethnicity rooted in a tribe. These writings and some missionary accounts tended to represent the aged as a unified category who resisted social change and were wedded to a traditional life cycle. For instance, they reported old people's complaints that wage labor in cities had attracted and spoilt younger persons. Older persons and old age as a distinct stage or category, typified as elders and "dependents," were therefore associated with the fracture of social relations rather than with retirement and social security as they were in the West. Later research in the form of social surveys conducted among old populations in urban slums in Zimbabwe, for instance, shows that a discourse of complaint regarding neglect and disrespect persisted and was partly associated with the poverty and deprivation experienced by older persons, irrespective of whether they were in the countryside or in cities.[68]

Anthropology from Within

Anthropologists associated with Bronislaw Malinowski, the pioneering social anthropologist at the International African Institute, and others who saw themselves as "insiders" termed the ongoing profound social changes a "compound" of two cultural influences or a "mixture of partially mixed elements," shaped by Africans but also by industry, missionaries, and colonial administrators who were no longer seen as external to African society.[69] Anthropologists who were not "outsiders" to Africa, working in emerging institutions—such as the Rhodes-Livingston Institute (RLI), founded in 1938—or who had themselves grown up in a constrained, racist environment gave a different color to their accounts of local societies and the place of elders and age-based hierarchies in times of industrialization and migration. These included Isaac Schapera, who was from a generation of Jewish South African social anthropologists trained in England; Max Gluckman (later director of the RLI); and Monica Wilson, who had been brought up in the Eastern Cape by missionary parents. They viewed these changes as marking not only a disjuncture with the old ways but also the connectedness of these societies with wider global processes. They also engaged with the histories of these societies rather than simply studying cultural contact, as earlier anthropological research had.

A major part of Schapera's work, primarily located in Bechuanaland among the Tswana, explored the socioeconomic changes introduced by the mining economies. Over time his research emphasis shifted from a somewhat ahistorical documentation of "old Bantu culture" in the 1930s to more historically informed accounts of the effects of colonial rule and labor migration in the 1940s. His early descriptions of traditional Bantu society noted that "age and seniority were of considerable importance in Bantu social life. The hierarchy of age was rigidly maintained. . . . This regard for one's elders was extended beyond the family towards the community as a whole. . . . Any insolence or disobedience was strictly punished."[70] In his later work, he argued that anthropologists needed to not only reconstruct the roots of tribal culture but also explore the historical nature of the contact with the colonizers; these changes, he argued, engaged colonial administrators, missionaries and entrepreneurs as much as they did the natives.[71]

Schapera's research in *Migrant Labour and Tribal Life* (1947) captured aging as a life cycle and generational movement of migration, assimilation, and return migration in a narrative that was specifically African in the problems it addressed: changes in Tswana society with migration, histories of the demands of mining industries, hut taxes, and the transformation of a self-sufficient economy. It was also perceptively linked and framed as a global story by his exploration of how the demands of a world economy were transforming local communities. Even though the Bechuanaland

Protectorate commissioned his study to understand how the flow of migrants to European centers of employment affected local society, he was unflinching in his analysis of the larger economic forces that had been unleashed by colonial rule, such as the encouragement of migration to mine gold as an "essential war service" from 1930 to 1935. By 1943, about 33,000 natives, he observed, were away from their tribal areas, seeking life in the mining townships mostly to explore the white man's world and finding more exciting occupations than the monotonous, unexacting life of herding and agriculture that was no longer interspersed with warfare, rituals, or ceremonies. Increasingly, labor migration marked the new coming of age, replacing older rites of initiation, and the "mark of maturity" (*bogwera*).[72]

In *Migrant Labour and Tribal Life*, the association of aging with dependence constantly underlay descriptions of youthful mobility. This is evident in Schapera's descriptions of the visits migrants made and the careful ceremonial redistribution of gifts and savings by migrants' parents or elders. Schapera's research on migrant labor and their moves to cities offers important insights into contemporary anthropological understanding of the place of older persons as a population rooted in a rural life and dependent on the young, migrant worker. Older persons in this narrative were not necessarily chronologically old, but consisted of parents, widows, and others, not absorbed in these new economic forces, who stayed behind in villages. The departure of young persons represented a dissolution of an old tribal life.[73]

In the same vein, Godfrey and Monica Wilson's *Analysis of Social Change* discussed the decreasing value of kinship in rural areas, the transition from primitive kinship to civilized society, and the expropriation of able-bodied young men, all of which resulted in falling agricultural productivity, malnutrition, and profound maladjustments in rural areas throughout Central Africa. In the Wilsons' work, "maladjustment" was a key concept reflecting the "oppositions" or "incoherence" affecting local social relations. They argued that social and economic changes, including race relations and segregation, were responsible for a disequilibrium in society, primarily because in "small-scale society," the total degree of dependence or the "intensity of relations" was high and not spread out, as in the modern world. Dependence on kin, neighbors, ancestors, and other such ties in a traditional society implied that a break in these relations could have a dramatic effect, and communities that had been focused on the past and its traditional dogmas were less able to negotiate change.[74]

The Wilsons offered a scathing critique of the oppositions and conflict that racism and unemployment produced in Central Africa, and they anchored their ideas in the coercion and contradictions of a colonial society. They also viewed the old in the villages as lacking in mobility and as representing closed age and sex groups. In a society undergoing rapid transformation, the old were deemed partly responsible for the disequilibrium; however, this occurred through no fault of their own, as the Wilsons pointed out. They observed, "young Bemba in Broken Hill [mines producing lead and zinc ores in Zambia] find it very difficult to support their elderly relatives (as by traditional custom they should do), yet the old people grew up in a society in which it was impossible to make provision for old age. . . . Similarly, their knowledge and wisdom is out of date, but they could not have acquired knowledge and wisdom applicable to the present. Schools were not available in their youth, and their experience is mainly applicable to a different form of society." In turn, the dependents— elders, women, and children—could not be supported on meager wages in town. The old—chiefs and parents—represented the symptoms of this maladjustment, the Wilsons wrote, as they were uncompromising "moral leaders of the countryside," representing resented values such as dominating "surplus women (who) usually live under the eyes of older relatives, whose influence continually presses on them the obligations of a traditional, or of a new Christian morality."[75] They believed these social and economic transitions offered a degree of autonomy to some (usually younger) groups previously constrained by the ideas, demands, and needs of an unproductive and dependent population of "old" persons in the villages.

Anthropological knowledge of old age and its status could also be used subversively, such as by fusing anthropological narratives with wider nationalist ends. Jomo Kenyatta, Kikuyu leader and founding leader of Kenya, was trained by Malinowski. In researching Kikuyu religion and ancestor worship, he used images of old age and the role of elders to reclaim an African cultural identity. "As a man grows old," he wrote, "his prestige increases according to the number of age grades that he has passed. It is his seniority that makes an elder almost indispensable in the general life of the people. . . . The elder in the community renders his services freely. He receives no remuneration in the way of a salary, but helps the community with advice and experience."[76] In Kenyatta's writings, the dependence associated with elders in the Kikuyu community was not a liability; instead, it marked the strength of kinship ties. Kenyatta not only interpreted the

Kikuyu past but also alluded to Christian ethics to build the loyalty of a wider community, showing, as Berman and Lonsdale argue, that Christianity could both support and undermine colonial rule once it became "domesticated" and allied with a unified cultural past.[77]

Anthropological Knowledge and Demographic Categories

Anthropologists also assumed the role of translators between fields of expertise, and they tried to deploy their intimate knowledge of local context to gain some leverage over demographers and local informants (such as census enumerators) in providing the government with accurate age data. Schapera discussed the importance of accurately identifying populations in the productive ages, and offered the translation of ethnological categories of age grades into chronological age to assist in estimating the actual numbers in the age groups of fifteen to forty-five and forty-five to fifty-nine, who were capable of providing strenuous or ordinary work. "The main difficulty in using a category like 'old people,'" he explained, "is its lack of precision. This unfortunately is inevitable when the majority of natives do not reckon their ages in terms of calendar years. Nevertheless, there is a somewhat more reliable criterion of age that could have been used for the adult population in place of the two categories adopted for the census. I refer to the age-regiment (*mophato*). . . . If a person's age regiment and the date of its creation are known, his approximate age can be estimated, since the usual age of initiation is from sixteen to twenty years." Schapera partly sidestepped the vital issue how useful chronological age is as a definition of aging. His interest here was in demonstrating that the anthropologist, or the authenticity of "insider" anthropological knowledge, could offer a precise account of "working" populations—and as a by-product, interpret, and define "old age"—thereby displacing the uninformed demographic enumerator.[78]

Also gaining prominence in these years was the "dilemma of social security." In the 1940s, there was a deepening of social security provisions; these had initially been extended to address the problem of white poverty, but had not encompassed colored and African populations in South Africa. Scholars have shown that in this decade, pressure for social security in the colonies had increased. White liberals argued that those excluded from the security of kinship networks needed support from the state.[79] Moreover, governments and companies began to extend welfare measures as a part of the "stabilization" of the worker populations at the mines. Sociologists noted that just as Poor Laws were followed by the Welfare State in English social history, a stage had been reached in Africa when the state must assume responsibility for social security, since labor could not be stabilized without permanent urbanization and social security. The perspective in terms of old age was that "the achievement of old age must be paid for either by distress among the aged themselves or out of the expanding economy of the country."[80] In comparative terms, they commented, the difference between the situation in the metropolis and that in the colony (in this case Central Africa) lay in the tempo. That which took centuries to achieve in Europe had to be accomplished in decades in Africa if the "achievement of old age" was not to "be paid for . . . by distress among the aged themselves."[81]

In the demographic and anthropological analyses of social change relating to urbanization in the colonies, the tempo of change was a critical theme laced with moral judgments and assumptions. The erosion of traditional institutions, traditional solidarities, and elder leadership was perceived as occurring at an accelerated and destabilizing pace. This fast-changing society was understood as too complex for the old people in Africa to adapt to by themselves, without expert intervention to "manage" the social tensions and the welfare resources. They contrasted the rapidity of these changes to the steady rise of cities and industrialization in the West, which had occurred at a stable pace over a long period of time. The history of modernization and aging in Europe was therefore a constant source of reference and a normative teleological model, in understanding aging, dependence and the need for social support from the state, even in the 1950s among the RLI researchers. Simultaneously, the future forecast of aging was of distress and decrepitude—a forecast very similar to the writings about maladjustment associated with older persons in the West.

Many liberal anthropologists regarded the progressive deepening of industrialization as irreversible and welcomed this "progress" as a new rite of passage for the young, with little or no mention of the old. Schapera argued that these changes migration and urbanization caused were not "a purely disruptive process"; they were crucial to the natives and the government, and were also of "psychological value in giving youths some tangible means of showing that they have reached maturity."[82] Old people—parents, elders, and others dependent on income from the young—were now generalized as part of this schema of social change but external to it, being located in the countryside, without capital, jobs, or security. They were, however, indispensable to the narrative about rapid, ungoverned change and a "maladjustment" that was as much moral and social as economic, where a prime concern was whether the modernization of "tribal" natives would be an "orderly march" or a "haphazard advance," since it was not likely to be gradual progress.[83]

Decolonization and Indian Village Hierarchies

While colonial ethnographers and anthropologists have been preoccupied with the biology, racial features, cultures, and the folklore of castes and tribes, anthropological accounts in new nations, such as India, began to shift toward ideas and concerns similar to those generated in a colonial context in Central Africa. In the late 1950s Indian anthropologists—many of whom had trained at the metropolis under intellectual gurus such as Malinowski and Evans Pritchard, as anthropologists at the RLI had before them—were undertaking fieldwork in villages and publishing village studies that marked a growing interest in social anthropology.[84] This went side by side with a focus on urban research in various industrial cities across India, even though caste and the "hierarchies" that were seen as central to caste, the immutable key to understanding Indian society, remained concerns.[85] These studies are interesting because by the 1950s to 1960s, despite differences such as a persistent focus on caste hierarchies, anthropological research in modernization and its life stages in the Indian context brought up similar concerns as those raised regarding African urbanization.

Narratives describing older persons located them in villages rather than in industrial cities, and surveys of industrial townships and cities consisted only of a working-age, young, productive population. The early work of well-known Indian anthropologist Dina Nath Majumdar is a case in point. In *The Fortunes of Primitive Tribes*, he explored a range of "tribal" groups, tracing their interdependence, changing cultural practices, and adaptations in terms of beliefs and sentiments based on threats from other cultures, labor demands, and urbanization. In these early studies, the old were crucial informants. They spoke about "how times have changed" and lamented the loss of the gods' and ancestors' power, exclaiming that the "youth had lost all respect for the old." In some tribes living near army settlements, parents and elders were seen as being dependent on the earnings of the young girls in their families.[86]

Later, in *Social Contours of an Industrial City,* Majumdar ventured on a sociological survey of the conditions that shaped migrant labor. He noted that the apathetic conditions in urban areas were "rooted in our caste structure which is a hierarchical system, and [prescribes] . . . the limits of social relationship[s]." Focusing on a young and predominantly male labor force, Majumdar and his field surveyors documented its occupational condition, social observances, lifestyle, and fertility-related practices. Completely absent in these studies of new Indian mill towns, just as it was from studies of the Copperbelt, was the population of older persons above the age of forty to forty-five years.[87]

In the Indian village studies initiated in these years, village elders were still important actors and informants, part of another hierarchy—that of the intergenerational family. In *The Remembered Village,* M. N. Srinivas's classic anthropological study based on fieldwork in a village near Bangalore in the late 1940s (but published decades later), Srinivas's main interlocutors were three old men in the village. As Schapera did, Srinivas commented on the young's uneasy and restless dependence on the old and referred to the lure of the city. Just as Schapera's account underscored the lack of challenges for youth, with occupations being limited to herding village animals and fulfilling labor obligations to the chief, Srinivas's account echoed tensions between the old and the young. He wrote of one of his interlocutors, a rich landowner:

> His sons respected him greatly but I had the feeling that fear was not far removed from the respect. Once his eldest son Swamy asked a boy to go and buy a box of matches from the family shop. He told the boy not to tell anyone that it was for Swamy. Nadu Gowda [the father] was sitting on the verandah in front of the shop. I asked him whether his father was ignorant of his smoking. He laughingly replied that he would be sent out of the house if his father came to know about it. He commented that his life was a miserable one—he scratched the land a bit (derogatory reference to agriculture), ate, slept, and reproduced, that was all. He lived in fear of his father. There were hundreds of others like Swamy in Rampura and neighboring villages, young men who were husbands and fathers, but who had to behave like children before the head of the family. They increasingly resented their dependence.[88]

Srinivas's account also traced how Nadu Gowda built his power in the village by a complex range of strategies. He deployed his caste superiority to demand a hierarchy of labor services, but was far from depending solely on the world of village- and caste-based authority. He had invested in a petrol bunk in Mysore and benefitted from the university educations, "brilliant marriages," and entrepreneurship of his sons.[89] The account gives us a glimpse of the resilience, rather than poverty and decline, of older persons operating within the framework of the intergenerational family in the village

Iravati Karve, a physical and cultural anthropologist, wrote widely on the Indian intergenerational "joint" family, its kinship networks, and the place of the old in the intergenerational family.[90] She argued that the "ancient" age grades in Indian society laid down in old Hindu texts had ensured that gerontocracy in the Indian village never became oppressive, as the old were urged to withdraw from worldly life.[91] She wrote, "Naturally any danger of clash of the old and the young for power, the good things of life etc. was sought to be averted. . . . Thus the aged were respected and cared for while they were prevented from dominating."[92] Karve's goal was not adding historical authenticity to vague generalized claims about a gerontological golden age or giving proof of who observed these strictures; rather, her writing mostly suggested ways to remedy current problems of social maladjustment relating to the economic, technological, and ideational forces "that were making rivalries between old age and youth rampant." The problems of old age, according to Karve, had to ideally be addressed by three generations living in mutual dependence, and norms of behavior had to be created for this.[93]

Even as anthropologists such as Karve suggested that the means to redress a social equilibrium disturbed by rapid social changes and urbanization lay in the family, she and her contemporaries were not overtly skeptical about national development and modernization as goals. Their analyses offered alternatives to understanding aging in a chronological frame by associating it with status and social change, but they also emphasized a politics of friction and disequilibrium, between rural and urban areas, between youth and old age dependence, and between tribal traditions, caste, and customs on the one hand, and city-based secular values on the other.

Christian Missions: Another View from the Field

In Africa, there were other observers of social change and custom trying to document the changing role of the aged and the process of aging across colonies: the missionaries. Interestingly, although ethnographic accounts by missionaries had a long history in the colonies, by the mid-twentieth century, anthropologists viewed them in increasingly derogatory terms, perceiving them as personifying a value-laden "ethnocentrism" and moral judgment that was seemingly effaced in anthropological writing, which strived instead for "listening and maintaining tradition."[94] In 1950, the French Catholic missionary society the Pères Blancs, or White Fathers, initiated an inquiry to gather ethnological data from its missions in West and Central Africa to increase their missionaries' familiarity with local customs and beliefs.[95] This dense inquiry consisted of about 750 questions that would trace a life cycle of customs, rituals, and beliefs relating to family, kinship, marriage, birth, and puberty. Questionnaires were sent to missionaries in each Apostolic Vicariate (consisting of many mission stations) spread across Mali, Burkina Faso, Ghana, Nigeria, Rwanda, Burundi, Uganda, parts of Zambia, Malawi, and Mozambique. Old age and death formed an important (and concluding) section to the questionnaire.[96]

The manner in which the organization of the White Fathers' inquiry (WFI) framed its questions was striking: the inquiry was organized linearly, in a homogeneous sequence of stages more proximate to contemporary social research on human development in the West (such as on the role of the family, notions of childhood, puberty, and old age as distinct stages) rather than being organized by the diverse cultural and religious understandings of the life cycle existing across the numerous ethnic groups and contexts where the inquiry was circulated. Questions about old men and women clearly asked the respondent priest to translate how "middle age" (âge mûr) and "old age" (vieillesse) were distinguished in local vocabulary.[97] It was not clear how the respondents understood and defined old age or who was an old man or woman (vieillesse and vieillard/vieille). They occasionally referred to old populations by chronological age based on demographic records; at other times, they simply based these references on the titles and descriptions assigned to the old or on the status and roles within households of old men and women. Some inquiries, such as "the aged (men and women) were relatively numerous or relatively rare as compared to the rest of the population in the villages near the [mission] station?" resulted in quotes from a recent census on the Yoruba. Others made no reference to how they arrived at their estimates aside from a headcount of small villages with populations ranging from about 200 to 300 residents.[98]

Missionaries still harbored anxieties about the perceived role and influence of older persons in the preservation of "pagan" beliefs still practiced
by Christian converts, and this may have influenced their focus on old age.
The WFI and its respondents tended to dwell on the "moral authority" of
the old in families and community. Questions were posed about whether
older persons missed the precolonial "good old days" when they (the elders) had played meaningful roles and "when everyone adored the family
idols." One of the questions was whether "the old complained easily or
are they happy that the customs of the ancients had been abandoned . . .
due to innovations and changes in the present?"[99] Respondents by and
large reported that the old did complain about a loss of power and fading
customs, but strikingly, many Christian converts continued to follow and
integrate older practices, and Christianity and the missions were not seen
as "outsiders" in African society. This accorded with anthropological evidence. Monica Wilson's research among the Christian Nyakyusa of South
Tanganyika in the 1930s had shown, for instance, that worship of the
"shades" or ancestors and seeing older persons as having afterlives was still
quite common among Christians who practiced what she termed an
"African Christian morality."[100]

More significant, the WFI in 1950–1951 was very much rooted in late colonial politics and concerns about old age in African society vis-à-vis Christianity. In poor, "undeveloped" societies, old age was initially related to the
politics of suffering and stigma that required the needy, including the old,
to be "saved" or protected with Christian compassion. In the mid-twentieth
century, old age and its destitution represented Africa's persistent social ills
that could not be attributed solely to the absence of Christianity or to
heathen savagery and ignorance, but had to be linked to the rapid and
ungoverned social transformation that left the sick, young, and old vulnerable. Scholars have discussed this emerging moral theme of Christian be-
nevolence in the context of missionary medicine.[101] The argument would
be refined later, in the 1970s to 1980s, when Christian NGOs and Jesuit
missions set up the first NGOs for older persons in Asia and Africa, and
"rescued" the old in times of famine and internal displacement; they were
pioneers in setting up social work programs and schools that addressed
the specific vulnerabilities of old age in young societies. They emphasized
supporting the "unproductive" old, who had been left behind by new capitalist forces and migration, but also emphasized the moral politics of seeing

old age as a distinct and vulnerable stage in societies undergoing rapid change.

It is important to understand the origins of these ideas and some of their contradictions when they were being articulated in missionary inquiries in the 1950s. Persistent concerns of the WFI questionnaire were whether old age was a time of decline (*déchéance*) and whether the aged were abandoned by families and communities. Respondents were repeatedly asked if children or collaterals were obliged by custom to take charge of their old when they were frail and incapable of looking after themselves. The question was followed up with: "In case of being abandoned can the old call for a family tribunal or the tribunal of the village chief . . . and can the tribunal deliver a sentence that is effective in practice?" The theme of abandonment was pursued over several questions, inquiring if, "In general, can we say that old men and old women are abandoned or ill-treated (dilapidated or run down huts, clothes, rags, malnourished . . .) or to the contrary? . . . Are there any exceptions? . . . Are there some who are totally abandoned and reduced to begging? Are there any specific differences between pagans and Christians?" Most of the responses from the missions tended to deny that the old were either abandoned or ill-treated, and even observed that "they were respected." Those without children were sometimes abandoned and lived on public charity, they admitted, but added that both pagans and Christians tended to look after their old with the same care (even if some noted that Christians devoted themselves more intensely and carefully to fulfilling these duties).[102]

Notions of the abandonment of the African old have a long history in missionary writing. Andreas Sagner's account of the Wesleyan Methodist and London missionary societies' nineteenth-century writings about the African elderly among the Xhosa records "dire portrayals" and atrocity stories of the Xhosa's treatment of the old. For instance, the legendary Robert Moffat, father-in-law of David Livingstone, had reported that, "The Xhosa carried their helpless aged to the bush to die, and extremely frail old women were almost entirely ignored . . . frequently left to starve or die of exposure or neglect." These ideas showed concern that the native old were simultaneously impediments to spiritual and material progress and also innocent victims of a primitive society. Missionaries certainly overlooked or neglected to mention the changing social patterns and poverty among the Xhosa in the wake of famine and disease in the 1770s, and they pressed forward Victorian notions of aging and dying as well as Western notions of intergenerational respect based on "civilized" behavior, which looked down on indigenous forms of respect (*intlonipho*).[103] Similar judgments of innocent suffering were also evident in social commentaries in India, by missionaries such as Reverend Peggs and others of the Serampore mission, regarding the Hindu practice of leaving the old and sick to die by the banks of holy rivers such as the Ganges, described as the "*Ghat* murders."[104]

But times had changed by the 1950s: mission values and interests were no longer only to catechize and civilize, and the missionaries associated with the White Fathers in the postwar period were not throwbacks to Moffat or Livingstone. Many had fought in France with communists and socialists, and some even entertained working class visions; they were conscious of growing pressures to make the Church more diverse. While they were often criticized for neglecting social problems, they did perceive the seriousness of problems of family life and old age in Africa, and they saw addressing these problems as part of an agenda of social progress. They framed their understanding of old age in the non-Western world less as a civilizational critique and more as a "lack," for it meant the old were not protected by "*le milieu familial*" (the environment of the family) and were made "visible" in society, representing its chronic poverty. Neglected by the family and state, aging was associated not only with the trope of abandonment in an uncivilized culture but also now with "destitution" and development.[105]

The White Fathers' ethnographic survey of the 1950s reveals that in the late colonial decades, missionaries were among several agencies that were simultaneously trying to understand, classify, and capture the changing characteristics of colonial populations, with a focus on the demand for and the impact of industrial wage labor, productivity, and migration. In these mission narratives, the old are accorded a separate section and place in the survey, giving them a stable and homogeneous identity. They are separated from the young. There are, however, few references to the other roles, religious or otherwise, the old played in shaping or initiating the life stages of younger members and in mediating ancestor worship; however, their respondents occasionally quoted local proverbs and sayings to illustrate the role of elders, hinting that the old and their place in society was always linked with other identities—of family, kinship, property, and gender. The missionary accounts across diverse societies, from the Yoruba to the Hutus, also indicate something the missionaries themselves failed to recognize: the "old" consisted of a small but significant population that was helping itself and holding families and communities together, even as village societies

reeled under the forces of capitalism, labor migration, and growing poverty at the household level—for colonial rule, as John Illife notes, had not
only preserved certain forms of poverty but also created new and resilient
ones.[106]

On the whole, missionary accounts and surveys reinforced the belief
that old age and aging were different in non-Western settings, and a perception or misperception of the misery and marginality of the old in that
world. Older persons were understood as being a population of dependents
in dependent colonies where the family milieu was disintegrating. These
ideas about aging populations as victims of chronic poverty and displacement would be repeatedly evoked a few decades later by international
NGOs (see Chapter 6), which sometimes worked with the missionaries in
the 1980s as moral and compassionate flag bearers for the old and vulnerable in developing nations.

Interpretations of Old Age in Young Societies

Old age as a marginal social condition, as an abiding mark of poverty, was
being linked with modernization in Africa and Asia as social scientists and
missionaries tried to understand, control, and manage the deep-seated social
and economic changes occurring in the colonies in these decades. What
impact did these demographic and anthropological studies have beyond
Asia and Africa, in the United States, in Europe, or in international population debates? Did this research in the colonies shape the making of gerontological knowledge in the West? I argue that gerontological writings
in the United States, for instance, began to be interested in comparing old
age in traditional and industrialized societies, but were steadfast in viewing
old age and elders in non-Western societies through a lens of "difference"
and through essentialized social categories, such as extended families. These
traditional societies were characterized as having historically experienced
gradual social change that had allowed for well-adjusted changes in social roles among the old, unlike in the West. These writers—and this is
striking—took little note of the contemporary anthropological and demographic literature on Asia and Africa that emphasized the unstable social
and developmental changes sweeping the colonies and young nations.

In the 1940s, there were some works published by gerontologists and experts on human development in the United States that drew on research
from missionary and anthropological literature. The social anthropologist

Leo Simmons's *The Role of the Aged in Primitive Societies* (1945) was widely circulated, with parts of it being reprinted in several important textbooks on aging—with changes in the title and referring to aging in "earlier cultures" (1956) and, later, to a more politically correct, "pre-industrial cultures" (1960).[107] Simmons's work, although published as early as 1945, was also evoked in canonical works on aging such as the *Handbook on Social Gerontology* (1960) and frequently cited by leading sociologists at the University of Chicago, such as Ernest Burgess and Robert Havighurst, as well as Clark Tibbits at the University of Michigan.[108] Apart from being quoted in later studies (1970s) on aging in developing countries, the book and its editions also enjoyed currency among leading biologists and psychologists. In short, between 1945 and 1967, Simmons remained the enduring spokesperson for cross-cultural gerontology.[109]

Simmons belonged to the first generation of medical sociologists trained at Yale during the Second World War, and his research reflected an effort to combine an interest in the biological and social sciences. Simmons's study method in the book consisted of identifying about 109 traits that he correlated in seventy-one primitive societies (comprising an arbitrary selection of tribes, of which sixteen were from North America, ten from Central and South America, fourteen in Europe, sixteen in Asia, and twelve in Oceania and Australia) to assess the differential treatment of old people. He employed an evolutionary framework based on ethnographic data compiled by George Peter Murdock at Yale, known as the Human Relations Area Files (HRAF), to offer "a report on the status and treatment of the aged within a worldwide selection of primitive societies." Simmons argued that there were differences in science, technology, and sociopolitical institutions that distinguished aging in primitive, pre-industrial societies where the old were a minority. In contrast, the fate of the aged in industrialized, civilized societies had led to a "helpless and hopeless period" among the old, when civilized societies were successful in keeping the old alive but did not know what to do with them.[110] Using the HRAF in his book meant Simmons chose traits such as abandonment, derision, or glorification of the old to assess their change in status. The appeal of his work was that even though it studied primitive societies, its lessons and message were aimed at the challenges posed by aging in the West.

Not all contemporary experts prioritized this approach. Some merely chose to use existing studies of families and kinship in pre-industrial settings, such as China, to contrast the plight of the elderly in the United

States with that in traditional societies. Contemporaries such as the Co-lumbia University–based sociologist Kingsley Davis used studies of family and kinship in agrarian societies in China as a contrast to bring out the les-sons of traditional societies, where the young observed a respectful attitude toward all old people; these societies were typified as representing a back-ward and feudal stage. Davis wrote, "In general the respect and power commanded by the aged is greatest in static agricultural and familistic societies. In China and the Orient, where these traits reach their extreme, the old have greater authority and prestige than any other age group." The authority of the old was revered in this familistic system, with the elder heading a "larger joint family" in life and being deified in death. He added, "To us the society seems to look backward rather than forward because of the stress laid on the aged as against the young. . . . *We dwell on the role of the aged in old China because it illustrates the opposite of our own situation.*"[111]

Simmons's work aimed not simply to bring out cultural comparisons and difference. He saw his study on aging as holding important lessons for "re-silient aging" as demonstrated by the aged in primitive societies. The se-curity and prestige achieved by the old in these societies were achieved through "personal initiative," and their condition and survival was charac-terized by an interplay between impersonal forces and "personal, conscious efforts" when they tried different expedients. In industrial societies, tradi-tional types of adaptation had broken down, and there were only planned and legislated forms of social security. In the industrialized West, there was a lack of roles and efforts on the part of the aged to maintain their place in the group and to ensure their support and care. Noting the challenges rapid change posed to the patterns of adjusting among the elderly, Sim-mons observed that the aging needed a lifetime to fit, adjust, and entrench themselves, but when conditions became unstable and change in the so-cial order occurred at a galloping pace, the old were likely to "ride for a fall" and be tripped up by the young.[112]

Studies such as Simmons's were popular because they addressed and il-luminated crucial domestic concerns about aging. Simmons's later work made a conscious effort to speak to contemporary debates, in particular anxieties about old age dependence and the growing "minority status" as-sumed by the old, as well as the associated political demands.[113] *Aging in Primitive Cultures*, with its images of sudden changes, migrations of fami-lies and tribes, and the threatened marginalization of the aged in primi-tive societies straddled between reverence and abandonment or violent killing, was a cultural and political analysis of the non-West; but with its message to the old to cope, to adapt over time, and not to be caught "off guard," it was also a lesson and judgment regarding the social and cultural changes overtaking American society.

Somewhat later, in the 1950s, in *The Aged in Rural Society*, sociologist T. Lynn Smith remarked that the relative position of the aged reached "its maximum in the most highly developed civilizations. That is to say that when the rural mode of existence reigns supreme, the lot of the aged is probably far superior to what it is in pre-rural (primitive groups), on the one hand, or in the more highly industrialized civilizations, on the other."[114] He dwelt at length on the patterns of aging in America, in particular the implications of aging in rural America. Much as Simmons argued in the context of primitive societies, Smith argued that the old were best off in societies that were "stable" and where change was experienced in a gradual manner. The rapid and accelerated transition of American society toward industrialization and a surge in the aging population had caused fractures leading to the old in rural areas being abandoned and to regions like the South becoming depopulated due to the migration to cities. Smith was especially worried by the heavy exodus of "negroes" from the South and the social costs of supporting the old and dependent in that population.[115]

The parallels with non-Western, primitive societies were close in terms of the challenges the old faced with devising ways to cope and make themselves relevant. Simmons had referred to new occupations being found for Polar Eskimos and Inca women attending to indoor chores or to scare off rodents in the field: none "was allowed to eat the bread of idleness."[116] Fears of old persons becoming "dependent" and of their idleness or lack of occupation after receiving social security were common anxieties among contemporary policymakers, and a range of social scientists contributing to studies on life after retirement wrote in these years about keeping older populations occupied and productive.

An interest in aging in primitive societies across the world, where the old were a minority and faced the challenges of being poor and marginalized, also resonated with a specific kind of social concern about aging. Smith argued that surveys on aging in the United States displayed important lacunae: they did not consider the expected sharp and continued rise in the numbers and proportions of the "Negro" aged. In the spectacular rise in aging that had occurred since 1930 in the United States, Lynn Smith noted that the increase in the "Negro" population was significant.[117] The problem of aging in the United States was far from uniform. Not only did it reflect the rapid growth in the black population according to Smith, it also had more important implications for resources such as old-age assistance, with certain states such as those in the Deep South more likely to be caught off guard by this growing crisis.

Smith's work had a wider resonance because he raised two interrelated questions. First, he questioned the multiplicity of meanings brought up in discussions of aging and its cleavages. Making aging out to be a new problem and that increasingly focused on urban white populations neglected to focus on its differentiation. It ignored the inequalities that underlay aging in the United States—the racial differences, the aging of "Negroes," and their deprivation. Smith also raised the case of state social security payments that would be brought on by paying and supporting an already vulnerable population of blacks if they were not kept back and tied to their lands in the South. This was the second issue his work highlighted, an aspect of aging that made it a growing domestic and international preoccupation: the question of "imbalance" within and between nations caused by migration, the perceived inactivity or dependence of those drawing state pensions, the maladjustment of the old to new social situations, and financial burdens. Smith's work on aging and migration was presented at the 1954 World Population Conference in Rome, where panelists were interested in the social and economic instabilities increasingly triggered by the movement of populations within nations such as America.[118]

His work demonstrated deep-seated tensions and racial disparities in the making of gerontological claims and worries in the United States. It offered an initial articulation of the idea that populations that were "different," such as African Americans in the United States and colored, colonial subjects in Africa, had a developmental trajectory and pathologies in common. The making of international gerontology with a focus on the biology of aging and chronic diseases further underscored these disparities regarding aging and its normative bodies and diseases.

2

Growing Old in the Time of Chronic Disease

In July 1954, the CIBA Foundation hosted a Colloquium on Aging in London.[1] CIBA meetings were known to focus on new and promising scientific agendas; this colloquium anointed the biology of aging as one such field.[2] Among the array of leading scientists, most from Europe and the United States, were two noted scientists who were the sole representatives of their continents: Vasant Ramji Khanolkar, the director of the Cancer Research Institute in Bombay, and Theodore Gillman, who worked in South Africa on malnutrition and liver cancers among the Bantu with his more famous brother, Joseph, a pathology professor at the medical school at Witwatersrand.

Gillman began his presentation by observing that his research contributed to understanding aging in "backward countries." He said, "The entire biology of backward peoples in Africa, the Middle and Far East, and elsewhere in this world, differs profoundly from that of Western civilized people, not primarily because of genetic differences (which cannot be easily assessed), but rather by virtue of a host of environmental factors."[3] Gillman's presentation at the CIBA conference made clear that research

among civilized, well-fed populations on aging and cancer was not generalizable to poor countries and among "backward" people. The risk of liver
cancer in these countries was not determined by fat intake and altered
blood lipids, as it was in white populations. Rather, the lifelong or "lifetrack"
exposures of backward populations to environmental factors such as malnutrition, poverty, heat, humidity, parasitic infections, and early adaptation
to urbanization caused a unique pathology of chronic diseases such as
cancer and premature aging. Since the Bantu suffered from liver cancer
in their youth, cancers among them were not a problem of late maturity
and aging as in the West. Liver cancers occurred earlier among the Bantu,
and other cancers were often not visible because the Bantu lived shorter
lives.

Gillman's talk signaled his resistance to the assumptions in contemporary
U.S. and European gerontological theories. In the late 1940s and 1950s,
aging was viewed primarily as a problem of senility, and interest in the
symptoms of senile changes and the potentially modifiable "wear and tear"
of organs in older persons grew. Western gerontologists were shaping an
agenda of aging research primarily around investigating chronic diseases
regarded as "diseases of aging." This priority had a significant rationale: it
was triggered by the growing problem of white, male, and middle-aged
bodies and their aging or their vulnerability to chronic diseases—a concern that resonated particularly in the United States.

These years witnessed the birth of international biomedical research
networks focused on studying the biology of aging processes. These gerontological experts actively searched for patrons and for intellectual support
to deepen their agenda. This led to a growing alignment between researchers
working on the biology of aging and emerging networks of cancer research, which were centered in the United States and Europe and rapidly
expanding into Asia and Africa. Ted Gillman's presentation at the CIBA
meeting and the extended research the Gillmans and V. R. Khanolkar
undertook separately relating to cancers in South Africa and India helped
recast the ways aging and its proxy in these decades—that is, chronic,
degenerative diseases—were viewed beyond the West.

Chronic Diseases and the Birth of International Networks

Since the beginning of the twentieth century, an emphasis on aging's links
with the effects of chronic, degenerative diseases had gained currency not

only among gerontologists but also among other prominent scientists, who argued that chronic diseases accelerated or distorted the "normal" course of aging. In the 1930s, the Nobel Prize–winning physiologist Alexis Carrel, working at the Rockefeller Institute for Medical Research, emphasized the usefulness of research on aging and its cellular development in particular. Investigations into "the nature of senility," he argued, "could throw vital light on nutritional diseases" and "such pathological problems of fundamental importance as sclerosis (hardening of organs), of premature old age, susceptibility to tumors and other unresolved problems of degeneration of the body preceding its time."[4] These notions reflected views, voiced in the interwar years, about aging being a disease potentially treatable by stemming its degenerative aspects. These views held that restoration of normal aging was possible with the right kinds of scientific interventions.

As war clouds gathered in Europe, the scientist Vladimir Korenchevsky, a Russian émigré in England who founded the British Society for Research on Ageing (1939), wrote to a group of American scientists suggesting the time was ripe to found an international association to propagate research on aging on a worldwide scale and "from all conceivable aspects." His pursuit was interrupted by the Second World War. But he did discover that a gerontological collaboration called the Club for Research on Aging (CRA) had been initiated in the United States with the support of the Josiah Macy Jr. Foundation.[5] By 1950, with prospects for an alliance seeming more promising, Korenchevsky visited several gerontological societies across Europe—in Belgium, Czechoslovakia, Denmark, Italy, France, and Spain—and encouraged them to fashion a common agenda, but he pursued American scientists most vigorously of all. He informed various foundations that his survey revealed nineteen societies interested in aging existed across the world. He also told prospective collaborators that he and his colleagues were organizing the first international meeting of gerontologists in Liege, Belgium to facilitate international cooperation in this extremely difficult area of research. He hoped that with steps such as these, "an international army of distinguished specialists in medical and scientific research . . . will be formed, and ready to attack, in [an] organized and cooperative manner, the problems of ageing," though he noted that funds were critical, because "an army without equipment was not an army at all."[6]

In particular, Korenchevsky directed his pleas to E. V. Cowdry, a Canadian-American biologist based at the Washington University in St. Louis. Cowdry, then chair of the CRA, had secured funding to establish the Gerontological Society (1945); he was also the author-editor of the seminal *The Problems of Aging* (1939).[7] Cowdry's experience of biological research went far beyond the United States, and his support was crucial to any plans envisioning an international profile for aging research. He had started his career working in China and South Africa on projects supported by the Rockefeller Medical University, and he was a prime mover in setting up international research networks and professional associations of biologists and medical researchers working on diseases such as cancer and arteriosclerosis. In the early 1940s, he had advised the Indian government on setting up a cancer research institute in Bombay. Cowdry's network and professional associations with international scholars were vast. In Korenchevsky's opinion, he could bring two crucial elements to this new initiative: an ability to translate scientific problems to a wider, interdisciplinary audience and access to resources in American foundations and government. During his trip to the United States, Korenchevsky met various members of the CRA, including Nathan Shock, the head of the newly established Gerontology Unit at the National Institute of Health (NIH). Korenchevsky's American contemporaries privately recorded their initial reservations in forging this alliance, but they admitted that research on aging in the United States was in its nascent stage, while Europe was decades ahead in the field. Some even conceded that an international collaboration would offer opportunities to explore European laboratories and exchange ideas.[8]

Following Korenchevsky's visit to the United States and a growing interest in collaboration, several American delegates and representatives of gerontological societies from about twelve countries attended the first International Gerontological Congress (IGC), held July 1950 in Liege, Belgium. The gathering was significant: it led to the formation of the International Association of Gerontology (IAG), consisting of European researchers and U.S.-based scientists, and it emphasized a primarily scientific agenda and program for gerontological research. Medical and biological research would reign in the IAG for a number of years before social experts began to predominate.

Most papers in the IGC's early years centered on the "diseases of aging," though scientists debated whether these diseases were actually related to and affected the aging process or simply affected a larger section of the older population relative to others. Some scientists even argued that old age was simply a stage when chronic diseases proliferated and were distinct from the afflictions of younger age groups.[9] Delegates focused in particular on arteriosclerosis, cancers, and heart disease—the "chronic diseases" becoming a distinct medical and policy category in the United States in the 1950s, according to the historian George Weisz.[10] Therefore, the study of aging and its diseases, including institutional support for health research and programs received in the United States, came to be rooted partly in the emerging agenda of chronic diseases.

This link between the agendas of gerontological research and research into diseases of old age was intrinsic to how gerontologists understood the aging process and aimed to "normalize" it. Korenchevsky, Cowdry, and other leaders of the CRA, such as Nathan Shock, wrote about aging as a manageable process. For aging to occur in a "normal" trajectory, the diseases that influenced the process needed to be controlled, because senility and death were not understood as "necessary" phenomena; they were contingent and could be caused by "pathological senility," when deficiencies or other dysfunctions occur.[11] Korenchevsky observed that gerontological research was still searching for what he termed "normal physical senescence" to understand how deterioration occurred in individuals. Present-day aging, he wrote, was a "pathological condition, a kind of disease that was abnormal." It was the duty of "medical gerontology," he advised, "to prevent the pathological part of aging" or to prevent premature and "abnormal" aging.[12] Gerontology therefore had to be constituted as a multidisciplinary field, involving experts in diseases of old age—those who understood changes in physiology and pathological processes—to explain how diseases affected various parts of the body, leading body parts and tissues to age in different ways and at varying paces.[13] The IAG was also working to build scientific legitimacy by distancing gerontology from dubious associations that had harmed its credibility, such as its ties with "anti-aging research" that aimed at prolonging life.[14] Korenchevsky was keen to project the biological aspects of gerontology and its disease-centered priorities as the primary and defining scope of the IAG's work.

The notion of aging as a problem had a ready answer in the promise of medical research. The president of the fourth IGC, held in Merano, Italy (1957), reiterated Korenchevsky's views, seeing aging itself as a new "factual condition" caused by eliminating the causes of early death, which resulted in an increased population of old people. The old, he added, were "relatively normal but more often suffering from ailments." Gerontology, he therefore surmised, had attracted special enthusiasm from medical men because old age itself was like a chronic disease, with "distinguishing marks of duration, progress, stationary phases and successive lesions." Its frequency and clinical causes in the form of various diseases needed to be investigated.[15]

The Subjects of Biological Gerontology

These disease-centered ideas also imbued gerontology with a unique and prophetic social mission tied to "human welfare." Korenchevsky summed up the social problems symptomatic of these biological challenges: "The problem [aging] has become of increasing importance for every civilized nation, because of the steadily progressing increase in the numbers of aging. The social implications are serious since a large proportion of the old people become a burden on the younger generation. . . . At present, old age, with approaching death, is a tragic period of human life."[16] The tragedy, as Korenchevsky and Cowdry interpreted it, had significant social dimensions, because the aging process and its abnormal onset affected men in their prime who were in posts of high responsibility. During the war, Korenchevsky argued, the pathology and physiology of aging had also become a war problem; transferring responsible posts to young men who lacked experience was not a solution.[17] Subsequently, Cowdry would underscore the issues of veterans' health and their disability payments and medical care; investigating their aging process would be vital to industry and to organized labor. Cowdry believed that international support for gerontological research was based on the shared fears in these societies of "progressive illness and economic dependency" brought on by the "problems of aging."[18]

These scientists were crafting a role for gerontology as a new field in the international arena by emphasizing it as "a science of consequence in human welfare" so universally relevant that it held the promise of becoming a "world movement" characterized by interactions that were "untrammeled by national boundary or professional status . . . to bring up the positive role of older people in a dynamic world and community."[19] These claims became the standard opening lines for many inaugural speeches at international gerontological meetings. At the First Pan-American Congress of Gerontology held in Mexico City (1956), for instance, attended by many IGC leaders, Cowdry, then chairman of the North American Committee of Cooperation, remarked that gerontology was "a subject in which the entire world has become interested."

Even as gerontological experts were building the IAG collaborations and scientific networks, they aspired to speak for the "entire world" from their newly created platform. The networks offered by chronic disease researchers, particularly those like Cowdry who straddled the research worlds of arteriosclerosis, cancer, and aging, offered an incipient field like gerontology a window to a more expansive scientific world. Cancer research networks provided a more cosmopolitan stage for gerontologists and their concerns to move beyond a largely provincial arena of aging in Europe and the United States. By the second IGC, hosted by Cowdry and his collaborators in St. Louis, the IAG committee had chosen a flower-like emblem drawn on a world map, indicating the scale of its vision and collaborations. The presence and contribution of collaborators beyond Western Europe and the United States was, however, limited in the 1950s: they occasionally joined the gerontological congresses, but they did not shape their agenda. Sometimes, international representation consisted of a token few countries; the IGC held in Italy in 1957, for instance, included delegates from Venezuela, Argentina, and Yugoslavia, some Polish and Greek representatives, and a few "observation" delegates from the USSR.[20]

Searching for Domestic and International Patrons

In the 1950s, experts affiliated with the IAG increasingly pronounced that aging was now a problem faced by every civilized nation, with gerontological research providing a worldwide panacea for its concerns. Prominent names such as Cowdry made these observations not only at international meetings but also at national aging meetings in the United States, where they tried to leverage domestic support for aging-related research and gerontological education.

In August 1950, after a summer spent attending gerontological conferences in Europe, the Federal Security Agency (FSA) invited Cowdry to the National Conference on Aging, which was being held at the special request of U.S. president Harry Truman.[21] Cowdry used the occasion to deftly interweave international and national concerns by listing common anxieties and problems, and underscoring the importance of funding new research programs to support the development of gerontological expertise as a career option for young scientists. He was quick to highlight what the government would reap from these initiatives, adding that the "return in human welfare . . . was so manifest" in this enterprise. American resources devoted to gerontology could contribute to the world's betterment through international cooperation while also establishing U.S. scientific leadership in an emerging field. He argued that new techniques made new directions in gerontology feasible, emphasizing both the possibilities of tissue-based research held for examining aging and the use of new electron microscopes to understand the aging process in various organs. Korenchevsky too had pointed to the promise held out if U.S. scientists stepped in to support gerontology. In one communication to Cowdry a few years before the IAG was founded, he wrote, "I have a strong feeling that our meeting will have some definite favorable effects on a more rapid development of research on ageing in all civilized countries. Every country is now watching the U.S.A."[22]

As a reputable cytologist, Cowdry was aware of the power and resources in biomedical research sourced from large U.S. foundations. From 1920 to the 1950s, biological research in the United States had received support to solve long-term political and social problems, with an increase in both funding and faith in science and its ability to solve medical and public health problems.[23] This patronage had guided the scientific agenda and careers of researchers in the United States, and had in turn brought international researchers to the Rockefeller laboratories.[24] Indeed, the Rockefeller Foundation had supported Cowdry's own career after he graduated from the University of Chicago: initially posted at the Peking Union Medical College in the 1920s, Cowdry worked at the Rockefeller Institute for Medical Research before he settled in St. Louis.

A Missing Link

However, as Cowdry noted in his presentation to the National Conference on Aging, the movement to mobilize scientific research on aging lacked support from the United Nations or "any financial bait or stimulation from the US"; it was distinctive in springing "from the grassroots." Cowdry's comparison of the IAG with other contemporary scientific endeavors highlighted a crucial gap in the birth of gerontology's international scientific networks: they were not overtly blessed by UN agencies, which otherwise supported a range of international scientific research in these years. Later, there was partial support (when many of the gerontological congresses were sponsored by UN bodies).[25] The third IGC in London (1954), for instance, was held with funding from diverse sources, such as the Council of the International Organization of Medical Sciences (subsidized by the World Health Organization [WHO] and the United Nations Educational, Scientific and Cultural Organization [UNESCO]), the Nuffield Foundation, and the CIBA Foundation.[26] The UNESCO, as historians have demonstrated, was a key UN agency in funding environmental and biological scientific research in the 1930s and 1940s; later, it sponsored research on population growth as both its "scientific" and "education" brief. In the 1950s, the UNESCO identified population growth worldwide as a source of cultural, educational, and scientific tension, and it supported projects exploring social tensions in industrialized and industrializing societies.

However, the IAG received no such resources initially, partly because the domain of gerontology and its biological framings were still viewed with ambivalence.[27] At the Merano IGC in 1957, the noted French demographer Jean Bourgeois-Pichat, who was employed at the UN's New York office, justified the world body's stance. Pointing out that specific agencies existed for many fields of social intervention, such as the United Nations Children's Fund (UNICEF), UNESCO, the International Labor Organization (ILO), and the WHO, he remarked, "There are no specialized institutions that are dealing with the aged. Is this a lacuna that needs to be bridged? I do not think so, since gerontology traverses many diverse fields." UN studies had demonstrated that life expectancy was still about forty to forty-one years in developing countries in the 1950s, in contrast to sixty-five to sixty-six years in the developed world. He argued that aging was still not an issue relevant to developing countries, for they had not succeeded in conquering infectious diseases, prolonging life, controlling fertility, and making a transition to an aging-structure population. Bourgeois-Pichat observed that UN priorities in offering technical support for aging-related programs had been focused on where population aging was most advanced, namely in Europe.[28]

Bourgeois-Pichat's voice needs to be situated as that of a representative of the Population Branch of the UN, who saw aging as defined by the universalizing models of demographic research. He was implying that aging was restricted to the West because in demographic terms it represented a linear, stage-wise transition from developing to industrialized countries that was explained by shifts in infectious and chronic disease as well as in longevity and fertility. His ideas, as historians have pointed out, assumed a social homogeneity that was not applicable or generalizable across all classes even in the West. The development of the Keynesian welfare state, with its support of social schemes and its justification for a large public sector in the economy led to growing rigidity in assigning and observing age thresholds.[29] Bourgeois-Pichat's criticism was that gerontology still lacked firm and standardized categories, and that its complexities needed to be compressed, to fit in with the demographic, normative frameworks espoused by the UN, where specialized agencies represented distinct life stages (such as UNICEF) or separate social and medical concerns (the UNESCO and the WHO, respectively).

Exploring Alternative Partnerships

With the UN failing to show much interest, IAG leaders looked for other sources of support. They noted that in the case of chronic diseases, both funding for research on them and institutional support were growing vastly, as several historians have documented.[30] In the mid-1930s, the U.S. Public Health Service surmised that diseases of childhood were largely under control, and long-term chronic conditions were the new disease burden and health threat in the United States.[31] The studies and pressure from scientific opinion in the country about the epidemiological challenges chronic diseases posed led to steps such as the establishment of the Cancer Institute (1937) and increased monetary and other support for work on such diseases. With professional ties being built across several areas of research, researchers who were founding gerontological networks began to work closely with pathologists working on chronic diseases. Cowdry and other CRA members were involved in efforts to build professional collaborations and research networks among researchers interested in debates on arteriosclerosis, nutrition, and cancer. The CRA found support from the Josiah Macy Jr. Foundation for both Cowdry's arteriosclerosis project and for organizing gerontological meetings.[32]

At times, the tendency to fuse the professional networks and membership of the aging and the degenerative disease associations was questioned, but often adjustments followed. Members of the American Society for Arteriosclerosis, for instance, resisted a common agenda with a conference on aging, since they wanted research that only related to arteriosclerosis to be discussed at their annual meeting.[33] Harold Dorn, a well-known demographer and cancer epidemiologist, who represented the FSA at the 1951 IGC in St. Louis, voiced a more serious criticism of the mingling of networks and agendas. Pointing to the somewhat motley crew of participants at the IGC in his report, he observed, "I have mixed feelings concerning the Second International Gerontological Congress. . . . My personal opinion is that the Congress exemplified the present confusion and lack of consensus concerning the problems of gerontology. . . . There seemed to be no clear cut idea of what was meant by the term aging nor what criteria one would use to place a meaning upon the word."[34] Dorn was referring to the multiple "problems" identified by gerontologists at the St. Louis conference, which ranged from debates about what constituted the process of aging and senescence, to the notion of aging as a pathological disease, to an interest in aging as a stage in late life that was associated with chronic diseases.

Most of the participants in IGCs in the 1950s were biomedical researchers interested in the "problems" of aging; they did not necessarily identify themselves as gerontologists, nor did most of them work in institutions fully devoted to aging research. Both international borders and disciplinary boundaries were transcended in gerontological meetings. Being at the margins of the UN's internationalist vision and lacking action-based support for large-scale research and programs implied fluid intellectual and professional boundaries that also held potential. Despite the lack of international patronage for their networks and plans, as Cowdry noted in his address to the National Conference on Aging, these experts brought significant advantages to a new field. They helped build networks across areas of biomedical research where aging research found sufficient scientific resonance.

Although Dorn critiqued the multiplicity of gerontological views and approaches evident at the second IGC in St. Louis, these characteristics could also become a strength in the form of the open and fluid networks in this emerging field. A good example of this is Cowdry's bringing to the conference a wide range of collaborators and researchers working on chronic diseases, in particular cancer and heart disease. Cowdry's private papers and correspondence in the months before the IGC are telling. They describe how he and his American colleagues on the IAG organizing committee used his older connections—through his work with the Rockefeller Medical University and his time at the Peking Medical College, as well as links through Harold Leroy Stewart, a leading force behind the International Union Against Cancer (now Union for International Cancer Control, UICC)—to reach out to scientists to attend the IGC.

Tackling the Problem of Premature Aging

Cowdry and others in the CRA, such as William MacNider, Clive McCay and Lawrence Frank, were among those interested in the effects of chronic disease on aging even before the efforts to build international gerontological collaborations began in the 1950s.[35] In his early and arguably best-known work, *The Problems of Ageing*, Cowdry summed up two conflicting views that existed about aging. The first view sees aging as an "involutionary process that operates cumulatively with the passage of time and was reflected in the modifications of cells, tissues and fluids"; the alternate view insists that changes in organs could be traced to structural alterations due to infections, toxins, traumas, and nutritional disturbances or inadequacies giving rise to degenerative changes. The pathological effects resulted from adverse environmental conditions or diseases and inadequate or "unwise nurture caused by poor care after an illness or surgery." The latter view indicated that members of the species of the same chronological age, who were assumed to constitute a homogeneous group, may be different, and that individuals "grow, develop and mature at different rates and therefore are biologically different despite their chronological age." Aging or early senescence, he wrote, "may occur in men and women who, chronologically speaking, are relatively young."[36]

The notion of premature aging—the manifestation of aging earlier, even before a person is chronologically old—gained ground in research because chronic diseases were seen as distorting the passage of chronological age. For many older persons, suffering from the morbidity of chronic diseases implied that they were physiologically older than their biological or chronological age. In a note prepared for the CRA in 1946, its chairman William MacNider noted that research on the aging process needed to focus on knowledge about middle age or the period when there was a degeneration of vital tissues. He added, "It would . . . appear that the present is the most appropriate time for funds to be secured in order to give an understanding of the ageing process and of those measures which may be instituted to prevent *premature ageing*, and, in a sense to stabilize the ageing individual."[37] MacNider was underscoring the idea that diseases such as arteriosclerosis and cancers destabilized the natural course of old age, aging the body before its time.

This, then, was the major current in the biology of aging that emerged in the United States and influenced the IAG: a growing interest in chronic diseases such as cancers and heart disease. According to reports submitted by FSA representatives, for example, at the 1951 IGC in St. Louis, the most attended session was on the "Diseases of Old Age" that explored the incidence of degenerative diseases in old persons. Its presenters were Leon Medalia, a pathologist who was an office bearer of the Gerontological Society, and Paul Dudley White, an up-and-coming cardiologist who would become closely involved with international cardiology conferences and the personal physician to Dwight D. Eisenhower. Medalia and White noted, "For the first time in history, the average expectation of the duration of life at birth has passed the biblical mark of three score and ten years. Coincident with our gaining control . . . primarily over the infectious diseases in the majority of persons, both young and old, a heavy responsibility has devolved upon us to study and to lessen . . . the progress and effects of the chronic, so-called degenerative diseases, mainly those involving the heart and blood vessels, in the earlier and old age decades as well as to combat malignant neoplastic disease." Based on studies at hospitals in Boston, the main abnormalities in upper age groups were identified as coronary sclerosis, arteriosclerosis, and cancers.[38]

The second major current in the biology of aging in the United States at this time was concern about the effects of chronic, degenerative diseases on a specific age group of older men and thereby on the country's "reservoir of manpower." During the war, Korenchevsky, in Oxford at the time, wrote about the urgent need to conduct research on aging in populations beyond the "old," since the war would take its toll on adult populations, including men who were leading military campaigns. He emphasized that aging was not a "matter of years" or a time-bound decline; it was stimulated rather by various deficiencies, and it could appear in the form of senility "prematurely" or manifest itself early through various pathological features.[39] Following the war, there was a shift in these anxieties, and gerontologists instead drew attention to the issue of the payments offered to disabled U.S. veterans as well as the challenges in obtaining domestic manpower to fuel America's growth ambitions within and outside the United States. In the 1950s, new Cold War challenges were mounting, and experts tended to associate aging with military concerns in challenging areas such as Korea. There was a perception that American ambitions overseas needed to be unfettered by domestic manpower challenges.

This was reflected in meetings such as the National Conference on Aging that Cowdry addressed, which was held two months after the situation in Korea had escalated. Federal Security Administrator Oscar R. Ewing made comments while inaugurating the conference that reinforced the links Cowdry and others forged between disease, aging, and manpower issues, as well as with the risks and diseases of a middle-aged and "mature" age group of men. Ewing observed that "the American people are growing up, in the most literal sense. . . . For the third time this century, the United States is passing through a time of crisis. . . . There is the danger of war that could go far beyond the action in Korea. . . . There is the danger of a long period—perhaps a generation—of concentration on military, economic and social strength without the test of war. . . . This situation calls for full exploitation of every resource we have, including our reservoir of manpower."[40] He added that the conference sought to rethink compulsory retirement and to find "a way of keeping people young as they grow old" in terms of usefulness.

CRA members echoed the anxieties voiced in the public sphere about the rising proportion of the aged. They shared particular concerns about premature aging and dependence in old age and recommended, as a means to restore the efficiency of older persons, their mitigation by careful examination of the role of chronic, degenerative diseases. The biology of aging, they argued, could help address the growing social anxieties concerning dependence. Lawrence Frank, a founder member of the CRA and vice president of the Josiah Macy Jr. Foundation, noted that the United States was passing from a large burden of child dependency to a large burden of old age dependency, especially an increase in the number of people in early- and later-middle age. While the large child population could be neglected, deprived, and exploited (as many children were) without protest or social reverberations, a large dependent group of aged persons in the population would have votes and could become a formidable pressure group.[41]

The views of American experts reflected contemporary concerns in the United States about the productivity of middle-aged males, the age of compulsory retirement, and in particular the tendency for chronic, degenerative diseases such as heart disease and cancer to strike the white male population. As Ann Pollock's work on race and science has revealed, heart disease was associated with middle-aged white men in their prime, while the African—American population was associated with a lack of modernity and with older disease paradigms associated with infections.[42] The emerging modern field of chronic disease research was seen as not germane to the poor health either of African Americans or even of American children. For instance, the infectious roots of heart disease and its association with young children were forgotten as heart disease began to be connected with a new, postinfectious disease pathology affecting those with complex lives of stress and strain.

The case of cancer and its disease identity, as Keith Wailoo and Baron Lerner have written about, was somewhat different.[43] It was associated with older women and their post-Victorian vulnerability, or "civilized whiteness," until the 1920s, even as it was increasingly clear that cancer in nonwhites was simply less visible and often underreported. Even in the 1950s, there was still "professional confusion" about its identity and racial distribution, often leading to conclusions, as in the Steiner study in Los Angeles, that white men of "Caucasoid" origin were its main victims.[44]

Experts such as Cowdry and scientists with a growing voice in international gerontological meetings, such as Nathan Shock, articulated views conforming to these assumptions. Their research did not cross the color line, and it also did not directly address the issue of aging and degenerative diseases in women except to consolidate ideas about the higher morbidity and mortality among men.[45] Experts perceived the biological and medical problems associated with old age as primarily associated with industrial societies and existing among populations that had conquered infectious disease and extended life expectancy. These societies were now faced with the degeneration associated with chronic diseases. Their research was primarily focused on the onset of these diseases and their effects on the process of increasing morbidity, dependence, and frailty. Both Cowdry and Shock, however, argued that the effects of chronological age and the process of internal aging of organs could be different. Shock observed that not all organs were functionally impaired by disease or degeneration at the same rate, with some being unaffected till the end, while Cowdry continued his early research showing that each organ degenerated with a distinct pattern and rate of senescence.[46] The onset of chronic diseases in different organs in each location and body could therefore vary greatly. This had significant synergies with cancer research in Asia and Africa where, as we saw with Gillman, experts claimed certain cancers, such as liver cancers, were associated with a "premature" aging of certain organs but had distinct causal pathways.

New Geographies and Horizons of Chronic Diseases

The association of aging with the agenda of chronic degenerative diseases had another crucial dimension: it compelled gerontologists to engage with populations, bodies, and risks that lay beyond the United States and Europe.[47] So far, biological aging had focused on the aging process in *individuals*; ideas about aging were largely formulated based on animal experiments and studies that were extended to human beings. An interest in the biomedical aspects of chronic diseases now paved the way for a movement beyond an overwhelming focus on colonies of laboratory rats and experiments involving cell cultures, to studies led by the UICC across Asia and Africa that began engaging with human populations and their environment.

The American cancer pathologist Harold Leroy Stewart, who occupied an influential position as Chief of Laboratory at the National Cancer Institute, began to work closely with Cowdry to make a case for studies that focused directly on human pathology and its environment while setting up a project to pursue international cancer studies.[48] In 1950, along with colleagues in the UK, Leroy Stewart planned a series of studies on the geographic pathology of cancer, with the support of the WHO and the American Cancer Society. At a symposium organized by the UICC in Oxford that year—later recognized as seminal in initiating comparative studies on cancer—Leroy Stewart and other scientists outlined an ambitious plan to internationally map the prevalence of chronic diseases such as cancers. They argued that demography and cancer pathology needed to intersect in order to demonstrate that cancers were conditioned not only by geography or genetics, as many experts earlier held, but also by patterns of life, habits such as nutrition and customs in various settings, and their effects on metabolism.[49] They framed templates for international cancer research based on exploring the role these "environmental stimuli" and "ethnological" factors played in influencing patterns of cancer morbidity worldwide.[50]

So far, gerontological congresses had assumed that studies on aging done in the United States and Europe that primarily focused on white male populations had universal relevance. There were very few studies of chronic, degenerative diseases such as cancers beyond "civilized" settings. Even within the West, research on cancer was beset with controversies about the incidence of types of cancers in different populations. In the United States, statisticians, physicians, and biologists debated the claims of racial difference associated with cancer and whether African Americans were less vulnerable to cancers but instead primarily afflicted by infectious diseases.[51] Even as these dominant images were being questioned and democratized in the United States during the 1940s, assumptions persisted about sameness/difference between the West and the rest in relation to the geographical distribution and pathology of cancers in backward countries.

As the debate around the pathology of aging and chronic disease, in particular cancer, grew in importance in these years, epistemologies and ethical questions from other societies began posing challenges to the universal templates of aging bodies and chronic, degenerative disease that had emerged from the West and the United States in particular. It was more difficult in the case of degenerative diseases to demonstrate what Dipesh Chakrabarty has termed "clairvoyance" regarding knowledge of other parts of the world based on the West.[52] It became important to widen the pathological gaze and to demonstrate greater flexibility in engaging with different contexts, as Leroy Stewart and others would now begin to explore.

Several questions arise here: How did experts living in societies dubbed demographically youthful and still caught in the throes of infectious tropical diseases, or still backward in terms of "social progress," participate in new agendas around chronic diseases and aging? How did "diseases of civilization," or conditions that Western experts associated with advanced industrial societies and a long lifespan, manifest themselves in primitive societies? Were backward people immune to or less susceptible to chronic, degenerative diseases since they were still not modern and had not controlled infectious disease through public health reform and seen a rise in life expectancy as the West after the Second World War?

Aging and Cancers in Asia and Africa

To pick up the threads of these issues, it is necessary to return to the July 1954 CIBA Foundation Colloquium on Aging in London where Theodore Gillman presented his and his brother's work on cancer among the Bantu in South Africa. Many of the CIBA conference participants had met at the landmark 1950 Oxford symposium to discuss research methods for exploring the geographic pathology of cancers worldwide. Gillman and Khanolkar, who had been present at that meeting, had concurred with leading cancer experts from the U.S. public health service and from the UK on the urgent need to map cancer incidence among colored and African populations. Joseph Gillman's notions of backward countries, chronic diseases, and of the age of cancer onsets were not framed simply as "different" from Western populations. Gillman and Khanolkar articulated a more complex view of the burdens of disease in Asian and African societies. They traced alternate models of age, disease risks, and premature aging caused by an overlap of infectious and chronic disease responsible for morbidity and mortality in countries that were not modern or fully industrialized.

To understand Gillman and Khanolkar's interests in leading these studies, it is useful to probe their correspondence with the UICC leadership, such as Cowdry. In 1952, Cowdry, who knew both Khanolkar and Gillman, tried to persuade the latter to visit Bombay and participate in an important research meeting of the International Union Against Cancer, which would be attended by delegates from more than forty-five countries. Gillman declined Cowdry's invitation, citing the deepening fascist politics that made South Africans unwelcome in India, but voiced the conviction that South African research would still make a contribution to "the world problem of cancer."[53]

Gillman was not the first to articulate this aspiration. Earlier cancer researchers in South Africa, such as Charles Berman, pointedly noted that cancer research could not be dominated by data and research from the United States and Europe alone. Gillman would build on these ideas as he wrote at length about the unique opportunities for research on cancers and other diseases among the ethnologically diverse population in and around Johannesburg.[54] Khanolkar felt the same about the role of his research on oral cancers, and he compared this data from India to East Asian studies and to cancer incidence in New York and London in order to establish the importance of understanding the unique patterns of pharyngeal cancers in India.[55] It appears that Gillman and Khanolkar understood that a decentering of medical research priorities, from infectious to chronic diseases, was occurring in the 1950s in the West, and the new spaces and subjects for investigations on malignancies and heart disease were now in the new scientific metropole represented by the United States. Thus, it was important to establish that Asian and African populations, especially productive adults, shared these susceptibilities.

Cancer and Aging in South Africa

Drawing from Berman's early work (1935) with Bantu mine workers and their vulnerability to liver cancer, Gillman argued that liver cancer progressed rapidly among the Bantu and had a far greater racial frequency than among other groups, including "Negroes" in the United States.[56] Apart from the role of climate and infectious diseases—both parasitic disease and hepatitis—Gillman also focused on metabolic abnormalities in the liver, in particular those relating to malnutrition, which may have influenced the onset of hepatic cancers or malignancies of the liver. This made the roots of cancer in South Africa and the population that it affected quite distinct.[57] Theodore Gillman, in his presentation to the CIBA meeting, emphasized the association between cancers and aging by playing on two notions: age and aging as a "life process" that was appropriate in Africa, where diseases and aging were affected by long-standing influences such as childhood malnutrition, and the focus on the chronologically old in the age-based studies of cancer in the West.

Gillman noted, "The estimated life expectancy of the African (there are no vital statistics available in our country for Africans) is extremely low—somewhere between 40 and 45 years. Associated with this low life expectancy we have found many indications of premature ageing and a whole series of reactions which differ from those usually seen among Europeans in South Africa and elsewhere." The incidence of cancers, he observed, were considerably lower in the African; and "about 90% of cancers in African males are cancers arising primarily from the hepatic epithelium." This could be attributed partly to the fact "*that the African just does not live long enough to develop the other type of cancers so common among Europeans.*"[58] The key reason for this tendency toward premature aging-related diseases and a low incidence of cancers also lay in the "life patterns" of people who differed "profoundly," as did their physical environments, due to climatic and socioeconomic factors.

Significant tensions lingered amid the efforts to assert a distinct paradigm of chronic disease and aging in backward societies. Even though these experts stated that cancer was a world problem that needed to be measured in its differences and sameness as compared to the West, they repeatedly used white Caucasian bodies and pathologies as models or reference points. One reason was that their engagement with surveys and studies financed by the American Cancer Society or other U.S. foundations called for their views and findings to partially align with some of the persistent concerns and categories dogging Western investigators, such as comparing Bantus and "Negroes" in questions about the increasing frequency of chronic diseases in old age.

Concerns about the onset of chronic diseases at a youthful age, their threats, and their differences had a specific political context in South Africa in these years, and research on malnutrition among black South Africans, as Diana Wylie discusses in her work, had a long and complex history in which the concerns of science, racial policies, and modernity overlapped closely.[59] The abiding concern with labor efficiency prompted research questions about chronic diseases; this was the case in India as well. In South Africa, health worries regarding cancer reflected dual concerns about white vulnerability to cancers and an enduring focus on understanding cancers among "pigmented" people. Cancer societies founded by urban white middle-class groups in South Africa sometimes consulted Gillman as they disbursed funds for research. Larger research projects found bigger funders: Higginson and Oettle, who set up big research projects in 1950–1960, were funded by Leroy Stewart at the NIH in the United States. The productivity of Bantu mine workers and their susceptibility to new chronic diseases, rather than the health of white populations alone, were important interests informing this research.

The studies relating to hepatic cancers and pneumonia among the Bantu workers had roots in liver cancer research by doctors employed by the mining industry and others who examined mine workers' disease pathologies, such as the vulnerabilities of "tropical workers" that Randall Packard's work has explored.[60] Packard, tracing the evolution of ideas regarding migrant Central African mine workers' susceptibility to pneumonia in South Africa, writes that medical researchers made the workers out to be a distinct social category and noted that their tendency to sickness, lack of efficiency, and early deaths were attributed to cultural and biological factors. This circumvented the need for reforming the living conditions of workers in these mines and also allowed medical researchers to focus on developing vaccine-based therapies for pneumonia.[61]

A few decades later, research on cancer among mine workers continued to emphasize inherent environmental causes over immediate occupational risks.[62] Medical researchers were reluctant to enter a debate about the conditions producing premature onset of cancers and differences in chronic disease patterns among Bantu miners. Joe Gillman's colleague Higginson's research on the Bantu and their tendency to develop cancer in their youth emphasized that dietary deficiency was important, but that liver cancer was not necessarily caused by malnutrition, as the Gillmans had argued in their research. He cited research by Khanolkar on hepatic carcinoma or liver cancer showing that malnourished populations in India did not demonstrate these risks, and that these cancers were caused by metabolic abnormalities during childhood.[63] In sum, he advised improved child welfare as a preventive measure and shifted attention away from the living conditions of mining labor. The identification of a complex range of extrinsic, intrinsic, and environmental factors as causing cancer in the early decades of life diverted attention from Bantu poverty, their malnourished diet during adulthood, and even their work and exposure in the gold and uranium mines.[64] Higginson and Oettle estimated that the last survey of the Johannesburg area was in 1947, which merely calculated the amount of food entering the city and might have been unduly pessimistic. In general, the diet was adequate and more varied than believed, and certainly not restricted to "mealie pap" and sour milk among adult urban Bantu. Previous life influences, such as "early life in rural area in times of drought" likely had lasting effects, and "orthodox western nutritional standards tended to overestimate minimum requirements."[65]

In the 1950s, Gillman and his colleagues faced difficult choices in their research in South Africa, and their writings reflected these tensions and an environment of mounting political pressures and suppression of liberal white opposition to an increasingly repressive state.[66] Even as the 1960s were characterized by a deepening debate about occupational cancers across the world, neither occupations nor exposures were even mentioned as Joseph Gillman's colleagues deepened their cancer studies.[67] By then, Gillman had moved to the new Institute for Medical Research in Ghana, which was promising to be a new center for African science and a model to project the status of scientific research in modern Africa.[68]

Cancer and Aging in India

Vasant Ramji Khanolkar shared Joseph Gillman's preoccupations regarding non-Western populations and their susceptibilities to cancers. Like Gillman, Khanolkar, who was president of the Cancer Research Commission of the UICC from 1950 to 1954, had led national-level cancer surveys for over a decade in India, focusing on an industrial population of millworkers in Bombay and its hinterland. He also led the geographic pathology of cancer studies in India. His networks in the Indian political establishment were deep and wide, ranging from close ties with Indian industrialists such as Naval Tata, whose family had set up a trust fund for cancer research in Bombay, to contacts in Delhi with leading figures in the Indian Planning Commission and the national leadership.[69]

Early in his cancer research, Khanolkar focused on challenging the persistent claims made about cancer and its geographical specificity. Even at the Cancer Research Commission meeting in Bombay in 1952, he stated in the press that although cancer was now recognized as a world problem, it still lacked a distinct, scientific name in India and was known only by its Sanskrit name.[70] Khanolkar's mission was to make the disease and its related scientific evidence visible, as well as to demonstrate that countries such as India could suffer from diseases and conditions of industrialized nations. No longer should these countries be associated only with the pathologies of tropical diseases also linked to India's colonial past.

His public health colleagues in India echoed Khanolkar's concerns. Writing in 1954, a senior public health functionary speaking at the Indian Science Congress observed that challenges like cancer were becoming increasingly prominent simply because "old problems are solved and new ones (have) arisen." He added that "tropical disease" was a concept that lacked wider purchase, since no diseases were peculiar to tropical climates. That category referred only to diseases of poverty, and "if taken in the sense of latitudes labels like tropical disease and tropical medicine were misnomers, since these diseases were not typical of tropical climates but of backward countries that had been banished from the west only because it had banished food deficiencies, industrialized and acquired colonies, improved sewerage, and introduced sanitary reforms."[71]

Khanolkar's research, presented at multiple meetings such as the CIBA colloquium, at the Oxford meeting on the geographical pathology of cancer and at other international meetings, was significant in challenging a persistent debate regarding the differential incidence of cancers in India. He argued that there was a "sameness" in diseases such as cancers across the world and noted that arguments that the cancer rate was "eight times as high among the 500 millions of civilized races as among the 1,200 millions of backward races including the 300 millions in India" were misplaced.[72]

However, establishing the incidence of cancer was by itself not a badge of modernity, since Khanolkar was aware that many developing countries were reporting an increasing incidence of cancer cases. Khanolkar also explored cancer's characteristics and social gradient in India, implying that vulnerabilities to different types of cancers varied greatly among the population. He therefore argued that cancer differed greatly in India based on "habits and customs and usages" among its social groups, depending on the impact of historical events over time that changed the environment of the people.[73] He identified two factors—environmental determinants and inbreeding or "endogamy"—as critical determinants for the occurrence and types of cancers in India.[74] In a widely quoted statement cited by Cowdry, Khanolkar argued that the more common types of cancers in India tended to occur above the chest, rather than below it, in contrast to Western populations in industrialized societies. By terming certain bodily sites or organs as more susceptible to cancers in environments such as in India, and some cancers as common in the industrialized West and rare in the Indian setting, Khanolkar was trying to align the differential development and modernization between countries.

According to him, cancers associated with specific customs and chewing habits were also distinctive of certain classes of people, such as the Deccani Hindus who worked mainly as gardeners, mill hands, stevedores, and policemen. These habits were in turn compounded by "ancillary factors" such as poor oral hygiene, malnutrition, and lack of adequate vitamins.[75] Tobacco chewing was common among lower classes and migrant workers in cities, who retained their traditional tobacco consumption habits; this implied these behaviors and cancer risks were typical of those who had still not adapted to modern habits and an industrialized life.

Khanolkar's research identified some social groups in India who suffered from chronic diseases in their older years and manifested the same susceptibilities as Western white populations. Parsi women, or those of the Zoroastrian faith who formed part of an urbanized, educated elite in Bombay, were an exceptional group among Indian women who had similar rates of breast cancer to those in London county hospitals and in New York, at the Memorial Hospital. The Parsis, he noted, were a tight-knit community with close inbreeding; they were prosperous business people. Their women were often unmarried or had late marriages and fewer children—very different from Hindu women "amongst whom the opposite conditions prevailed"—which caused Parsi women to suffer from higher rates of breast cancer.[76]

Even as Khanolkar wrote up these last conclusions in the early 1950s, he was aware that his own professional support for cancer research had originated from the Parsi community and from the interest of its leading business family, the Tatas. After Lady Meherbai Tata died from leukemia, her husband had endowed in her name a trust for cancer research in Bombay.[77] Both Cowdry's visit and recommendations on planning cancer research in India and Khanolkar's own career at this point were supported by this largesse. Leukemia and breast cancer in this case were feminized diseases in the West, associated with white women. Their occurrence among Parsis, who were associated with Westernized, liberal, modern life-styles and endogamy, reinforced ideas about their being modern and mimicking white populations in their disease susceptibilities.[78]

In these years, cancer research was beginning to generate interest in other Indian cities, such as Madras, among an urban middle-class public that was founding cancer societies due to growing concerns for the number of lives lost among their young professional colleagues.[79] In this case, chronic, degenerative diseases such as cancers were affecting a productive and socially significant population—and felling them in their middle rather than later years as in Europe or the United States. Khanolkar was aware of these trends, and he used the association between an earlier age of cancer onset and the implications for development and productivity in India to good effect. The ominous challenge posed by cancer in Indian life, he noted, lay within the "age composition of the Indian population." He observed that too much attention had been focused on one age group and its premature deaths in India, such as the deaths of infant children, of whom "roughly a quarter die during the first year." Their plight had drawn public attention "mainly due to the excellent propaganda by infant welfare organizations on the matter of deaths in infanthood. However, the mortality of older age groups had been overlooked."[80]

In India, Khanolkar wrote, unlike in the West (where higher mortality occurred later in life due to longevity and child mortality rates had fallen), high mortality occurred during infancy and continued to be four to eight times higher until the age of fifty-five. "Considering the short life expectancy in the country relative to the west, this had serious implications because it implies a forfeiture of nearly half of its population during the most productive period of life or the period of their greatest effectiveness," he wrote. "These are the people for whom the family, the community and the state make the biggest sacrifices and who in other countries live long enough to prove of inestimable value by attaining the full span of their usefulness. It is the age group which supplies in other countries men who rule over the destinies of institutions, armies and empires." This did not preclude attention to older groups in the long run, he wrote, since cancer "occurs most often in people more or less advanced in years and that mortality from it rises as the number of elderly people in a community increases."[81] This would happen eventually in India through the elimination of "avoidable disease" and a reduction in mortality, but the immediate challenge was different from that in the West.

Toward a Social Approach to Aging

Both Gillman and Khanolkar were engaged in research that required them to address developed and backward nations' demographic politics, disease politics, and typical disease typologies at a time when these notions were being increasingly questioned. By the 1950s, calling certain chronic diseases such as cancers "diseases of civilization" was less tenable than earlier in the century, because civilization as a concept—in this case with its demographic and epidemiological attributes—had new and changing connotations. Prasenjit Duara's work explores how civilization was not only associated with Eurocentric notions of race and culture but was also increasingly being freed from the "cosmology of progress." Ideologues in Asia and Africa were viewing civilization as an "ethnographic concept" that allowed a multiplicity of traditions that conceded new and alternate passages to modernity.[82]

Experts in international organizations however, continued to identify chronic diseases and aging with mature, modern societies and were less willing to recognize their onset through other pathways in nations that were still undergoing complex social and disease transitions. In a speech to the Western Pacific regional committee of the WHO in Manila in 1954, an expert from the UICC noted the rising incidence of cancers in countries such as India, China, Pakistan, Indonesia, and the Philippines. "This finding [of rising cancer incidence] is a sign of your success because you are preventing death from epidemic diseases as you are lowering infant mortality in these countries[;] you are also successful in increasing [the] number of old people in this region. But unfortunately, the increasing number of old people in a community you have produced is expanding the field of cancer patients which are alarmingly noticeable at the present time."[83]

His speech is interesting in that it reflected enduring attitudes regarding the association of chronic diseases, such as cancers, with the Western models of modernization and old age, both as a biomedical notion and as a developmental category. Although chronic diseases could temporarily be experienced in a youthful population, the desirable long-term vision of modernization was to project similar patterns as in the West. This model implicitly saw older persons in the West and the distorted development of non-Western societies and their youth as an "expanding field" for certain diseases. In turn, this model did not recognize chronic disease in other sections of the population at all.

Conclusion

Despite evidence that medical experts tried hard to understand the place of aging and chronic diseases through alternate histories of disease transition and development, and even contested the dichotomies of backward and civilized societies, the legacies of these international debates are difficult to map forward. Asian and African researchers such as Khanolkar and Gillman, and the succeeding generation of cancer experts such as Higginson and Oettle, and Premnath Wahi in Agra, continued in international cancer research networks linked to researchers in East Asia and other parts of Africa. However, Khanolkar increasingly began to see his cancer work as divorced from the winds of change that blew toward development-related agendas such as population control.[84] Development, food resources, and birth control gained interest among political leaders and experts, and chronic disease research was confined to progress in cancer-related pathologies such as tumor registries. On leading India's medical research agenda, Khanolkar focused on supporting a new generation of cancer research scientists in India's scientific research centers in Bombay and elsewhere; he also succeeded in involving leading politicians, such as the Indian President Rajendra Prasad, in cancer campaigns. But his research did not get translated into integrating cancer programs with the emerging focus on social and community medicine and other public health programs in rural areas.[85]

Further, the growing bifurcation of approaches to control and check infections and noncommunicable disease was getting wider, making it more difficult to make connections between and across different age groups and diseases as attempted researchers attempted in the 1940s–1950s. This led to increasing silos in research and programs between infectious and chronic diseases. Aging was increasingly seen as a distinct arena, separate from youthful populations and reproductive health, in terms of government priorities and its health policy interventions.[86] In a meeting of the WHO Regional Office for South-East Asia, for instance, it was stated that the Indian population was passing from the "growing to the ageing group," and this shift implied the need to establish a separate "cell" to study the latter. Further, with increasing disillusionment with disease-focused campaigns and their debacles and with the dawn of the historic Alma Ata declaration in 1978, when the social goals of health, such as primary health care through preventive strategies, health promotion, and community-based approaches were proclaimed by UN member states, the enthusiasm of the 1950s to solve world problems through control of chronic diseases was fading.[87] By the 1960s, views of aging as a social problem increasingly focused on social maladjustment and other issues. International gerontological networks no longer saw the biology of aging as a key issue, and social workers, psychologists and human development experts began to interact less and less with the worlds of biomedical researchers.

3

The Emergence of the
International Gerontologist

Clark Tibbitts sensed an opportunity. In 1964, when Tibbitts was posted at the Office of Aging in the United States, the UNESCO office in Paris invited him to edit a special issue of the *International Social Science Journal* that would introduce social gerontology to an international audience.[1] For Tibbitts, it was an acknowledgment of his attempts, with other members of the International Association of Gerontology (IAG), to project social gerontology as an international social science. The UNESCO's step gave social gerontology an international stamp of recognition.

It was significant in other ways as well. The UNESCO issued the invitation to a U.S., not European, expert. In his article for the journal, Tibbitts chose to herald the arrival of what he termed a new and critical social discipline by citing Ernest Burgess, the University of Chicago–based pioneer in aging and human development studies. In this fashion, the influential role assumed by U.S. experts in social gerontology was reinforced. Moreover, the UNESCO's invitation to Tibbitts underlined the ascendancy of U.S. experts' espousal of the social aspects of aging, a view that began gaining ground in the early 1950s as the focus shifted from the biomedical interest of earlier years. Tibbitts and his colleagues set out to project aging as a worldwide social and psychological agenda that was not tied only to demographic shifts but reflected a larger sociological problem of dependence and infirmity.

Social Adjustment in Aging

In 1950, when the noted sociologist-demographer Kingsley Davis, known for his work on the population of developing countries, addressed the problems population aging posed in developed societies, it signaled a transition in aging research's major focus from chronic diseases to aging's social aspects. The setting was a conference on the social and biological challenge of aging, held at Columbia University in New York City. Davis opined that the "problem" of aging had become numerically greater than either the "Negro" or the adolescence problem in the United States. He also said that the statistics of the future should not be used to spread alarm; the looming specter of mass senility could be averted if medical science succeeded in slowing down the aging process and making people organically younger in relation to their chronological age, just as it had successfully curbed death at younger ages. Conversely, the problem and its solution, Davis hinted, was fundamentally a social one, because whether the old were viewed as a problem or not depended "not only on their number and physical condition but also on their social situation."[2]

In the 1950s, social research on aging was attracting unprecedented interest and funding from a range of researchers and foundations, and it was further supported by debates in the public arena relating to social security reform (1956) and retirement. Social scientists began dominating IAG partnerships, and its leadership too, and the social aspects of aging—in particular the field of social gerontology—became an area of growing interest. Writing in 1952, Oscar Kaplan, an eminent social scientist, commented on the increasing influence of social science research in the United States and the need for the IAG to recognize this shift to E. V. Cowdry. This presaged the expanding role played by social scientists in deciding the agenda and priorities of the gerontological association. Kaplan, a pioneer of geriatric psychology and one of the earliest behavioral scientists appointed to the gerontology section of the National Institutes of Health (1946–1950), observed that "One of the major difficulties confronting our committee is that most of the available speakers are medical persons, whereas most of the institutes . . . in this country have a social science accent."[3]

Ethel Shanas and other social scientists from the University of Chicago, and Tibbitts, who joined the United States Department of Health, Education, and Welfare as part of its special staff on aging, were influential in challenging the long-standing agenda of the International Gerontological Committee, set by its scientist founders like Vladimir Korenchevsky. With support from the National Institute for Mental Health in the United States, Tibbitts had initiated the first project to train professionals in social gerontology, and for many decades, he remained in a strategic position for influencing policies relating to older Americans.

Ethel Shanas, who had a long career in social gerontology in association with the University of Chicago, communicated with Nathan Shock, a founding member of the IAG, pressing on him the need for sessions in the 1964 IGC on new research in sociological and psychological sciences, rather than having a program centered overwhelmingly on the biology of aging. Shock accepted the request without hesitation.[4] Shanas would later become a key representative of the United States to the Department of Social Development, a division of the UN Economic and Social Council, in New York in the 1970s, when an agenda for a worldwide assembly on aging began to be planned. The seeds of social gerontology, sown by the American experiences of aging with a focus on ensuring productivity and adjustment, would later set the course of a worldwide agenda on aging.[5]

The social world and ideas generated around aging and its social and psychological aspects and implications were concentrated at the University of Chicago. These intellectual networks shaped international comparisons and brought together a range of researchers who drew different but mutually reinforcing conclusions about aging populations and the wide political implications of these changes. In these years, the study of social and psychological aspects of aging became a well-funded program of research and teaching at the University of Chicago supported by the Social Science Research Council (SSRC) and led by Ernest W. Burgess, Robert J. Havighurst, Herbert Goldhamer, Ethel Shanas, and others.[6] Institutions such as the SSRC and foundations such as Carnegie and Rockefeller also began supporting the work of social scientists on aging. Burgess and Havighurst, for instance, received generous funding to conduct surveys to track the changing attitudes and behaviors of retired persons. They began collaborations supported by the SSRC, and in the 1940s they led research, centered in the Committee on Human Development at the University of Chicago, on the problems of the elderly, including teaching and research focused on "social adjustment in old age."[7] The studies emerging from Chicago emphasized, through simultaneous investigation into different families, ethnic groups, and social classes, the need to understand older persons' attitudes toward themselves, their perceptions of aging and of who was considered "old," and the behaviors associated with aging. They also touched on deepening public and policy concerns about the need for the growing population of older persons to cope with retirement.

The project on social adjustment in old age attracted widespread attention, and its participants understood and addressed the challenges of adjustment and adaptation in old age in diverse ways. The project found acceptance and support from the National Institute of Mental Health and, after 1964, from the newly founded National Institute of Child Health and Human Development. Some biological aspects of gerontological training remained a part of this perspective, and the faculty often worked with differing views on aging, ranging from Havighurst's Kansas City Studies that emphasized an "activity theory of aging"—that most people readjusted to their roles in society—to other findings by Elaine Cumming and Warren Earl Henry, who argued that aging implied a "finitude." Old age represented an inevitable disengagement, and there were nine postulates in the process of lessening interaction or disengagement that was associated with old people.[8]

From his base at the University of Michigan, Tibbitts, one of the earliest social science experts to engage in studies related to the social adjustment of the old, worked closely with Havighurst and Burgess, both pioneers in studies of life stage-related adjustments. Tibbitts argued that science and technology had produced a new element in society, a generation of middle-aged and older persons who were "increasingly detached from traditional society responsibilities and rules."[9] These influences and this new generation of older persons was in danger of threatening the middle generation's well-being and likely to affect American institutions and ways of life.

Tibbitts and his colleagues worried that the old's lack of "adjustment" would affect national productivity, and they thought a new approach to aging was required. Their pamphlet, "Productivity at Any Age," reflected these views: "While the first half of the twentieth century has been called the age of the child, during the next fifty years, we will be directing our efforts to make the period of maturity more useful."[10] Just as older persons needed activity, paychecks, and a feeling of independence, the authors of this pamphlet argued, the nation needed to understand and focus on its stake in their usefulness and productivity rather than fostering older persons who were "dependent on others for their livelihood and care." There were compensations for physical aging in terms of long-term skill and judgment. In a society that had long placed an accent on youth and conflated aging with disability, these capacities needed to be fostered. This interest in "adjustment" was drawn from studies reporting that personal adjustment was "routinized" in stable societies where cultures could adapt to the individual's needs. However, in societies subject to the "disarray of industrialization," where social organization was rapidly changing, not only did older persons experience a loss of roles and vitality, but the social set-up, mostly the family, was unable to mediate the adaptation that coordinating among existing social networks and institutions required.[11]

The social gerontologists and demographers exploring adjustment in old age in the United States were not evoking a novel set of problems: the occupational risks of industrialization to bodies and their susceptibility to new diseases were familiar in medicine. Aging experts tended to view the maladjustments of the nineteenth century, such as the threat of infectious disease, as terminal, but the imbalances of the mid-twentieth century differed. The growing numbers of the aged attracted an inordinate amount of state resources and services. These seniors were likely to invite other forms of social disorder and pathological conditions, since their need for social benefits was viewed with undue sympathy by the public, and their growing needs would, in turn, cause long-term societal maladjustments.

Europe as a Social Laboratory of Aging

Initially, these researchers conducted their studies primarily based on surveys in American towns and cities. At this point, knowledge about aging in the United States had still not acquired the self-confidence and belief that it could offer universal lessons in other settings. The United States was still something of a demographic laggard, seen as trying to catch up with the "Old World." Sociologists, psychologists, and demographers such as Burgess, Tibbitts, and Hauser at the University of Chicago understood that the United States was a latecomer to problems of aging already being addressed by other "civilized cultures," and through the IAG, they built support to conduct cross-national studies aimed at investigating the lessons that might emerge from aging in European nations. These social experts framed aging as a "world" idea because it marked a common social and civilizational condition; in this linear trajectory, Europe was in the lead and the United States "adjusted" to its new national status and transition. Population aging represented the maturing of civilizations and marked the West as different from other "backward" nations. European experiences were seen initially as a benchmark and even a political and social forecast of a trend yet to be experienced in the United States.

Burgess observed that the United States had experienced an "initial early lag" in industrialization and urbanization, followed by a later, rapid forward thrust in economic and industrial growth. The early lag, however, resulted in the United States' "backwardness . . . in meeting the needs of older persons who were trapped in the vortex of the acceleration of economic change." Due to these "unplanned" and "unforeseen" social changes, old populations were increasingly stranded in a phase of economic transformation, and children were able to accommodate their parents less and less, whether in-home or in paying for their assistance. Burgess added that between 1900 and 1950, the average number of adult children decreased, the proportion of grandparents doubled, and destitution and the insecurities of an industrial society followed. Understanding Europe was a means of anticipating the challenges ahead planning for America's future, since rapid industrialization and urbanization in the United States was leading "to unplanned and unforeseen changes" affecting families and labor.

The third IGC held in London (1954) offered U.S. experts—both scientists and social scientists—the opportunity to probe the situation in Europe more closely. Some extended their itinerary, visiting nine European countries to gain a better understanding of aging programs in there.[12] On their return, Tibbitts and his colleague Wilma Donahue explained the rationale behind their travels: "the appearance of large proportions of older people in the populations of European countries occurred about a generation earlier than in the United States. Hence, it is natural that these countries should have done a good deal of pioneering in meeting their needs."[13]

Over the next few years, Burgess led an effort to compile a detailed review of European social research and social programs, in order to probe and compare the social aspects of aging in Western countries. Burgess's painstakingly compiled work, *Aging in Western Societies* (1960), was widely

cited and remained a classic in comparative studies of aging for many decades.[14] Europe, Burgess observed, presented itself as "an unintended laboratory in social gerontology" for this project, and both continents shared
the experience of industrialization and urbanization transforming families
and communities.[15]

Other initiatives included cross-country surveys and comparative studies
supported by the UN, including the *Old People in Three Industrial Societies* study (1968), led by Shanas, working with European colleagues. Contemporaries viewed these efforts as a step toward studying the elderly, a
neglected social group in the population who offered "no potential contribution to social output" but "consumed social resources."[16] Shanas and her
colleagues, such as Peter Townsend in Britain, were criticized for neglecting
to focus on the heterogeneity of the old in these societies, especially the
poor condition of the elderly in custodial care. These comparative studies
were pioneering, however, in challenging persistent assumptions about the
old and in highlighting that the elderly were created partly by industrial
society and its social actions, in particular the enforcement of retirement
and the segregation of their formal relationships.

The comparative work by Shanas, Townsend, and others was pathbreaking among aging studies in the early 1960s. It questioned assumptions about the absence of family and isolation associated with old people
and raised fundamental questions about the nature and transformation of
Western society and its implications for old age. This represented a break
from past scholarship, as others had argued the family was a relic of rural
and stationary society, a barrier to occupational and technological change;
therefore, it was not and could not be a source of support for the old.[17] Collaborating to bring together research in the United States and Western
Europe demonstrated the differences within and among social gerontologists, as they argued that studies needed to follow older persons and families over several generations to understand how "adjustment" and support
in industrialized societies was devised.

Making Aging in America Exceptional

The political implications of aging had already been a concern among European experts even in the interwar years, and as we have seen, demographic pessimism relating to populations in the metropolis had emerged
in Britain. These projections and anxieties in Britain and France inevitably

influenced Burgess and his demographer colleagues, such as Philip Hauser and Frank Notestein, who interacted closely with Richard Titmuss, an expert in social work and old age, and Alfred Sauvy, the well-known French demographer.[18] By comparing dependency ratios in the United States, Canada, and West European countries between 1850 and 1950, Hauser explored the links between demography and the social and political fallout of aging. The economic and social burden represented by old persons was illustrated by France, which had the highest ratio of older persons (age 65 and over): 49 for each 100 of intermediate age (45–65). The United States, with 40 older persons per 100 of intermediate age, was among the "lowest of countries in this respect," but Hauser warned that it (along with the UK) was one of the countries where the old age dependency ratio had rapidly increasing between 1900 and 1950, "adding 5.9 senior citizens to her population for each 100 persons of working age." Though there was not sufficient research on the associations between the ratios of young and old, Hauser observed that a growing population of the old might have implications for the social and political conservatism of society and might limit opportunities for the young to advance and innovate.[19]

Kingsley Davis and Philip Hauser both dwelled on the example of France, since its specter of potential national depletion could represent America's future. Becoming like France was a frightening prospect for these American intellectuals, because French society, with the highest proportion of old persons in the world, was characterized by a "stagnation of industry and agriculture" due to the welfare dependency of the aged.[20] "The army of the aged" Davis argued, could be diverted however, if the United States did not adopt a "Maginot-line attitude and take up the paraphernalia of functionless social security." Luckily, old Americans did not share this attitude, Davis surmised; they wanted to keep active and productive, and therefore only needed to be shown how to achieve this.[21]

Wider implications and fears based on perceived threats to security were also associated with aging. The United States continued to age, and aging Western countries, under conditions of declining fertility and mortality, increasingly resembled the demographic profile and age-structure profile of the French. This was likely to polarize the Cold War world into "old" industrialized countries and "young" developing countries, a new demographic divide, congruent with fissures in the world political order, that posed a "political question" regarding whether Western nations could keep their lead over young nations. Hauser and his collaborator Raul Vargas

argued that national differences in aging reflected the alignments of contemporary world politics. In particular, they tended to coincide with the
UN classification of nations by age structure comprising "three distinctive
political groups, the 'free world,' of which the United States is the leader;
the 'Communist world,' of which the USSR is the leader; and the 'neutral'
or 'uncommitted world,' of which India is probably the key nation." Vargas
voiced a concern that if youth meant vigor and age meant debility, the
Western nations faced a future of being "handicapped in the intense competition" in all spheres: economic, social, political, and even military. The
aging of nations was therefore represented as an agenda necessarily allied
with not only demographic and economic concerns, but political ones as
well.[22]

Confining Aging to the West

The impulse for comparative surveys and engagements with European experts reflected the need to explore social and demographic likeness or
proximity, but in the 1950s, the notion of aging in civilized societies was
mired in Cold War social science politics, and did not take nations beyond
Western Europe into account on political-ideological grounds, even if they
fit other "criteria." In the introductory sections to *Aging in Western Societies*, Burgess noted that population aging's uniqueness lay in its mature features being shared principally by the culture in Western Europe and the
United States. The four countries that merited comparison with Western
Europe—Australia, Canada, New Zealand, and the United States—were
peopled by Europeans; they were pioneer areas that transitioned from agriculture to industrialization later than Europe had, as they took time to
pass from colonial to independent status. However, they now fully measured up to the criteria of membership in their urbanization and industrialization, viewed as an "outstanding characteristic of Western culture."[23]
The comparison with Europe was made on careful grounds, and just as
society and demography were matched and pronounced as being in
tandem in these societies, these groupings reflected other political and
economic polarities, beyond demographic features, of the Cold War world.

Population aging in studies such as Burgess's *Aging in Western Societies*
charted the emergence of early ideas associating aging with the linear
stages of progress toward modernization, with those "ahead" and "catching
up" in industrialized nations, and "outsiders" in those nations, such as

Eastern Europe and Soviet Russia, who had not followed these norms. Burgess and his colleagues had to confront the dilemma of whether to include communist countries in their comparative survey of research on aging in Europe. Havighurst noted that while aging represented a stage of human development and adjustment in all individuals, aging in populations was closely linked to cultural maturity and political evolution in nations. The last, in turn, legitimized how and why the Soviet Bloc remained peripheral to these emerging networks.

Contributors to the project, including Chicago-based demographers such as Hauser, made the case that aging was a consequence of the Industrial Revolution. If aging was a by-product of the technological, social, and economic changes that traceable to industrialization, the study needed to include societies beyond Western Europe. Burgess responded by observing that aging societies were defined not only by their economic advance, but also by their political values. Aging was a feature and trend shared by and discerned in "Western civilization"; implicit in that were not only demographic features, but also the political and ideological prerequisites associated with population aging.[24]

The "Communist dominated countries," he wrote, "do not meet our criteria for membership in western culture . . . not only universal suffrage and the guarantees of free speech, free press, and freedom of movement and of association but also industrial democracy." Because the Soviet Union, its satellites, and Yugoslavia differed widely from Western culture in their economic and political values, there was as little to learn from their experiences as from the experiences of economically underdeveloped countries in Latin America, Africa, and Asia.[25] The "countries of Western culture" shared certain notable social trends in aging that defined their uniqueness and comparability: not only had their industrialization process led to urbanization based on migration and population density—it also created certain essential characteristics of the modern world in the West, including a specialization of personal interests, goals, and roles in cities, decreased sentimental judgment, and a matching increase in "rational attitudes."

Aging reflected and brought together the attainments of modern societies. In these studies, the original aging subject was European, and the features of model societies used to understand aging were of European origin. The United States was seen as closely following the West European model. The pace of change and modernization in these societies was viewed as "normative," as was the way key sections of their populations adapted to these changes. European nations had experienced aging over 150 years of modernization, followed by the United States catching up in the mid-twentieth century; this posed the question of other laggards. Communist countries had been left out of the equation, but what of Asian and African countries and their modernity? These too failed to meet the "criteria of membership in western culture." Additionally, in Asia and Africa, different concerns prevailed: the onset of urbanization, migration, and industrialization was rapid and disorderly, family life was rapidly dissolving, and new diseases and welfare burdens presented further complexity. This contrasted starkly with the West, where aging occurred after industrialization was complete, and public health, welfare provisions by the state, and technological advances had led to both longevity and a fall in fertility. Aging as a developmental and demographic stage in Asia and Africa could not be considered as on the same scale and criteria as in the West. For separate reasons, both Western experts and social scientists in Asia and Africa would advance notions of "difference" regarding age and aging in non-Western settings.

Looking Inward

Comparative studies and surveys on aging, such as those initiated by U.S. experts, were driven primarily by domestic concerns or by experts and leaders being confronted with the dilemmas of a newly aging population. This becomes evident from the tepid response of U.S. experts when they had to identify concrete "lessons" from studies such as *Aging in Western Societies*. Burgess observed that although Western cultures shared a common trajectory from agricultural to industrialized life, the implications of the European experience had to be approached with "considerable caution" in terms of using findings for U.S. issues. "It is true," he wrote, "that our country is part of western culture. Therefore what happens in Europe in the field of aging has meaning for us. But the value to us of European experience must be viewed in terms not only of our likenesses but also our differences." The differences he identified were the vast difference in scale between the United States and the countries of Western Europe, the density of population, higher mobility and migration across the United States, allocations of state-level responsibility in the United States, its cultural diversity, and lower levels of income in Europe.[26]

Interestingly, Burgess's observations hinted at ideological barriers and differences rather than differences relating to faults and flaws in European aging programs. When American experts observed aging-related policies in Europe, one of their key concerns stemmed from their discomfort with the ideology of welfare itself. European countries, Burgess noted, had historical and traditional backgrounds that informed their thoughts and actions in aging policies; this did not exist "in the young United States," a nation without the baggage of traditional commitments and contracts that impose obligations toward dependent groups in society. Burgess, Havighurst, and Davis emphasized the need for studies and research promoting independent and productive behaviors and activities among older persons. They also called for evaluating all existing and future projects to test if they resulted in increasing dependency or promoted independence among older adults, rather than allowing public sympathy for the old to lead to support for untested new social projects.[27]

The American experts were making a twofold case here. In their critique of welfare sentiments, they debunked the tendencies of the public to let altruistic sentiments instead of scientific objectivity shape their attitudes to the old and thus influence political attitudes and policies. This underscored the potential of social gerontological knowledge and its experts to represent and relocate this field. Further, their expertise offered an antidote: they could help depoliticize these currents by lending the debate an alternative vocabulary and frame that would divert the debates to scientific rather than moral and political issues. In these statements, we can discern the use of the language of expertise to cast objective perspectives on issues; expert knowledge was deployed in an attempt to withdraw issues relating to aging and its social policies from popular views and pressures so that it could be understood as a separate and distinct terrain. These politics in aging perspectives presaged the magnified political tensions and divisions that would emerge in the representation of aging as a world-scale development and humanitarian agenda in the 1980s.

Other differences with Europe, according to the U.S. experts, was that their work focused on different key problems than work from other Western countries did. In England, for instance, early surveys on aging by Charles Booth focused on welfare and support for industrial workers, with the principal emphasis on poverty. On the other hand, research in France was typified as focused on families and fertility in the face of *dénatalité* (declines in fertility).[28]

Further, the United States still saw itself as a young society with an emerging "problem" of aging focused on labor productivity and participation rather than concerns about falling fertility and family structures (as in Europe). The main concern for U.S. experts was the low labor participation rate, since the population of those aging had doubled but the number of workers continued to be static. The main fear about becoming "a nation of elders" was that older workers seemed to have the highest unemployment rates and had difficulty finding reemployment.[29] Kingsley Davis, for instance, observed that employment was a "major ingredient of satisfactory social and psychological adjustment." He also observed that older persons' relations to labor markets was key and that—despite the fact that the number of persons 65 years of age and over had quadrupled 1900, while the U.S. population had only doubled—"The proportion of all workers to be found in the older age groups, 65 years of age and over, remained about the same throughout this period—4.0 in 1900 and 4.8 in 1950."[30]

For the emerging rank of social experts on aging, their research was increasingly relevant, with potential to reform and regulate the old, to offer ameliorative studies of aging crucial for integrating older persons into U.S. society, and to help older people adapt to retirement and to independent, active aging. They offered social solutions in the realms of both individual adjustment and institutional means and connections. Some researchers in the United States alleged this emphasis came at the cost of more theoretical work on aging; social gerontology and its practitioners, they noted, saw it as their mission to provide solutions to bridge the perceived gaps in social institutions, such as the family. This was the act of combining sociology with amelioration, as Howard Jensen noted in his remarks on the implications of aging: "For humanistically inclined researchers, the biological objective of gerontology is to make old age attainable. The sociological objective is to make it satisfying [that] medical progress has increased the proportion of the aged, technological progress has reduced the proportion of meaningful roles available to them, while the cultural lag of the social sciences leaves us as yet ill-equipped to deal with the resultant problems of personal and social adjustment."[31]

Through their comparative studies, Burgess, his colleagues at the University of Chicago, and their network of psychologists, demographers, and sociologists, were reinforcing their role in shaping the intellectual agenda and priorities of international aging research in these years. By studying aging populations outside the United States, they could strengthen their claims in the domestic arena. They also saw a significant role for themselves in leading the incipient field of social gerontology.

Disseminating Social Gerontology

In the UNESCO's *International Social Science Journal*, Tibbitts prefaced his master narrative of social gerontology's emergence for the journal's international readership by quoting Burgess, who called social gerontology an "emergent field . . . that was not directly concerned with the biological aspects of ageing but concentrates rather upon its economics, social psychological, sociological, and political aspects . . . [on] the status and roles of older persons, their cultural patterns, social organization, and collective behavior as they are affected by and as they affect social change."[32] He also elaborated on Burgess's perspective, tying it to the effort to disseminate social gerontology internationally, by linking the study of old age and its relations with social structures to the evolution of societies.

Based on this idea, Tibbitts and his contemporaries claimed the problems of older persons and the progressive changes in their status reflected the historical development of their societies. Therefore, the problems of aging were not typical of industrialized Western societies alone; they were "age old," reflecting the scales of change and development in all societies in the world. Societies over time, ranging from hunter-gatherers to preclassical civilizations, from the Middle Ages until modern times, showed a changing accommodation of the old. In the modern age, changes in technology threatened the social participation of the old the world over, resulting in their displacement from traditional positions in the economy and family in industrialized societies.

Tibbitts's writings for the UNESCO journal defined aging in society by its behavioral and psychological aspects. Aging was a "problem" that needed to be remedied by changing the behaviors and attitudes of older people, who sought different degrees of engagement and disengagement with their living environment. The old represented a social and psychological problem, and they faced challenges that needed different forms of individual social accommodation. Social gerontology and its research offered a solution "to the individual and social problems of ageing." The task of social gerontology was managing the inevitable decline and dependency. Experts such as Tibbitts, and research and teaching produced by other social psychologists, aimed to make both individuals and social systems better adjusted to this inexorable social process, to deal "with the impact of older people on the social system and with the nature of societal responsibility for them," now that older people had emerged in larger numbers.

When discussing the societal aspects of aging, Tibbitts was careful to include a wider range of countries beyond the United States and west European societies. The arc of aging was not geographically restricted to countries in Western Europe or other countries that had inherited its culture and development, such as the United States. He mentioned Australia, New Zealand, and Japan as joining the ranks of those that needed to solve the problems of individual and social aging, and he left the way open for new entrants from developing countries. He also inserted a role for an emerging rank of social experts such as himself, who would provide "rational guidance in the solutions of problems arising out of extremely rapid increase in the number of older people and out of their displacement."

Support from the UNESCO also provided Tibbitts with an occasion to assert the formidable research lead the United States enjoyed in social gerontology, speak about state funding in the country, and display European gerontological partners, in particular institutions in the UK and France. His survey discussed several sites and networks across Europe where social scientists were leading studies of aging: research in England supported by the Nuffield Foundation, programs at Bristol, research at the London School of Economics (which had built vast training programs and curricula relating to aging) and centers such as the Centre de Gérontologie in France.[33]

A Field of U.S. Influence

American social experts' ascendancy in mobilizing international networks and research collaborations in aging was readily evident. American experts were influential in pressing for social expertise's greater role in the IAG's annual meetings, and social science and social welfare research on aging had increasingly occupied prominent positions. At the fifth meeting of the IGC, held in Merano in 1957, an important shift occurred when a social research committee, led by an American and a European expert, was founded and immediately requested that Robert Havighurst, president-elect of the American Gerontological Society, be invited to deliver the plenary address.[34] The next congress, held in San Francisco (1960), was hosted by Robert Kuplan, an expert in social welfare. American social practitioners and welfare experts in aging thus increasingly found professional space at the IGC meetings. Until then, many European members had resisted the entry of social workers and aging-related practitioners on the grounds that the IAG and its congresses were centered on gerontological research alone.[35]

The invitation to anoint social gerontology among the ranks of international social sciences in the UNESCO special issue was itself no accident. It had been carefully planned by social scientists in the IAG, who had requested funds from the UNESCO to support a research meeting on aging held in Sweden just around the time of the sixth IGC in Copenhagen (1963).[36] As demonstrated in correspondence preserved in the Clark Tibbitts and the UNESCO archives, the IAG leadership had carefully cultivated networks with the office of the director-general of the UNESCO and received a grant based on the claim that their research would "bring answers to such questions as have arisen as a consequence of the fact that the population in many countries to an ever increasing extent . . . consists of aged people."[37] After this, as an article in the UNESCO special issue on old age documented, the floodgates of social science research on aging were flung open, with each IAG conference raising the bar with an increasing number of papers on diverse themes. The diversity in panels and paper themes was, however, somewhat limited; they would mainly have interested experts in the United States and Europe, as they addressed concerns about social security reforms and the retirement and displacement of older workers, and discussed standards of living and income security in developed nations.

The influence of U.S.-based research and the leadership of American social scientists in the emerging social gerontological enterprise was unmistakable. It was reflected not only in Tibbitts's account in the UNESCO special issue but also in other articles in that issue referring to research conducted in the United States. Despite the fact that the leadership of the SSRC was shared between an American and a European social scientist, who both decided on papers and panels, sessions at IGCs such as in Merano consisted overwhelmingly of American scholars presenting their work. Even at the UNESCO-sponsored research meeting mediated by the Swedish government, the suggested panel and participants were mainly American social scientists.[38]

This growing overlap in international social gerontology's visions and agendas, with ideas originating from the United States, resulted from the new patterns of support for aging research and academics emerging in the country since the early 1950s. Easily accessible funding for their research and the publication of a large number of social gerontological studies in the United States, including textbooks that marked the scope of this emerging field (such as Tibbitts's), meant that a first generation of sociologists and psychologists (such as Burgess, Havighurst, and Tibbitts) was quickly succeeded by others who now assumed a growing international profile. Shanas aided by a range of her students led multicountry comparative studies that found funding in the United States and from UN agencies interested in social welfare. Others such as Walter Beattie, who had trained at the University of Chicago and become involved in building networks of gerontological educators in the United States and beyond, led such studies as well.

Extending the Arms of Europe to the United States

That Europe was now reaching out to a U.S. leadership was clear at the first meeting of the Paris-based International Center for Social Gerontology (ICSG), held in Lisbon (1970), where an international course in social gerontology was inaugurated. These meetings were reminiscent of Korenchevsky's early efforts to contact Cowdry and others in the United States, but the focus now was on disseminating gerontological education and advocacy rather than on biomedical science and research. The organizers of the ICSG course worked closely with Tibbitts and other Americans, such as Walter Beattie and Wilma Donahue, who were part of its executive committee, and they echoed the argument, made earlier at the UNESCO forum in Sweden, that the science of gerontology had evolved from "a biological discipline and an object of research" to a clinical discipline and then matured to produce social gerontology. This was termed an "inevitable development" that arose "when a civilization, due to an immense need for human and social justice, seeks new ethics and new truths." The meeting itself, the organizers noted, was geostrategically located in Lisbon, presenting the message of a civilization that had "reached its height" and representing "the arms of Europe extended towards the effectiveness and thirst for knowledge of the American continent."[39]

The norms and standards of this emerging field and its new questions relating to aging were thus clearly located in European values. Further, based on this past, these experts aimed at leading forward another march, "the triumphant development . . . of gerontology." They aimed to offer what was termed "futurology"—or to shed objective light with scientific evidence and methods, thus establishing a "taste for prediction" related to aging that would help mobilize government support.[40] Allusions were also made to the critical timing of the meeting, as it occurred during a "revolutionary demographic situation" throughout the world, a reference to the rising challenges posed by aging populations, but using the metaphors of population control and explosion that were predominant on the international agenda at the time.[41]

Although the ICSG founders did not elaborate on these claims, we can discern a few significant ideas in these opening overtures. These interactions pointed toward a strain of social gerontological thought emphasizing not merely a welfare services–based debate or approach to aging, but also speaking of older persons' rights to work and support. Less convincingly, the ICSG also claimed that its aims and agendas were lofty and transnational, and that social gerontology was relevant to all "civilized" societies in the world, though its wider membership was still limited.

Alfred Sauvy, the eminent French demographer who had coined the term *tiers monde* (1952) or *third world* to refer to the exploited populations in "underdeveloped" countries, captured an inequity that was closer to home: the exclusion of the old within welfare societies.[42] His essay, included in a volume commemorating the first international course on social gerontology in Lisbon, allows us to understand that social gerontologists were evoking the language of human and social justice because they believed there was an urgent need to redress and restore the universal right and freedom of individuals to choose the length of their working career and job options and to receive a retirement pension. They were concerned with and challenged what Sauvy termed the methods and procedures adopted in contemporary society to "eliminate" old people.[43] The elimination process, he noted, may take two different forms of undesirability: elimination from the economically active population and elimination from sight by segregation in specific areas and communes. In industrialized countries, this arose out of the fear of unemployment and the stigma of "social condescension," and it led to the inactivity of active men.[44] In effect, Sauvy wrote, the present system of retirement "acts like a guillotine" as age-based retirement and a lack of social integration would lead to psychological stress and eliminate older persons due to their rapid decline and death after retirement.[45]

Gerontology's Travel to the Rest of the World

By the 1970s, the ranks of the IAG were growing more international and diverse. A history of the IAG, written by long-time president and early founding member Nathan Shock in the early 1980s, meticulously documented this swelling of the ranks. Experts and societies from countries Asian countries, such as Thailand and India, and Latin American countries, in particular Mexico, Argentina, and Brazil, were new entrants in these years.

Observing these changes, Tibbitts claimed that social gerontology was expanding its institutional and expert networks among those who shared common goals and perspectives of old age. As a field, it was of growing relevance to the world, because in both developing and developed nations, social interventions led by the state were increasing, as was the assumption of collective responsibility for service functions. Irrespective of demographic shifts or population aging, social gerontology could inform welfare policies relating to old people in these settings.

These experts were representing old age as an issue linked not simply to the demographics of population aging or development, but to social change and behavior. By emphasizing the uniformity of aging and the aged across the world and its causes in a lack of familial and societal "adjustment" in the face of social and technological change, these experts laid the grounds for this research's wider applicability in Asia and Africa in the next decade. In 1978, Beattie, in a well-known briefing to the U.S. Senate Committee on Aging, argued that even though regions such as Asia were still facing the problems of high fertility and a youthful population, the sheer number of the aged and old in these nations posed a problem. In this case, he was not referring to the politics of retirement from the labor force and social policy (as in the West), but to development and the rapid social changes such as migration.[46]

However, the UNESCO research meeting and the publication that followed reflected interactions among experts primarily from Western Europe and the United States. The grant application to the UNESCO mentioned that the gerontological research meeting to be held in Sweden would include participants from Asia and Africa, but it seemed to have remained mostly on paper. More significant, there was no representation from Eastern Europe or Russia, even though the ninth IGC was to be held in Kiev (1972).[47]

French Networks in the Metropole and Beyond

There were alternate pathways for aging research and advocacy to reach non-Western societies. Gerontology in France, in particular, followed a different route, developing more slowly in the demographic and social fields, but this research deepened in the 1960s and later.[48] This growing interest in social gerontological research and the links forged by French gerontologists with U.S. experts and UN bodies such as the UNESCO and the International Labour Organization (ILO) in these years was crucial, because it would soon lead to seeding new networks in aging-related research in Francophone Africa.

In the IAG meetings and in UNESCO-supported meetings on aging, participating French experts expressed their interest in old age primarily in terms of its demographic and economic implications, although their views shifted somewhat after *A Social Policy for Old Age* (1962), the Laroque report that shaped postwar thinking about aging in France, was published.[49] The report characterized aging populations as tending to social isolation and related old age to poverty relief. The report's associating aging with *la dépendance*—either in terms of the need for medical relief or of retirement—implied that psychological research in aging was slower to emerge, partly because the focus remained on economic productivity, but also because there were limited state resources available even in later decades for large studies in social gerontology.[50]

In the late 1960s, Paul Paillat authored the earliest studies focusing on the social condition of the old in rural France. A demographer who trained with Sauvy, Paillat continued to be the sole French representative in international meetings of social gerontologists. Others active in the field included Jean Auguste Huet, a socialist politician interested in aging and social policy, who observed that "studies in the social aspects of aging are at the top of the national interest." Huet recognized the importance of developing an international plan for gerontology so that universal standards of language and measurements could be established. Huet hosted meetings of the IAG in Paris in the 1970s, but noted that, while the organization gathered about 2,000 specialists every three years for an international congress, "these meetings have only a scientific character." Reflecting on the new leanings of gerontological research in France in the 1960s and early 1970s, he argued that the role of social studies in gerontology was to understand the economic and demographic implications of old age and to link the challenges of birth and old age.[51]

Huet and a collaborator, Joseph Flesch, established the ICSG in Paris. The stated aim of the center was to reach out to practitioners, social workers, "promoters, directors of establishment," nursing staff, and politicians "who seek to solve the problems of the years of retirement." In an application for affiliation to the World Health Organization (WHO) in 1983, its leadership claimed that it "unites 11,000 individuals of 90 nationalities" through teaching, seminars, conferences, and work with UN agencies and NGOs interested in aging. These networks were still mostly focused in Europe, in terms of the ICSG leadership. Although the ICSG membership was widespread—ranging from Senegal, Sudan, Cameroon, Burundi, Guatemala, and Nicaragua to China, Pakistan, India, and Sri Lanka—none of the reports of the international meetings the Center organized between 1970 and 1980, such as in Mohammedia (1978) or Quebec (1980), discussed the role played by these members.[52]

The ICSG made efforts to set up meetings in the late 1970s and1980s in Francophone colonies in Africa. It was more flexible than the IAG in collaborating with UN agencies to hold meetings to familiarize countries in Africa with gerontology. Through the 1970s and early 1980s, WHO and ILO representatives attended ICSG meetings, and ICSG representatives in turn participated in WHO meetings held after the UN's landmark World Assembly on Aging (Vienna, 1982).[53] The ICSG also received advice from two U.S. social scientists—its long-time board members Beattie and Donahue—while Tibbitts participated in their first teaching programs, such as those in Lisbon. Its ideological roots and the political interests of its leaders, such as Joseph Flesch, were allied with French pension funds. This implied that, unlike American experts who focused on labor productivity and employment, they continued to retain a focus on aging, dependency, and welfare debates.

A Porous Curtain?

In the 1970s, old stereotypes of a geostrategic nature seemed to be eroding, though lingering Cold War alignments persisted even as international meetings among gerontologists began to proliferate. Notions that gerontology was a product of and relevant only to nations that had liberal, democratic societies, thereby excluding communist nations in the 1950s and 1960s, seem to have been set aside by the 1970s. In 1978, the eminent Soviet gerontologist D. F. Chebotarev, who had been president of the organizing committee of the IGC held in Kiev in 1972, was also invited to testify at the significant hearing of the U.S. Senate Committee on Aging.[54] At the Senate hearing, Chebotarev's statement was useful mainly to highlight the extent of geriatric services and social provisions available in the Soviet Union, and for U.S. gerontologists to underscore the need for more resources and support in some of these areas. Ideologically, however, these meetings and rapprochement did not always reflect common ground, mostly highlighting the continued interest of Soviet researchers in the biological and physiological sides of aging rather than its social aspects, although some research on retirement and inactivity was presented at the IGC in Kiev.[55]

For a view of the tensions and the nagging politics that shadowed the growing circulation of gerontology on an international scale, let us look at the ninth IGC in Kiev, a significant event in the annals of the IAG, jointly organized in the USSR in 1972. Delegates from the United States, Western Europe, and Japan attended the conference, which began with an impressive and lengthy program.[56] Ideological differences and grandstanding were evident even in the inauguration ceremony. In the inaugural address, Chebotarev traced the beginnings of modern gerontology in the USSR to Kiev in 1938, identifying its origins as marginally preceding that in the West and as having evolved simultaneously with gerontology in the United States. He noted, "Most wonderful changes have occurred since the first . . . world major gerontological conference, sponsored by academician A. A. Bogomolets, and since the publication of Cowdry's book in 1939" (which had offered a summary of the literature on various aspects of aging).[57]

The papers presented were almost all based on research from the USSR and Eastern countries, on the one hand, or from Western Europe and the United States, on the other. Comparative work was absent, with some exceptions in the work presented by Shanas, who examined and compared aging in Poland and Yugoslavia with a few Western European countries and the United States.[58] International controversies were never far from the surface, and tensions festering since the Stalinist years spilled out into the open, demonstrating that the networks of cooperation IAG members had built were easily disrupted. This was mostly because support in the form of expenses, such as the travel of many hundreds of delegates to these meetings, originated from researchers' respective governments.[59] The Soviet Organizing Committee refused to allow the Soviet biologist and dissident Zhores Medvedev to attend the meeting in Kiev, causing many U.S. gerontologists to protest, since the former's work was well known among age researchers.[60] Israeli delegates, in what Nathan Shock termed a "continuation of politics" at the conference, were not encouraged to attend by the Soviet side, with U.S. support of Israeli delegates causing increased tension.

Interestingly, even though the IAG was a privately formed professional association, it reflected political controversies and geostrategic tensions in the Middle East that assumed wider proportions in international bodies, such as when aging began to be discussed at UN meetings in the 1980s. During the 1982 UN World Assembly on Aging in Vienna, for instance, a motion on the "Israeli aggression against Lebanon . . . and the vulnerability of the elderly in armed conflict" was repeatedly brought up for discussion, asking for "immune protected areas" to be established for Arab refugees over sixty years of age. A speech made by the representative of the League of Arab States emphasized that even though the Arab world had protected its old from the "violent jolts that had taken place as a result of the onslaughts of development and modernization," the Israeli aggression was now endangering the situation of the aged.[61] This brought up an argument and a new vocabulary concerning the old that would deepen in later decades: that aging was potentially an international issue that was not only compounded by development and modernization, but was also subject to vulnerability because of trauma and violence (as Didier Fassin describes in his work on the "politics of suffering").[62] Even here, however, the issue of whether the old were a separate group from the rest of the civilian population that needed protection from trauma was repeatedly raised by countries that abstained from bringing political issues into a "subject-oriented" conference on aging.[63]

The rapprochement of gerontologists across the Iron Curtain did last beyond individual conferences, mostly due to the links and initiatives maintained between leading experts. Chebotarev in particular remained the face of this cooperation for some years, through various positions he held in the IAG while also the director of the Kiev Institute of Gerontology. As a close reading of Nathan Shock's bibliography of geriatrics and gerontology demonstrates, Western gerontologists were in close touch with the biological and experimental research on aging being conducted in the Soviet Union and socialist countries long before the meeting in Kiev (1972). Increasingly, when demographic worries had begun to grow in the USSR in the 1950s and 1960s due to a lowering of the birth rate, social and demographic research too began to deepen.[64] The Kiev conference, despite its limited attention to a social gerontological agenda, revealed a common set of interests that aligned the challenges of aging with those of retirement. Delegates noted that retirement or the "pension disease" was the chief social gerontological problem shared by all developed countries.[65]

The sharp edges of Cold War rivalries did not play themselves out strongly in gerontological meetings, especially since cooperation in life-prolonging research and the biology of aging had been an early, shared interest. But the dissemination of the gerontological gospel to developing countries by social scientists, rarely, if at all, involved any Soviet researchers. By contrast, gerontological enterprise was coopted into the larger U.S. mission of cultivating and supporting social science in young, developing nations in the Cold War years with the aim of checking the spread of socialist influences. U.S. experts also felt a growing need to disseminate gerontological knowledge beyond the West, to circulate, test, and compare the relevance of their work in social gerontology. In an indirect manner, their views underscored the significance of Western gerontology as a universal reference point, a claim that was sometimes subverted by social workers, sociologists, and development experts in developing countries, who either denied the relevance of gerontological research and teaching or offered alternative priorities in understanding aging.

The opening and closing of the minds of American social experts and gerontologists occurred during their visits to Europe, over the course of their research and conference partnerships on the continent. These engagements and encounters demonstrated the uncertain, contested, and ambivalent nature of social gerontological theories in the West. They also reinforce that the Western gerontological enterprise was made and unmade by Cold War politics and its inclusions and exclusions, and colored by the insecurities American experts voiced regarding the implications of aging for their society. There was considerable self-doubt and debate, even as the norms and models of aging were being examined: What did it mean to be "ahead" of other societies in aging? How relevant was Europe (and in this case, France) to aging in the United States, and what were the politics (of aging, but also of security concerns and rivalries) that weighed on these anxieties? Was it possible to learn from the "mistakes" of those who were "ahead" in terms of demographic changes? Was a catching-up process possible, and if so, how could it be achieved? Interestingly, these same questions are being posed today in societies in the global South looking to "catch up" with the West.

4

~~~~

New Frontiers:
Aging Experts in Asia and Africa

IN THE EARLY 1970s, the world of aging beyond Europe and the United States remained in the shadows. Individual experts from developing countries, such as India, Pakistan, and China, sometimes negotiated their membership in the International Association of Gerontology (IAG), but their experiences were still seen as distinct from those of Western industrialized nations, and their participation in the IAG and its congresses was mostly sporadic. However, interest in gerontological education was growing in the United States at this time. Walter Beattie and the sociologist Donald Cowgill established a group of gerontology educators at the state level. They and others wanted to understand gerontological knowledge's reach in other developed and developing countries, and they began planning its dissemination further afield.[1] With the close involvement of Beattie and other social gerontologists, such as Clark Tibbitts and Wilma Donahue, the Association for Gerontology in Higher Education (AGHE) was founded; in 1978, after Beattie took over as president, the association initiated a survey asking experts in a few countries in Africa, Asia, Latin America, and the Middle East about gerontological teaching and research in their countries.[2]

Cowgill was chosen to conduct this survey, partly because, by offering a model of development and modernization across time and by forecasting the development of gerontology in societies worldwide, he had drawn significant attention from sociologists. Cowgill and Lowell Holmes had introduced perspectives of modernization into gerontology when they offered what they termed a cross-cultural theory of aging—based on factors such as migration, urbanization, the shift of parental care from families to the state, and changes in family resources and ownership—to explain large-scale social changes and their effects on aging.[3] Gerontological development varied based on industrial, social, and economic indices shared by the West and the rest, they claimed, but how aging emerged in non-Western nations that were latecomers to aging differed significantly from how it emerged in industrialized, Western nations. Cowgill and Holmes's work, even apart from later criticism about how their arguments typified and oversimplified complex social and political processes in developing nations, was not always well received, and several contemporary U.S. sociologists argued that they displayed a naïve handling of the "concept of modernization" and assumed that chronological age, "rather than public conceptions of old age," was the "arbitrary cut-off for old age" across societies. In their effort to demonstrate dramatic shifts from a "pre-modern gerontocracy" of powerful elders to a modern-day dependency of the old, they confused key terms and categories with each other, such as kinship structure with household composition.[4]

But Cowgill and Holmes's forecast of gerontology trends in developing countries provided an interesting insight: in the West, aging was initially stigmatized as a problem or burden, and the adoption of more progressive attitudes concerning retirement and social security followed. This in turn was followed by writings and movements that resisted ageism and supported the rights of the old. All this had a gradual, sequential trajectory in the West, primarily in Western Europe and North America. Cowgill and Holmes predicted the same for developing nations, many of which, in their "model," were lingering in early, formative stages in their concerns about old populations.[5] However, they pointed out that "social" concerns arrived before biological or medical concerns in developing countries. Social perspectives and policies on aging, in particular relating to poverty and social support for dependents and the destitute, were visible early on, but medical and biological research—an early manifestation of aging-related expertise and research in the West in the 1930s and 1940s—was yet to emerge in settings beyond the West. Although Cowgill and Holmes's narrative offered new slants on some peripheral aspects of aging in the developing world, gerontology and aging in non-Western settings continued to be derivative in these years, demonstrating gaps in comparative framing.

"Situated Knowledge" and Surveying Education

Donald Cowgill initiated his study for the AGHE by writing to sociology departments in various universities and institutes across the world. Based on the responses he received and a survey of the literature at these sites, he concluded that awareness of gerontology as a separate and distinct field of research, teaching, and policies was absent in most parts of the world. Clearly, a world of outreach still awaited American gerontologists.

In some cases, his survey shed light not on the limits of gerontology in other societies, but rather on his thin knowledge of contemporary research. One letter Cowgill received from Japan, an Asian nation that had held some hope for gerontologists because it showed an early decline in fertility, informed him that gerontology was not a well-developed field. It is interesting that Cowgill displayed no surprise at this response. His quest to promote social gerontology never turned up prior research about demographic decline and fertility in Japan conducted by well-known American social scientists. He also assumed that aging research in other countries would intersect with and replicate research in American sociology departments—and be in the same discipline (sociology) rather than other fields of knowledge.[6] Where he did locate local interest in fostering gerontology, it seemed to have emerged not due to urgency over demographic shifts or developmental challenges; rather, it was simply spurred by sporadic contacts with U.S. academia. The latter implied that occasionally, a local expert had taught, been trained in, and researched in gerontology in the United States before returning; this presented the possibility of developing research programs and curriculum in those countries in the near future. Cowgill noted this was characteristic of Kuwait, and an ex-student expressed the same hope in Thailand, where there was "transplanted interest."[7]

In Nigeria, the response was far more categorical: the head of department at the university wrote to Cowgill that aging-related research was unlikely to be a priority since the focus was still overwhelmingly on youth and population control.[8] Sociologists in Egypt responded that aging research was closely associated with their commitment to poverty research, including urban destitution and widowhood, but gerontological research by itself was absent. These responses were complex, contingent, and diverse, but Cowgill's analysis was definitive and his findings somewhat pessimistic. He concluded that the only geographically proximate countries, such as Canada and Samoa, were influenced by U.S. programs. By contrast, he explained, developing countries "are still struggling to keep their 1. Population under control 2. Youth in good health therefore there is little interest in the aged."[9] Cowgill's study provides a detailed table where he scored "advances" in gerontology such as teaching and research. He demonstrated that most nations in the developing world lacked even the core features he identified as signposts for the development of gerontology.

How does this survey and its conclusions relate to our narrative about aging's emergence as an international agenda, as documented through international gerontological congresses of the IAG and new international NGOs such as the Paris-based International Center for Social Gerontology? Cowgill's correspondence with academics and social experts across many developing countries offers a narrative that conflicts with claims made in these years and earlier about the rapid expansion of gerontological knowledge and training and its reception in many developing countries. For instance, in 1956, at the grand opening of an international gerontological conference in Mexico, E. V. Cowdry thanked the organizers for allowing the meeting to be held in Mexico, signaling the worldwide influence of gerontology. He was echoed by the U.S. state representative, who promptly followed this up with an outline of the impressive range of aging programs and policies in the United States, implying the country's leadership in this upcoming international agenda.[10] Although state departments in the United States had begun to recognize aging and its research field, gerontology, as an international issue of some merit—the United States Department of Health sent their representatives to most international gerontological conferences— it was difficult to concede that aging was a global agenda waiting in the wings to succeed population control, as the well-known French gerontologist Joseph Flesch claimed in 1969.

Even as the 1970s witnessed American gerontologists' growing need to disseminate gerontological knowledge beyond the West—partly to circulate, test, and compare their work's relevance in social gerontology—some American gerontologists also felt the need to make their research more relevant and accessible to the developing world. Beattie articulated this in 1977 at a U.S. Senate hearing:

Social policies and practices in regard to aging individuals, and community and social responses to their aging members have been based mostly on stereotypical information. Scientific knowledge has only begun to emerge. Much of this where it is available, is based on studies within the more developed countries of the world. . . . Despite this recent development of gerontological research, a body of knowledge is developing which requires dissemination and utilization. . . . The present knowledge and methods for gerontological research [should] be organized in such a manner as to provide their being transmitted from those more developed regions where they are currently in use to the developing regions of the world.[11]

Studying the Aged in China

Walter Beattie's vision of gerontology's way forward in the developing world found few takers. Even as Western gerontologists claimed to be challenging persistent mythologies about aging in these years, their insights were still limited to their own societies, and they failed to question norms or stereotypes about aging in Asia and Africa. Donald Cowgill's visit to China in 1978 and his inquiries there constitute one of the rare attempts by a leading American gerontologist of the 1970s to study the situation on the ground in a developing nation. Over a few weeks, based on the access allowed him by the Chinese government, Cowgill conducted interviews and meetings to plumb the state of family life, the relations between generations, and the "Homes of Respect" nursing home care offered to the aged without families. Cowgill visited China a few years after it was allowed back into the UN (1971); by then, its experts were beginning to participate in World Population Conferences and its demographic policies were becoming better known.[12]

After Cowgill's visit, the opening of China to gerontologists was reported closely in the United States. In papers and reports where he was quoted, Cowgill took for granted the essential features of what were perceived as "traditional societies" still defined primarily by "filial piety." These features comprised an unchanging, homogeneous family structure and the domination of old over young due to cultural status and entrenched social and moral codes. Cowgill had expected the communist government's critique of Confucian principles, the collectivization policies, and migration would have eroded these ties; however, he "couldn't see it. They mainly still have influence. They mainly are revered, cared for as far as rural areas are concerned, supported financially." Traditions, he added, had endured decades of revolutionary change. At the same time, Cowgill looked within China to define and engage with the problems of aging familiar to American readers and policymakers: retirement, the perceived dependence on social security, and the social withdrawal and inactivity attributed to retired persons. He observed that while the Chinese had mandatory retirement, he had not seen a single person jobless or retired: all continued to work at jobs ranging from crafts to teaching, often "six hours a day, six days a week."[13]

Cowgill's narrative of aging and family relations left China's intensified and ambitious birth planning programs unaddressed. Although old-age support through government programs for the infirm and for aged and retired workers existed, state priorities lay elsewhere. Increasingly, state focused on regulating the family for the purposes of controlling "biological and social life."[14] In the early twentieth century, radical Chinese leaders had spoken about reforming traditional family life in China as a means of effecting "national salvation," but by the 1970s, state intervention tied the path to modernization and national progress to planning births.[15] Cowgill overlooked the impact of population control, focusing instead on collectivization policies and the association between modernization and long-term changes in land possession and status. Aging in China was an adjunct of family life, he thought, but Cold War preoccupations regarding communist ideology's effect on family- or filial piety-centered societies colored his views.

Filial piety represented an age-old social institution in his analysis, and his writings are problematic in tending to conflate its practice and discourse, which consisted mostly of Confucian tenets in his work. He and others did not recognize that intergenerational ties, rather than being eradicated, were undergoing transformations.[16] The constant reference to "traditional" societies as characterized by filial piety and male-dominated, patrilocal relations was common to Cowgill's writings and well-known earlier works on aging; the sociologist Kingsley Davis wrote, "In general the respect and power commanded by the aged is greatest in static agricultural and familistic societies. In China and the Orient generally, where these traits reach their extreme, the old have greater authority and prestige than any other age group."[17] Davis saw filial piety in agrarian societies such as China and India or the "Orient" as a mark of static culture. It was to be found in cultures of memory and was dominated by religion; new technologies and

ways of life had not appeared in these societies. The difference, a few decades later, was that Cowgill, aware of changes under Mao and his succes-
sors in the 1960s and 1970s, was trying to assess continuities and change.

Generalizations such as Cowgill's and Davies's had further implications.
The sociological essence of the aging process was captured only by the
male relations of landowners, old fathers, and young sons who were central
to these intergenerational ties. This account decentered women, bachelors,
unmarried daughters, orphans, and other socially marginalized people, such
as prostitutes, who were not part of this gendered narrative of Confucian
hierarchies. It took little note of those who resisted or diverged from these
norms, including for instance the rural poor, who often migrated to cities
without forming large, co-residing families and parts of China, including
rural Taiwan, characterized by mother-centered families.[18]

Cowgill noted that there were distinct, ongoing changes in family relations and functions in China, yet he concluded that once modernization
processes such as migration and urbanization intensified and lifestyle
changes occurred, China might follow the path of the United States and
"face some of the same issues in aging."[19] In other words, his analysis had
serious limitations, as he was writing as an American gerontologist visiting
China rather than as a sociologist with long-standing insights into Chinese
society. Almost as an afterthought, Cowgill privately admitted to a colleague that he was unsure of the accuracy of what he and his gerontologist
companions had observed, for they had been dependent on what the Chinese government had selected for their perusal.[20] Although he and others
increasingly saw family interdependence in China as governed by communist politics and state policy, which directed social changes such as land
laws and collectivization, they did not reflect on the consequences of demographic policies themselves.

Gerontological knowledge traveled to sites beyond the West, and, to
move beyond the history of international gerontology narrated through
American expertise and even beyond a Eurocentric viewpoint, we must
understand how the prevailing ideological currents were translated and received in non-Western contexts. Cowgill's visit to China may have been
fleeting, but what effect did it have on his readership, or that of his gerontologist contemporaries? Did these works on aging and modernization
circulate and shape gerontological expertise in Asia and Africa? Gerontological writing in China began to appear in the 1980s, soon after the seminal World Assembly on Aging in Vienna (1982). The first generation of

Chinese experts based in China began to identify themselves as gerontologists in the 1980s. They had read the biologist Cowdry's writings, Cowgill's
and Holmes's modernization theories, and Clark Tibbitts's work.[21] Access
to these writings and discussion of these works was more frequent after
the Gerontological Society of China was established (1986) and a Sino-
American Conference on Ageing (1986) was held.

Gerontological Exceptionalism in China

Gerontological writing began to appear in China in the 1980s, soon after
the seminal World Assembly on Aging in Vienna (1982).[22] In the career of
Wu Cangping, one of China's leading gerontologists, we can see both the
excitement of founding a new field and the continuities with older demographic beliefs and nationalist projects. Regarded as the father of China's
social gerontology, Wu studied in the United States as a youth and returned
for gerontological training at Columbia University in the 1990s. He shaped
gerontological training throughout the Deng era, and many of his colleagues regard him as a living example of productive aging.[23] The influences that shaped his ideas on aging, according to Wu, include important
meetings such as the international population conferences organized by
the UN and gerontological conferences such as the World Congress of
Gerontology (1996). He visited India and parts of the Middle East during
his career to observe population policies and meet experts. These visits, particularly to India, which was suffering from scarce resources and overpopulation, helped him understand how China had to continue implementing
its birth-planning agenda to control its population while facing new challenges such as aging.[24]

Wu referred to Western gerontological studies in his writings, but
asserted that they served merely as a starting point from which to adapt
gerontological expertise to Chinese needs.[25] Gerontology in China, he
added, needed to address important legacies, such as Mao's thoughts and
Deng Xiaoping's theories on China's development; Marxist thought had
been relevant in those early years, he stated emphatically, when considering the applications of gerontology in China.[26]

Wu opined that in China, gerontological learning included values, such
as the needs of "social harmony" and sharing collective resources, which
would be Chinese gerontologists' unique contribution to the field. The
notion of social harmony Wu evokes does not, by itself, usefully convey

precisely the distinctive contribution gerontology aimed to offer society in the Deng era. Rather, in Chinese political cosmology, it referred generically to Confucian values regarding the continuing importance of a collective identity and the importance of maintaining stable rule without the instability of individual values. But Wu was developing his ideas about aging in China and the need to maintain an active, aging population in the Deng era, when the state was pressing forward a model of "socialism with Chinese characteristics," as Dengist ideologues termed it, and this colored his ideas.[27] He emphasized that Marxist materialism—the primacy of the material "base" and economic reconstruction over "ideas"—was critical. So the challenge aging posed needed to be addressed not simply through ideas about individual adjustment and through attitudinal and behavioral factors, as reflected in the work of Robert Havighurst, Ethel Shanas, and others, but also by following wider social, material goals of national development.

In the years after the UN Assembly on Aging, as Wu and others wrote more prolifically on gerontology, they elaborate their ideas in more detail. Wu Cangping emphasized that his early career as a demographic expert helped him speak with greater confidence about gerontological knowledge and the challenges posed by aging in China. These lessons from population policies, he noted, taught him that the country's aging problem "has to be dealt with in the context of China's particular situations."[28]

For Wu, as well as for the other demographers he cites as contemporaries and mentors, China's poverty and backwardness were rooted in overpopulation. As a developing nation, China could not explore the same options as developed countries: their death rate was still higher and life expectancy still lower than those of developed countries. These views—including the notion that China was growing old before growing rich and would have neither the universal social security supported by a welfare state nor the high standards of living among the old characteristic of the West— inevitably shaped Wu's gerontological writings.[29] China's planned birth programs also played a part; these policies were intensifying toward the one-child policy that Wu describes as a "macro-developmental goal, for which it incorporates family's fertility activity into the network of state planning and social management."[30] The country's aging problem, Chinese gerontologists emphasized, had to be handled in the context of its particular scenario, in this case its birth control policy. Wu's early ideas evolved at a juncture when population policies were a cornerstone of China's developmental visions. Without criticizing these policies, he argued that their implications for falling fertility and rapid aging were inseparable from gerontology. Gerontology in China had to acknowledge the historical importance of these policies and thus also assume a role in maintaining social stability: this implied taking responsibility for older persons who had sacrificed for the sake of China's future and had only one child.[31]

On what basis did gerontologists such as Wu build their authority, apart from offering comparative perspectives gained from traveling on an international circuit of prominent gerontological and demographic conferences? Wu himself built it primarily via internal Chinese politico-scientific authority. Qian Xuesen, the politically powerful long-time director of China's space research program, a crucial scientific leader and patron, was instrumental in this process. In August 1984, Wu published the article "Ageing and Our Solutions" in *People's Daily*; more publications in scientific journals followed.[32] A few years later, in 1988, the Renmin University journal published an article that shared an open letter from Qian Xuesen. In the early 1980s, Qian had supported Song Jian and other experts in propounding a scientifically informed birth program focused on a one-child policy, marking a shift, according to many, from a Maoist leadership focused on ideology to science under Deng.[33] Qian expressed his appreciation of Wu's writings on gerontology and his efforts to introduce it to a Chinese audience. Inevitably, this interest from Qian and other powerful scientists of China also resulted in a more specific critique of Western gerontology, and indicated where Chinese studies should lead.[34] Qian advised Wu to emphasize the positive aspect of aging rather than following the Western trend of viewing aging as a problem.[35] Wu noted that, in the years that followed, his approach of advocating a Chinese way based on principles such as active aging (endorsed at a later UN assembly) was becoming increasingly popular. The notion that China had to look beyond seeing aging as a problem and to integrate it with its existing developmental goals persisted over the years.[36]

Gerontological Exceptionalism in India

In the early 1980s, experts in South Asia were evoking earlier studies, such as those by Burgess and Kingsley Davis, as a starting point from which to reflect on the differences between how developed and developing countries understood aging and the old. Familiarity with Western gerontology, and indeed its spread in the years soon after Cowgill's study, catalyzed these researchers to reflect on the category of old age and its implications. As in China, the immediate concern for South Asian experts was the absolute number of the aged, which had increased due to longevity. Indian demographers such as Ashish Bose demonstrated that many countries in South Asia had reduced mortality, with life expectancy increasing in 1980 from thirty-five years to over fifty years, but efforts to reduce fertility and infant mortality were still ongoing.[37] Only Sri Lanka seemed to be heading toward reducing infant mortality, and its population pyramid varied from others in South Asia, as its life expectancy of about 70 years was closer to Western countries'.

Another urgent concern for South Asian experts was the disturbance and dependence caused by modernization among older adults. A delegate at a conference on aging in South Asia (1982), citing the works of Western experts such as Kingsley Davis, noted that the latter had emphasized "the main problem of the aged [was] their marginalization after their retirement and the need of re-integrating them in the political and cultural life of the country and helping them get over loneliness caused by the loosening of the parent-child bond. . . . In the South Asian and other Third World countries [however] it is a question of the economic survival of the family as a unit."[38] Walter Fernandes, a sociologist and activist, summed up these concerns in his introduction as Wu Cangping had done, noting that industrialized countries could afford the type of social security that was beyond the reach of poor countries. The latter accounted for 75 percent of the world's population but less than 25 percent of its wealth, and the condition of developing countries reflected the marginalization of their aged as these countries were marginalized "in a neo-colonial economy . . . in the world scene."[39] Their old did not suffer as much from social and psychological isolation because family ties remained. The main problem for them was economic survival.

Even among aging researchers in South Asia, there were significant differences in perspective. Urban sociologists, activists, and planners at the meeting on aging in South Asia referred to most of the early studies of the aged as focused on the retired. They saw their own work as diverging from that on urban "middle-class" based concerns such as retirement. As Lawrence Cohen's work demonstrates, some of the pioneers who wrote about aging in India discussed senior citizens or those employed in the formal sector; for these experts, aging was foremost an issue concerning the "senior citizen" or retired employee who had worked either in the Indian government or its public sector enterprises—and who was most likely male, urban, and Hindu. Kirpal Singh Soodan, who trained in a social work school in India, wrote one of the earliest works of gerontological research based on a social survey of the "aged" or pensioners in the north Indian city of Lucknow.[40] He emphasized that aging was a "new" problem to India, and he repeated the trope of aging as a devastating family crisis that spelt the breakdown of what was regarded in the past as an ideal, intergenerational family. As Cohen points out, apart from a narrative of a "fall" that assumes a golden past, these gerontological studies made the "pensioner" out to be a "disadvantaged elder." According to Soodan, the pensioned individual (most likely male) was suffering from a "loss of social status, a diminished income, and psychological stress."[41] Soodan added, "It is paradoxical that while the number of the aged the world over is increasing . . . it has resulted in a large number of aged who are ill, defective, socially and emotionally disturbed, and economically dependent. . . . They may become either an asset to a nation or a social menace."[42]

The views and focus of later Indian gerontologists would vary greatly, even as they quoted and employed Western gerontological writings. The experts at the conference on aging in South Asia, for instance, intertwined gerontological literature with several critiques of development and health programs. They referred to aging emphatically as primarily an issue of poverty and subsistence (unlike Soodan, who spoke of aging as a proxy for retirement), and they emphasized the need to convert the old or retired into a national asset rather than leave them as dependents or a "menace." The former approach allowed Fernandes, De Souza and the others hosting the South Asia meeting to speak of aging as primarily an issue of marginalized older persons who worked in the informal sector; when locating the rights and needs of older persons, they invoked development's national and worldwide failures vis-à-vis older persons. This approach was also a search for an alternative vision of development for the powerless, and it transcended politics to claim a moral space: "any discussion of the aged, to be meaningful, has to begin by demanding a change in the international unjust economic order. . . . This is not a question of social welfare measures for a few aged persons but of the human right of three fourths of humanity to live a decent life."[43]

There were growing echoes of these views in the 1970s and 1980s, because severe critiques of the international economic order and the failures of development were emerging. These ideas reinforced the claim that aging was a broad-based humanitarian issue beyond the realm of national, political ideologies. However, this idea did not necessarily resonate when aging and the cause of national development became intertwined. Social workers at the local level attempted to "indigenize" issues relating to the young, the old, and the vulnerable, and from the 1970s through the 1980s, the field was recasting its subjects. At the same time, the priorities of development, whatever its failures, shadowed the expectations of these social workers from developing nations vis-à-vis supporting older populations and, in turn, their expectations that families resume their "traditional" responsibilities.

Social Workers, Development, and the Aged

The AGHE international survey led by Donald Cowgill was initiated partly to try to gain greater political ground domestically but also to demonstrate American experts' widening professional reach. Despite the survey's forlorn conclusions about how little gerontology and, in effect, aging-related training counted in many developing countries, it did underscore that experts such as Cowgill and Beattie could assume intellectual leadership of the international aging agenda. They premised their claim on the theory that the few gerontological education and incipient aging programs visible in developing nations owed their origins to the West, as Cowgill suggested when he summarized his reports on gerontological education in Kuwait and Thailand; in these places, he noted, interest in aging had been created by a few students he had trained or supported for training in the United States.[44]

Gerontology as a distinct field of study and expert knowledge was absent in developing nations. However, as Cowgill's efforts to assess its spread by inquiring at sociology departments across the developing world indicated, gerontology did have other proxies in the growing number of schools of social work in the developing world and in the ranks of social workers trained in them. Social work schools in the developing world often owed their origins to missionary enterprise. Two of India's earliest schools were established by American missionaries, as had schools in Africa such as the Jesuit-supported schools of social work in Zimbabwe.[45] These social workers formed a growing army of field experts to address the problems of social development of Asia's and Africa's expanding cities, which were in the throes of rapid urbanization, migration, and the social fallout thereof. Aging was only one of the "welfare" challenges they addressed, and they rarely focused on it as a distinct issue, linking it with the breakdown of families, youth problems, and changes in social and economic structure.[46] This cadre of social workers is a significant link going forward in our narrative, for in the 1980s and 1990s, when opportunities arose to implement the first national-level aging plans in developing countries and participate in UN or international NGO-led local and regional meetings on aging, these social workers took up the assignments, drawing from their experiences of urban social services.

These years saw a significant shift from the 1940s and 1950s, when training in social work education had been imported from the United States to developing countries, often facilitated by UN support of these schemes.[47] By the 1960s, social workers were being trained by experts at sites beyond Europe and the United States and were evolving their own critiques of Western social work pedagogies, in particular of the American approach to social work. U.S. influences were being diluted in other ways. In the 1970s, East African social workers were being trained by Israeli experts, who helped them build new professional literature and teaching materials that were relevant to Kenya; by 1970, nearly 150 graduates had been produced at this new school of social work.[48]

Influential networks that sought to coordinate the materials and approach used to train social workers in developing countries were also emerging. Records of meetings from across both Anglophone and Francophone Africa reveal that the Association for Social Work Education in Africa (ASWEA) led these efforts in the 1970s and 1980s to "decolonize" the field. Many case study booklets and innovative, context-sensitive curricula for rural and urban social services were produced, and meetings among educators and practitioners were held, so that social workers could align with the national development plans and goals of many countries in the region. Some of the programs and new training were for community workers in rural areas, with a focuses ranging across maternal and child health; nutrition; containment of "social plagues" or health risks; community improvement programs to build water projects, mosques, and community centers; fostering youth groups to train them for employment and service; and even adult education services.[49]

Aging as a separate field was not discussed in the materials produced by the ASWEA network, but the curricula of the training programs emphasized stages of "human development" and linked various life stages in their framework. It focused on enforcing family support and community responsibility for the needy, disabled, or aged. The training situated the problems of old persons within the problems of family life, urbanization, and rural-urban migration. Particular attention was paid to disability, destitution, and the needs of vulnerable groups in times of famines and disasters.

In terms of teaching and course material, separate modules on aging as a later life stage were included in syllabi covering urban and rural sociology as well as psychological and developmental theories. For instance, the Unit of Social Administration in Ghana, the Social Service School in Tanarive, the Higher Institute of Social Work in Cairo, the Institution of Social Training in the Central African Republic, and even the government administration school in Mauritius listed social psychology, genetic psychology, or human growth and development as subjects taught; these aimed "to enable students to understand the biological and psychological development of the individual from birth until old age [and] the relevance of modern theories of personality to each phase."[50]

Notably, these courses and their content did not hesitate to bring up wider issues such as the politics of international development and its programs. This explains why many social workers writing on aging, such as groups at the Indian Social Institute in New Delhi, also referred to the inequalities in the world economy, which was aligned in favor of developed countries.[51] Social work training in South Asia and Africa addressed the politics of modernization, and leading schools of social work that served as models for others in Africa, such as the School of Social Work at the Haile Selassie University in Ethiopia, taught urban sociology courses that explored the growth of and changes in urban populations, demographic changes and their significance, and urban stratification and the distribution of power in these spaces. An interview with Father Joseph Hampson, a Jesuit missionary and the director of fieldwork at the School of Social Service in Harare in 1985, revealed that these syllabi set by the ASWEA, and in particular ideas emanating from the Ethiopian and Egyptian social work schools (which linked the social work mission with bringing about social change), inspired other schools in sub-Saharan Africa.[52] Modernization, its precarious assumptions, and the hardships inflicted on various vulnerable groups in society were often emphasized, and it seemed the only ones who could deal with these issues were the social workers who could reinforce family and community bonds.

In a set of guidelines issued for course development in Africa, for example, a leading social worker bemoaned the introduction of new, unfavorable social developments due to a "capitalist money economy" and
urged, "Social work must be adapted to the African way of life including
the African concept of the family. . . . Since we cannot turn the development clock back it is up to you social work practitioners, administrators and
educators to develop relevant techniques. . . . When providing family welfare services every effort should be made to enrich family life and assist
families [to] maintain their cohesion. . . . Similarly in rendering services to
the aged and the handicapped, communities must be made to accept their
responsibilities towards these categories of fellow-citizens so that what is
done for them is so done in the context of community life and they do
not feel that they are unwanted."[53] The approach to social and welfare
work and services was taking a turn from a "remedial" and curative approach, aimed at picking up those who had fallen by the wayside, to offering
development-related mobilization that reinforced community responsibility and emphasized "preventive" approaches. Social workers saw aging
in developing societies as being embedded primarily within social structures,
such as family and community, and they aimed to act as local intermediaries
assisting in development programs for social change, such as allevi-
ating poverty, rather than to simply help their "clients" adjust to existing
structures.

From Rural Abandonment to Urban Displacement

The meager fruits of international development helped create a new role
for social workers in the 1970s; they also made urbanization and its malcon-
tents a crucial site requiring intervention. In these years, urban sociologists,
environmental experts, and UN agencies were worried about accelerated
growth and rapid change in habitat: as they saw them, a crisis in urban life
in developing nations exerting pressure on cities' fragile social and economic fabric. These posed a "world problem" of "human settlements" in
developing countries.[54] This demanded urban planning and programs to
regulate the so-called urban environmental equilibrium by initiating
means to relieve growing population congestion in cities and by identifying the social services required to mitigate the urban poverty and dependence that resulted from the failures of development policies. A cadre
of cosmopolitan urban experts, mostly from the United States or the UN,

who forecast upcoming problems and fieldworkers, such as social workers working in slums and squatter settlements, were engaged at different levels to address these new worldwide complications in urban social and economic life.

Social welfare concerns relating to problem adolescents, families, and social evils such as "beggary," all viewed in the context of labor welfare, were gradually effaced in these centers. By the 1970s and 1980s, social development issues focused primarily on urban areas were prioritized.[55] In the 1980s the Madras School of Social Work, for instance, shifted from its earlier focus on urban indigents and beggars, including old and abandoned persons, to reporting on the condition of the old in "new" habitats such as slums and shantytowns and discussing their integration and "livelihood strategies."[56] Increasingly, the priority was emphasizing aged individuals' own roles and volition in rehabilitation and assisting voluntary agencies in integrating the denizens of slums, rather than deepening state welfare responsibilities.

These studies' content and recommendations were not entirely surprising. Social work tomes that often read like policy directives from the Indian government, such as the *Encyclopaedia of Social Work in India*, which was routinely published by a government department, had stated this emphasis even in previous decades. During the Partition of India and its resultant violence and exodus, the aged and the infirm had been rescued by social workers and housed in refugee camps. Subsequently, vulnerable groups expressed heightened expectations for care and social security that frightened social policymakers, who emphasized the resurrection of family responsibilities for care as an alternative, projected family as the rightful place and refuge of the old, offered to support only the destitute, and attempted to regulate and set standards for voluntary agencies to take over. With the accelerated urbanization of the 1970s, during which experts deemed human settlements a "world" problem, international development and its fallout was critiqued, but the emphasis on individual and family contributions in terms of social protection for older persons was only reinforced.

Social workers were key consultants in mediating "local" knowledge; this is implicit in the UN's development priorities changing to urban environments and habitats, social work schools' expressing growing interest in contributing to social development, and experts in social work schools contributing to UN-led studies across various regions compiled in the *Report on Aging in Slums* (1977).[57] In keeping with the ideology of "social development" now being espoused in the arena of social work and aging, the report recommended community engagement from below that would emerge from these slums. At the same time, the report displayed a limited sensitivity to the plight of the old. The UN report noted that studies conducted in Peru and in cities such as Jos in Nigeria had shown that the problem of dependence—especially of old women and widows who had migrated from villages or of old workers who stayed back in cities—was likely to escalate in the coming years.[58] UN experts surmised that the spaces old people occupied were lacking in developmental promise. These views were clearly articulated in the earlier UN *Report on Improvement of Slums and Uncontrolled Settlements* (1972), which had emerged from a meeting in Colombia in 1970 attended by delegates from twenty-seven countries. The report cautioned that "a distinction should be made between 'dead-end' slums, those with a minimum of economic potential where old and socially unadapted people live, and the 'open-end' slums composed of relatively young families, with potential for economic growth. The economic potential of the open-end slum community plays an essential role in the total urban development process." The UN report's parting advice was to regard the aged and their communities in these sites as "pilot programmes." It was suggested that "The ideal role of government in regard to slums and squatter settlements is the stimulation, mobilization and direction of resources and energies found in these areas towards developmental ends."[59]

In Africa, in addition to welfare and development training, emerging issues relating to humanitarian relief, drawn from experiences in various African countries, would be strengthened in these years. Experts trained in refugee-related relief work were vital in reinforcing national-level networks that worked with international NGOs (such as HelpAge International) to provide relief to old persons in refugee camps for those fleeing civil war or drought. Deliberations among African church organizations in the 1960s and later, along with support from Scandinavian resources, led to an emerging concern for the aged among the humanitarian relief organizations that would gain prominence in later decades in Africa.[60]

Social Visions from the Locality

Social work leaders in developing countries were trenchant in their critiques of international development and the fallout of modernization projects. These experts, however, perceived those who were dependent or needy—such as adolescents, the "handicapped," and elderly—as the responsibility of the family and community. In many cases, this reinforced existing inequalities and deprivations. For instance, the elderly of African origin in Zimbabwe were made dependent on local and community re-sources; this conveniently excluded them from formal social security sys-tems that had so far recognized only the needs of white citizens.[61] Social workers also asserted that since newly independent countries could only afford limited schemes of social security, they were not in a position to as-sume the responsibilities shouldered by Western welfare states. The plans for welfare reform for the aged were ambitious, and its real prospects in developing nations were not immediately feasible. The limited number of social workers in these countries therefore carried a "difficult burden."[62]

How did social workers perceive and frame the old in their urban habi-tats? They reinforced old age as a social category divorced from chrono-logical age. The latter was perceived as inconsistent and unfathomable in Africa and other developing countries, where the state could be arbitrary when it came to deciding who was "old" and "deserved" social entitle-ments.[63] The new social forces of urbanization threatened this category. Most social workers charged with looking after the new urban poor (such as the unemployed, the aged, and the destitute) viewed Africa's rapid ur-banization through a moral lens. To them, the city represented the intru-sion of disruptive social evils and the erosion of an essential and traditional Africa. The "community" and its "tribal approach to obligations" were still central, as emphasized by William Clifford, who produced A *Primer of Social Case Work in Africa* (1966), "the first handbook on the new profes-sion of social case work in Africa," which remained an important reference for social work curricula in East Africa for many decades. The "African" was a "social being" who was used to group thinking, and this identity could not be ignored in training for social casework techniques that needed to be sufficiently adaptable "to meet the special needs of the continent."[64]

Social workers in both Asia and Africa continued to see old people as "group objects." This was brought out in the family case studies that sometimes illustrated experiences with old persons. Clifford's casework, for instance, described his experiences with rehabilitating old persons and destitute persons. These old persons were described as those "who had broken under the stresses and strains of community life . . . and now were no longer self-sufficient."[65] In his description of a case of "destitution and old age," he wrote, "Ada was an elderly woman. She was said to be about sixty years of age but may have been much older. With no records of birth in Africa . . . ages are often in doubt." Clifford described the caseworker's record detailing Ada's condition: she was living in a car near the locked residence of her son when she was found by a city council worker.[66] Ada's case was one of abandonment by her auto mechanic son, James, who was difficult to trace "without complete country-wide coverage of social work services." Clifford noted that the case raised the sensitive issue of whether (as believed), "by tribal custom Africans look after their dependents. This is generally true but in this case we have the kind of exception which is likely to increase as the towns grow and dependents are separated from relatives." Ada represented a severe problem, it was noted, of the homeless aged as found elsewhere in the world; she typified the problems of old age, but she also reflected the "fierce independence of the aged" as she wanted to stay in a familiar location. The case illustrated that "her age and circumstances make it difficult for us to talk to her about self-reliance, but the principle was not lost sight of."

Ada's abandonment represented a break from previous "traditions" attributed to "tribal custom"; she also broke from tradition simply by being an old person and a woman lingering in a public space in a city. She was "out of place." Controlling her and trying to return her to family or "tribe" marked efforts to reorder the urban environment and renew traditional patriarchy—and to erase the social defilement of both. Her return could restore the equilibrium of both her personal conflicts and public dilemmas of urbanization, even though she displayed a lack of adjustment and a stubborn independence as well as an indifference to her lack of any means. All this was traced partly to her matrilineal tribe and partly to a possible resistance to the rhythms of capitalist forces in the city, as old people were often seen as being slow in adjusting to new values.[67] Ada's odd behavior outside of her family was not acceptable; it was seen as pathological, calling for a caseworker's intervention. Other studies showed that eccentricities and quirks of the aged within the family were tolerated.[68] The approach to the "problem" of Ada appears to demonstrate that even the newer strains of social work, more attuned to Africa or the developing world, had biases, persistent colonial assumptions about primeval identities—of caste, tribe, religion, and other group identities—and of the concomitant need for social work experts to rationalize these tendencies.

There were, however, new priorities and values associated with these interventions. Another manual on social casework, produced by the Oppenheimer

College, reflected on casework experiences in Zambia for Africa as a whole. It noted that social group work in emerging countries had to have a "stress on nationhood and nation building," and that the approach should not be about either remedying the individual or concern for the country, but about bringing together and reconciling both objectives.[69] Even though the youth population was central to this preoccupation, worries about both the young and the old were linked, and anxieties regarding their expectations were a source of worry. The young, the writer of a social work manual warned, could have "an unrealistic appreciation of what the nation owed them; an exaggerated idea of their own worth . . . or a value system out of step with the country at large" that needed to be corrected.[70] In the case of the old, there would be a growing difference between those who had lived under colonial rule and those who followed; the latter would have been more individualistic in their youth and would subscribe to currently pervasive values of equality, self-dependence, and social justice, which would lead to different expectations of their families and nation.[71] An Indian social worker from a school of social work in Rajasthan wrote that the old and attitudes toward them were determined by the young who determined the former's social status. In no case, he added, should traditional authority infringe on democratic and secular values. The implication was therefore that aged persons needed to be supported and cared for, but achieving wider national goals of modernization was vital, and could not be compromised.[72]

The debates in these decades demonstrate that social experts faced significant challenges in reconciling their interests in the changing structures of families, urban poverty and destitution, as well as remedial welfare services within the behemoth that was social development. Social development called for them to reconcile the maladjusted individual or the groups that had lost their social identity and role, with broader goals of national development. Development and its programs in developing countries were overwhelmingly youth-centered enterprises that focused on the dependency of children and the disruptive powers of juveniles and youth. To insert the old as a distinct group into the paradigm of development was immensely challenging, even in the 1980s and 1990s.

5

The Birth of Global Aging and Its Local Afterlives

In July 1982, the UN hosted a World Assembly on Aging (WAA) in Vienna and anointed population aging as a global problem. Population aging had been of immediate concern only to developed countries, but now the issue was an agenda that linked the developed and developing worlds and was projected as representing a shared future.[1] At the WAA and in its echoes in subsequent years, policymakers from developing countries and international and national experts would unanimously declare that population aging was now a "universal phenomenon." Between the 1950s and 1970s, "old age" as a distinct social stage with particular roles and needs had become a category of analysis and the subject of a new field of international research and practice. It had increasingly caught the attention of social workers in newly founded social work schools and departments and among sociologists studying urban social change in families and communities.[2] Although aging's reach as a wider welfare concern spanned many developing countries, neither studies on aging and social adjustment nor meetings held by networks of international gerontologists alone could have created the momentum for a transnational worldview of aging.

In the arena of population and development between the 1950s and the 1970s, experts referred to future and probable demographic shifts in developing countries, but no significant interest was expressed in this subject. In August 1974, at the United Nations World Population Conference held in Bucharest, the who's who of population control, including heads of government, met to review a decade of contentious population control programs and goals.[3] The Bucharest conference declaration was significant for unambiguously aligning population control with development and asserting that demographic change could only be brought about through the equitable sharing of world resources and by fostering socioeconomic development.[4] The conference report observed that "the population of the developing countries is basically [a] young population, which needs a more just, equal and human world and calls [for] social change," implying that the problem of aging was distinct to developed countries.[5] These passing references aside, the conference in Bucharest in no way presaged the "birth" of world aging.[6]

Neither the Eurocentric nature of international gerontological networks and aging associations nor the interest in aging, displacement, and poverty displayed by social work schools in Asia and Africa offers a credible explanation for the making of an international discourse or its mobilization. How then did the "world" become the designated field of inquiry to represent aging populations? Which impulses shaped the appearance of a new world agenda, and what kind of international consensus did this represent? Once a diffuse "world" agenda was articulated and largely left adrift without resources, what were its afterlives? How did experts in various parts of the world redeploy the WAA in Vienna and its plan to assert various other alignments? This chapter focuses on debates before and after the Assembly, particularly tracing the processes that led to the Assembly to understand how networks and competing visions about aging were being articulated, and examines how groups of experts and activists in developing countries saw and translated these events.

My interest lies in situating the origins of the WAA in the context of development politics and the failures associated with modernization and developmental visions in the 1970s and the 1980s. Aside from their surface significance, debates around aging were also articulating pessimism and anger at the challenges and roadblocks on the path to a promised modernization in developing countries. In developed nations, the economic crises of the 1980s necessitated rethinking the implications of neoliberal policies and state responsibility toward older persons, such as responding to the retrenchment of welfare benefits. In some cases, such as in the United States, this political status quo in domestic aging policy led to pressures to turn outward, toward international efforts.

For many observers, the proposed agenda of the WAA and its many manifestations—such as its regional preparatory drafts, advisory committees, and the innumerable iterations that emerged from the WAA declarations and plans (and I examine only a fraction of these produced over a decade)—offered a fluid space to confront what was not easily explicable or reversed: the changes that were occurring in social and economic lives worldwide. Debates at the WAA also marked an attempt to link this failed narrative of UN-led modernization and urbanization to certain growing challenges: old-age dependency, labor, and delinquent families and youth. In various statements about the WAA, one can also hear echoes of these economic failures in the lived experience of affected families and communities in regions and nations across the world. These experiences and voices were means of confronting and resisting these developmental changes rather than accepting them.

This chapter first traces debates among UN experts and international demographers regarding populations, longevity, and falling fertility. Even though these debates forecast an eventual fall in fertility, demographic forecasts and anxieties by the 1970s were still not pressing for a "world" agenda that represented the challenges posed by aging populations. Next, it turns to the question of how experts shaped UN agenda—particularly the mobilization among experts in the United States that shaped the making of the WAA—and also anticipated its tensions. The chapter ends by examining the debates at the WAA and their recasting and "afterlives" across sites in Asia and Africa follows.

Demographic Forecasts for Asia and Africa

At the outset, let us continue to follow demographic research and debates in these decades and to review the roles population experts played, focusing in particular on the expansive demographic and social data UN agencies generated. Even though, in comparison to their concerns about birth control and high fertility, the UN's World Population Conferences paid little attention to aging populations, they generated comparative demographic surveys, social development reports, and data that were significant in shaping a growing interest in worldwide aging.

At a meeting of the second IGC in St. Louis (1951), a participant noted, "Chronological aging is a characteristic of the peoples of Europe, northern America and the British Dominions in Oceania. In Asia, Africa, and Latin America, there is only a small proportion of aged persons in the population. This small proportion moreover has shown no tendency to rise."[7] The difference was that in Brazil or India, for instance, only one person in forty or almost fifty, respectively, was sixty-five years old or more, while in France, one person in nine was of this age. East and West looked as though they would never meet, with the former characterized by high fertility and mortality. The conclusion was that "the proportion of the aged was small and continued to remain small in these societies." In the late 1950s, and increasingly later, experts captured these demographic binaries in more persuasive ways. Demographers and policymakers were beginning to represent the demographic differences between developed and developing countries via fertility change models. The forecasts of progressive fertility change across societies served a range of functions over these years, the most central being their use by the population control movement in its attempts to effect fertility decline, with high fertility being viewed as a barrier to economic progress and modernization.[8]

In the early 1940s, demographers at the Princeton-based Office of Population Research articulated the classic formulation of these forecasts: the "demographic transition." This evolutionary and linear theory was reformulated in the 1950s as a forecasting tool offering the means to understand how a society transitioned from a preindustrial to a postindustrial state of demographic equilibrium by controlling fertility and consequently transforming themselves into modern, industrialized nations. Simon Szreter argues that even though flaws in this model and its limitations had been pointed out, demographers and experts at the UN and the World Bank made it more policy-aligned or "contaminated" in these years to make predictions about long-term patterns of change and their resulting fertility decline in developing countries.[9]

Some Asian countries, particularly India and China, were perceived as influential cases where this transition was much awaited due to their population control policies. India had already been the subject of U.S. studies and support, as Matt Connelly's study demonstrates.[10] Alison Bashford points out that Japan in the interwar years and for some years after the Second World War also became a focus of attention: its birth and death rates were seen to be changing during the American occupation, and Japan's politics of needing territorial space due to population expansion was a cause of concern. By the 1950s, the country was of less interest as a replicable case of fertility decline for the rest of Asia, but debates about Japan helped to endorse population policies that prioritized fertility regulation rather than migration or population transfers.[11]

Eagerly awaited though they were, fertility declines were slow to materialize, and some perceptive experts, such as the American demographer Irene Taeuber, were skeptical about the transition occurring uniformly across all developing countries along the evolutionary lines Frank Notestein's articulation suggested.[12] Increasingly, in the 1960s and later, it became evident that population-control programs were not yielding the expected results, and that the best contraceptive was perhaps development itself.

Taeuber, an expert at the Office of Population Research at Princeton University, had started her career waiting hopefully for Japan's declining fertility to be a model for others. She was keen to emphasize that family planning programs by themselves would not achieve dramatic results. Nor was it helpful, she thought, to view the world as being simply divided into high- and low-fertility countries ranging from the developing to the developed world. In a paper presented at the Second World Population Conference in Belgrade (1964), Taeuber said that "historical replications of the demographic transition are not likely." Although the latter had occurred in Europe, among European peoples overseas, and in Japan, which had modernized earlier, it could not be made a basis for predictions in countries that were currently in earlier stages of developments, simply because the future of mortality and fertility in these countries was different. Science and technology were being borrowed rather than invented, and there were many deterrents to economic growth. Other missing factors included a commitment by the government and the people to the goals of modernization and the democratization of concepts of need and welfare.[13] Taeuber observed that even as mortality was responsive to technological and scientific advances, fertility still continued to reflect traditional values and folk practices.

Yet the UN persisted with projected fertility estimates for the whole world, even if their tentative nature was recognized, as it especially was in the case of mainland China, where both data and technical adequacy in making projections were lacking. The UN assumed that fertility would decrease by half its original level within thirty years of the beginning of a decline, but this expectation and its promise of changes in the broad social and economic development of the nation was not a reliable panacea for population growth.[14] Estimates of future fertility were more complex than those of declining mortality, one of the achievements of modernization, for the former involved social and psychological dynamics.

Many other experts among leading Western and Asian demographers agreed with Taeuber about the difficulties of making, as the UN was compelled to, long-term future predictions regarding fertility or estimating a worldview of projections for the years 1980 or 2000. But the general agreement was that many less-developed countries would see the start of a fertility decline toward the end of the century, for, as Taeuber noted, "The future of population growth is primarily the question of the future of development," and the latter was to have a consistent effect on declines in fertility.[15]

Asia was the focus of the largest population control programs in these decades, and India had been the subject of the earliest forecasts regarding the implications of high fertility and dependency, in works by American demographers such as Ansley J. Coale and Kingsley Davis. At the Asian Population Conference in 1964, participants noted that even by conservative estimates, the population in the Economic Commission for Asia and the Far East (ECAFE) regions was poised for substantial increases through the 1970s.[16] A decline in birth rates was unlikely to halt this growth, although the ratio of dependent children would fall progressively, allowing for an improvement in living conditions.[17]

Developmental over Demographic Anxieties in Asia

Discussions at the Asian Population Conference underscored that in Asian countries, population aging, or a rising proportion of older persons, was not a critical demographic concern since the proportion of older persons in the ECAFE region relative to that in developed countries was low, and fertility continued to be high even though mortality rates were declining. "Nevertheless," the conference report noted, "small percentages in the large populations of individual countries represent great numbers of people." This raised issues about the social implications of development rather than demography.[18] Experts' recognition of aging as a problem in Asia was prompted less by perceived demographic risks of aging and falling fertility, and more by a concern about social welfare and support for vulnerable populations affected by rapid, imbalanced development. The main challenge in the Asian region was the ongoing demographic revolution, caused by population growth due to declining mortality and persistently high, relatively stable fertility. The difference with the West, the ECAFE report argued, was that in the West, the decline in mortality had been achieved along with industrialization and the growth of cities in both size and numbers, so that population growth had been supported by urban industries.[19] Expanding urban opportunities had been balanced with technological advances in agriculture to produce more food despite a diminished agricultural population. In Asian countries, the density of the agricultural population in relation to agricultural resources, or the pressure on land, resulted in migration to cities that lacked employment opportunities, housing, and other utilities; this led women and older persons in rural areas to become increasingly dependent on young, male, urban migrants.[20] Some nations, like Japan, had achieved a high percent of urban population, but these were not representative of the region as a whole.[21]

The demographic problems intersecting with old age in Asia were perceived as emerging from the extended family system—relatively stable in rural areas—and its threatened disintegration into nuclear family units with urbanization. In India, for instance, migration to cities was accompanied by an outward migration of older persons to rural areas. Thus cities had a youthful population, but with mortality declining very fast in urban areas, city populations were only likely to grow. However, the report noted, the city-states of Singapore and Hong Kong were reporting a rapid transition toward the nuclear family, which was related to "rapid economic development and modernization. . . . [In] other countries this transition towards the nuclear family was proceeding at a slower rate." These rapid social changes affected older persons, who needed social protection and welfare support as urbanization and migration were weakening their authority and traditional ties. The loss of social security within the family, in other words, required a counterbalance in the form of social programs.[22]

UN Data and Fertility Debates in Africa

Regional demographic data for Asia in the 1960s and the 1970s failed to stimulate a discourse on population aging caused by demographic transition, but such a discourse was even more marginal to debates in Africa. At the First Population Conference, held in Ibadan (1966), an expert noted that only about 27 percent of the population in tropical Anglophone Africa lived in countries covered by demographic inquiries including fertility, mortality, age distribution, and migration (Ghana, Uganda, and Congo). Predicting vital demographic trends was thus a challenge.[23] Experts pointed out that countries such as India had initiated a national population control program more than a year prior, and that so far population control policies had focused on Asia. Although Africa continued to face the problem of poor data, especially in determining fertility due to age misstatement, research by the Princeton Office of Population Research and data from the life expectancy tables compiled by the UN Economic Commission for Africa together projected a demographic picture of very high fertility in tropical Africa, "even if not uniformly so."[24]

In response to whether a demographic transition was underway in Africa, demographer John Caldwell wrote that a mortality transition was clearly taking place and steepening since the Second World War, in patterns similar to those Asia and Latin America.[25] "No major fall in fertility had been experienced but [it was] . . . afoot" as pressures on the family were likely to occur due to government population policy measures and child survival. Demographers emphasized that more than two-fifths of the population in tropical Africa was below age fifteen and that this dependence needed bigger investments.[26]

A Sought-After Predicament

In all of these writings, the final stage in the demographic transition represented a much-desired equilibrium and modernization for developing countries rather than a stage of anxiety over a new and perilous stage of aging. A UN report that assessed achievements in what was termed the second development decade (the 1970s) observed that many developing countries remained at the threshold of the demographic transition. There were enormous differences in demographic attributes across developing countries; some were beginning to display attributes of more advanced countries, while others had not begun the transition to lower birth and death rates.[27] A fall in fertility held the promise of government-led development no longer being dissipated in low levels of capital formation and development; it would also be accompanied by the strong, distinct social changes that prompted these demographic shifts. As notions of reducing fertility and child dependency trickled down and India's popular press interpreted them, demographic transition was understood as a promising "type 4" stage when the country would evolve from the high birth and death rates that prevailed in the 1940s to a transition stage with a high birth rate but a fairly low death rate; in the last stage, fertility would had been controlled through family-planning programs.[28]

The beginnings of a fertility transition also reflected the difference between elite and poor populations within developing countries, making the onset of chronological aging and a growing proportion of older persons a problem of certain classes. By the 1970s and 1980s, in discussions at international population conferences and national debates in India, the demographic transition was mostly viewed as a devoutly desirable distant end increasingly mired in what had been termed at the Bucharest conference "demographic inertia," which was caused by a lack of support for the wider social and economic development that could bring about fertility change.[29] Meanwhile, in 1975 at the National Population Conference in Delhi, some researchers argued that differentials in fertility also measured the divide between the poor and the elite, since "The elitist class in this country are already in a state of demographic transition. . . . What we need is a people's plan, a demographic plan for the masses."[30] Achievement of low fertility and the onset of population aging, it was hinted, signified not simply a difference between developed and developing countries in equity and development but also the schisms within a nation itself. This would in turn lead to seeing and interpreting the needs of the aged in distinct and often contradictory ways.

These wide heterogeneities between and within developing countries and the differences in demographic development between the First and Third Worlds implied a complete lack of wide international consensus on an emerging agenda for the aged and elderly when it was voiced in the 1970s. Aging was not an easy proxy for the developing world's problems, as demographic writing was still speaking of demographic aging, or an increase in the proportion of those beyond the age of sixty years, as a development scenario of the future—of the long term—rather than the present. It is worth noting that in the 1980s, environmental agendas made inroads in international negotiations (such as the Montreal Protocol, 1987) by growing out of overlapping networks of atmospheric scientists and policymakers who framed an "ozone discourse" that addressed threats that lay in the distant future.[31]

However, in the case of global aging, demographers did not take the lead in shaping a political or scientific discourse encompassing the world in their claims regarding risks and crises; basically, middle-level UN bureau-crats and social gerontologists led the early campaigns toward the WAA in Vienna. In later years, some international NGOs and social experts forged loose epistemic networks in Asia and Africa, in the interests of advocating for a revision of the Vienna Plan of Action (1982), but their influence on state interests was and continued to be limited in the 1990s and 2000s, when they deepened their local support.

In his critique of international development, the anthropologist, Arturo Escobar has written that the Third World has been framed through "common signifiers" such as overpopulation, poverty, and other problems.[32] I argue that in discourses advanced before and after the WAA, aging was repre-sented as a developmental issue and associated with challenges in devel-oping societies, because, in international and national engagements around modernization and developmental issues, these vocabularies, policy path-ways, and political constituencies were already in use.

To represent aging as a new demographic problem implied longstanding challenges, as it brought up the question of the relevance of ongoing pop-ulation policies. Jason Finkle describes the inertia of population policies at a national level after the pathbreaking points of the Cairo Declaration on Population and Development (1994), when targeted family planning was condemned by all nations. Finkle also documents its persistence in India, a state-level signatory to the Cairo Declaration.

Fighting Two Battles

Responses in China in 1984, soon after the Vienna WAA declared aging a new world problem, illustrate a similar preoccupation. A first genera-tion of gerontologists in China, including Hong Chang Ping, cautioned that mitigating the threat aging posed in China did not mean the gov-ernment should "loosen its population policy." That had to remain the first priority, while Chinese people ensured that the population aging problem was not ignored.[33] As dense scholarship on the one-child policy in particular has shown, local implementation of population control policies in China varied, as did their effects on reducing second births among Han Chinese families, but the need to check fertility and "the goal of limiting the population under 1.2 billion by the end of the 20th century" was also closely tied to visions of development and resource distribution. These priorities persisted and overlapped, even as gerontological research and the challenge of an aging population would begin to be accepted in the 1980s.

Some Chinese gerontologists did not unequivocally accept demographic projections regarding an aging population and a rapid fall in fertility. Hong Chang Ping, for instance, argued in writings published after the World Assembly on Aging in 1982 that China needed to find its own, different model in addressing the problems of aging and that striking a balance between aging and the one-child policy was possible.[34] The same concerns emerged in an interview with Wu Cangping, regarded as the father of Chinese gerontology, who observed, "At very beginning nobody understood gerontology. I was one of the pioneers to suggest that we should learn about aging, we should study aging. . . . They thought I was crazy at that time as they didn't know anything about aging; it was a new term for China and its [gerontological] terminology began to be more familiar in China, only after 1982. . . . At that time the family planning people even came to talk to me, they said you shouldn't suggest that there is an aging problem, it will affect our family planning program, but I think it's inevitable, we must face these problems."[35]

Finally, attitudes toward both population control and aging programs reflected similar beliefs that China's problems stemmed from needing to keep pace with development and productivity, and thus were distinct. Wu Cangping summed this up:

> [In the West] since they have a developed economy, they are only thinking of elderly people, but in China we are fighting two battles. One is to fight [for] development and the other one is to fight with the elderly issues. Therefore in China, we should take the development as top priority—that means development in high labor productivity, so that one person can work very hard and even support a high dependency ratio. . . . We should develop our economy first to find the material basis to cope . . . with aging, and then think of aging strategies that will integrate families. And . . . we should choose from all the experiences that we have studied abroad such as in the United States, Russia, India and any other country, to fit with the Chinese national condition.[36]

As we shall see in the following section, the Chinese delegation at the WAA echoed these tensions, but the developmental vision underlying the

population control programs at this stage still prevailed over any acknowledgment of more complex challenges in the offing.

Prelude to Vienna: Worlds of "Difference"

Demographic policies and scientific forecasts at international or regional
levels, as we have seen so far, did not necessarily motivate a political consensus around aging as a distinct and pressing agenda. In the 1980s, as the
WAA approached, instead of policy makers and experts being unified, the
fault lines among them were widening and growing polarized. The WAA's
vision even suggested "difference" rather than worldwide solidarity. An
analysis of international NGOs' and gerontological associations' responses
to the UN draft agenda for the WAA attests to this, but it also suggests that
expertise on aging and mobilization led by NGOs outside the UN was
growing, presaging a "world" agenda based on decentralized, loosely aligned
communities of social experts, activists, and organizations working in the
field of aging.

In May 1980, large civil society organizations working on aging met in
Vienna with UN officials from the Centre for Social Development and
Humanitarian Affairs (CSDHA) (associated with the UN Economic and
Social Council [ECOSOC]), based at the time in Vienna, to discuss their
views of the work plan and ideas being proposed for the WAA and to ensure their contributions to the outcomes of the Assembly being held two
years later.[37] On the civil society end, the meeting was coordinated by the
International Federation on Aging (IFA), a North American NGO founded
about a decade earlier; at this point, the IFA leadership reflected a somewhat narrow range of partnerships spread among mostly European, Australian, and U.S. pensioners and geriatric medicine associations.[38] Even at
the outset, those articulating "the UN's point of view" at this meeting
made clear that the time had come to think broadly about aging policies
and to lead aging into international policymaking arenas. This in turn required aging research and its categories be situated within "certain realities in many societies of the world."[39] Gerontological science that had so
far rested on the activities and networks of scientists, activists, and social
workers was going to be disseminated to a new audience and shaped as an
"international action program."[40] The chief adviser to the World Assembly,
Tarek Shuman, who was trained in social work, summed up its plans: "Our
hope is that [the WAA] will be a meeting of decision makers. We do not

want to duplicate the efforts of yourselves and other gerontologists in the field who are holding national and international meetings and discussing the various issues of aging on technical and scientific levels. We do, however, feel we need to start talking to decision makers in a language they will understand. We feel that gerontologists, like other scientists, have been talking among themselves for a long time. It is now time to take the opportunity to start translating."[41]

UN experts such as Shuman, who formed a small constituency in an incipient social program within the organization, were creating a space for themselves to spread the political agenda of world aging to an international audience and to governments. These initiatives introduced and deepened a new axis in the realm of aging between UN bureaucrats associated with the CSDHA and state representatives. Political tensions and the economic downturns of these years colored their vision, as we shall see. Further, ideas on aging and society (such as the WAA plan of action) were shaped not only by these groups and their dialectics, but also by diverse interpretations in local societies.

At this stage, international expertise in aging policies was still limited, but UN officials were keen to make aging part of a larger set of contemporary concerns and in order to impart greater relevance to the WAA plans among developing nations and their policymakers. Shuman and his colleagues therefore explained that making concerns about aging relevant across the world necessitated emphasizing both developmental and humanitarian perspectives in understanding the problems of the elderly worldwide.[42]

Including Europe and Excluding Diversity

The views UN officials voiced were not always well received. Certain prominent invitees at the WAA were quick to assert that aging as an international agenda tended to overwhelmingly concentrate on perspectives from the Third World. Even as aging was widely identified at the WAA as a challenge both developed and developing countries faced, some groups found the UN's recommendations at odds with their approach to aging and to fields of current interest in Europe.[43] They complained that UN rhetoric was marginalizing the concerns of the aged in developed societies in order to foreground the interests of the old (consisting of the poor and destitute) in the global South. Eduard Pumpernig, the European Federation for the

Welfare of the Elderly (EURAG) representative, confessed frankly that the Federation, a body representing the interests of 40 million elderly persons, had reservations even about the UN's preliminary program and plans for the WAA. He was of the opinion that international campaigns should focus on "the false image of age" and its stereotypes, as these notions interfered with the elderly achieving the full independence, dignity, and productivity.[44]

Instead, the UN was turning to focus on the "problems of the elderly" in different settings. Commenting on the WAA report, the EURAG general secretary wrote, "It was further regretted that the whole structure of the report gives predominance to the certainly very urgent and necessary development of the countries of the Third World—this seems to be justified from the humanitarian point of view. But it is feared *that the problems of the elderly in the developed countries will be omitted completely in this World Assembly.* At least it seems absolutely necessary to differentiate more between the problems of the Third World and those of the industrial countries."[45] The EURAG therefore suggested that a separate group be created, with a focus on "the problems which are characteristic of European peoples."[46]

I argue that the North–South differences the EURAG emphasized actually masked old and new interests that were shaping Western gerontological ideas. In the 1940s and 1950s, both in the United States and Europe, in discussing aging and its close association with chronic diseases, scientists focused primarily on a population of white, older males and their health and productivity. This perception partly lingered in EURAG interests in the early 1980s. The EURAG was focused on ensuring support for a similar social group, prioritizing the continued productivity of older men and their access to a labor market, as they made up its main constituency. Older workers from male-dominated fields in industry formed the largest part of these affiliations and interests within the EURAG, and there were concerns that they should not get marginalized or left behind.[47] It was these groups and their labor and employment concerns that preoccupied them, rather than the WAA's focus on rescuing the aged poor in the Third World through social development schemes and improved social services.

At a EURAG meeting held a few years earlier in Belgrade (1976), these gendered notions of aging, employment, and productivity were frequently voiced. Delegates at the meeting from many parts of Western and Eastern Europe focused on the aging male worker, as they mused about his adjustment after retirement. One delegate noted that a person was "as old as his ability to adapt to his surroundings."[48] Pumpernig spoke about older employees' potential, and it was clear, when he spoke of their capabilities in comparison to younger workers' capabilities and further participation in the social process, that he was speaking about male labor efficiency. He observed, "The calm shown by the older manager, whose coolness as a leader is seen as a consequence of *his* greater knowledge of human affairs, is complemented by the qualities of patience and perseverance is acquired and proven in the settling of conflicts and quarrels. . . . This . . . should be given greater recognition by the older person *himself*."[49] In similar concerns voiced about older workers and pensions, women were mentioned, but only as dependent widows due to their longer life expectancy and place within the family.[50]

Newer challenges due to the worldwide economic downturn of the 1970s, in particular the crisis of welfare in the 1970s, made many agencies and policymakers turn away from underscoring continuing state and public responsibility for older persons in Europe. The EURAG representative observed that the "problems" and issues raised by the WAA, such as housing and health, had been discussed ad nauseam in Europe already; he dismissed them, noting that these "past" concerns of the First World were now preoccupying developing nations in the "present." He was, however, expressing an implicit priority of minimizing state role and intervention. These perspectives on aging spurning state-inspired developmentalism and growth resulted from a nascent neoliberal mindset that was deepening in the 1970s. The EURAG, for instance, prioritized changing social behavior and attitudes toward the elderly over addressing the structural and embedded causes of vulnerability among older persons, such as poverty. Its general secretary highlighted the need to address negative images of aging, to abolish stereotypes, to preserve human dignity, and in particular to focus on improving "life after retirement," when many older persons experienced marginalization.

The EURAG and its partners were focused on creating opportunities for the old to thrive and survive as liberated individuals in a free market, and therefore they aimed at addressing policies to save them from social stigma that would prevent their social and economic participation. They were less concerned with the problems of the elderly that required intervention and resources, even in industrialized societies. The EURAG representative conceded that the North and South shared the issue of the family's importance, which was worth investigation. In addition, the family was a resource for older persons only if it did not need excessive support from outside.

A Lifespan Approach

Not all of the views expressed at the meetings in Vienna drew a binary between the interests of developed and developing nations, or the West and the rest. Some emphasized a more decentralized approach to aging than that suggested by the WAA. In a section of the meeting devoted to knowledge gathered from Austria, the UN social development division hosting the WAA invited Leopold Rosenmayr, known for his contribution to lifespan research and studies among the old in Vienna, to speak.[51] Rosenmayr offered a veiled criticism of the UN approach, noting that it seemed to focus on a somewhat "one-sided" perspective on old age as a distinct stage of loss and decline. He argued for a longitudinal lifespan perspective emphasizing that aging needed to be addressed even in mid-life, and that a historical understanding of generations and their experiences could reveal a diverse perspective on issues of aging, since the conditions people experienced in their youth shaped their attitudes to hardship and physical and material limitations.[52] Rosenmayr also did not see a concomitant reduction of government responsibility or a reduction in public services with this approach; rather, he recommended "supplementing those of the welfare state," implying a greater role for grassroots initiatives, regional nongovernment services, and private organizations.[53]

Rosenmayr noted that social conditions for exerting autonomy and self-help in old age needed to be created. At the same time, there was a need to reflect on social engagement for the elderly in advanced industrial societies where capitalism had perceived old age as an unproductive life stage. Indirectly, he also responded to Shuman's claims about the expertise offered by UN experts in translating research and scientific claims that were somewhat opaque and theoretical to policymakers, asserting that "empathetic" scientists could mediate between those offering social services in the field and senior administrators.[54] This view emphasized local context and the development of habits and practices built throughout life, rather than at the end.

Voices such as Rosenmayr's were not heard much in UN circles beyond the Vienna meeting, and his work and ideas remained centered on issues of aging in industrialized nations even though his work was influential in social gerontological critiques that attempted to look beyond chronological age as a life-stage and focus on lifespan research. From the point of view of our narrative, his ideas are of interest as his research (following pioneers such as Ethel Shanas, author of a comparative study of aging in three industrial societies) emphasized the need to look more searchingly at the "universal" assumptions about aging in western societies and its givens, such as the decline of family support with growing modernization.[55]

Decentering a World Agenda from the Locality

Rosenmayr was skeptical of the plans UN officials mounted to build an international edifice for advocating aging concerns around the "problems" of aging, and also skeptical of the UN's focus on aging as a distinct stage tied to either dependence or lack of productivity. His views resonated among other social experts. In this case Ingrid Gelinek, a leading office-bearer from the International Association for Social Work (IASW)—an organization founded in the interwar years consisting of worldwide voluntary associations and linked to social work schools worldwide—conveyed her doubts over whether the WAA would yield dramatic progress. She emphasized the need to integrate social workers, practitioners, and older persons from across the Third World to plan the steps ahead.[56]

In other words, the UN's vision and that of its advisory NGOs was being criticized for not being sufficiently inclusive. The IASW representative was suggesting that the UN was stepping in to advise on aging worldwide based on idealized models of aging in the West and possessed insufficient knowledge of both humanitarian and developmental aspects of aging in the global South. She observed, "I have been in international organizations long enough to know that no international meeting ever *solves* any problems. However, I do believe that our sessions illustrate that there is a very valuable exchange of information going on which may lead to the beginning of cooperation among the often cited non-governmental agencies which—contrary to what they claim—have great difficulties in cooperating, and to the beginning of vital coordination between the United Nations . . . and the so-called non-governmental groups."[57]

The International Council on Social Welfare (ICSW) was known for its strong ties with social work schools in "developing countries" and its close links with experts in social policy and practice at national levels.[58] Its national chapters had been involved in efforts to address the social and health challenges older persons faced in communities across Africa and the Caribbean, and Ingrid Gelinek pointed out that although these efforts were nascent, they were significant because they were generated from national and local settings such as Kenya and Jamaica. These efforts were addressing the challenges faced by the aged in newly urbanized areas, particularly their health problems, and focused on the short-term humanitarian aspects of aging (as distinct from the long-term developmental goals related to aging), such as improving service delivery to older adults in Kenya, where a Standing Committee on Relief of Distress among the Aged (1967) had been formed.

According to Gelinek, the UN needed to keep other pioneering examples in mind, too, especially instances of integrating care and health services at the community level that were fused or integrated with existing development programs. The ICSW drew attention to the work of their national partners, for instance those in Jamaica who formed a committee to address issues of aging in the Caribbean. The example of Jamaica was particularly resonant both for this meeting held before the WAA and for subsequent years, as it became an example for offering social development schemes that integrated aging programs with a history of long-standing community development projects. Sybil Francis, a leading social worker with an early background in rural land settlement, rural housing projects, and the establishment of child development centers, worked closely through the government and with local communities to strengthen social assistance and health projects for older persons, especially relating to nutrition. Building on a model that drew from primary care and on local human resources, her work was aimed at extending the interest in aging-related issues to providing support universally rather than targeting only the most needy and frail.[59]

For Gelinek, such examples represented the integration of aging as a policy issue with the broader priorities of community development. This approach aimed at preventive method, rather than viewing the old as physically dependent and aging as a stage of inevitable marginalization caused by modernization and rapid development in developing nations. Gelinek noted that the WAA was expressing a "limited view of the world," and added that the UN, its allies, and NGO advisers such as the International Federation on Aging working with it on this vision were reflecting the "situation and problems of older people in Europe, or in the United States, or in the so-called Western Hemisphere."[60] Instead, the so-called developing and developed world had plenty to mutually learn from each other about old people, she argued, as every society was "developing."[61]

The difference in perspective between these EURAG and the ICSW spokespersons regarding their expectations of the WAA is interesting. Both sets of experts conveyed their differences with the framework of goals and perspectives the WAA was introducing in Vienna, even before these aims had been formally showcased and endorsed by the UN member states. Their views marked the contradictions and tensions that characterized the mood in the international arena in the 1980s, which colored both social gerontological research and the scope of social programs. The EURAG's views on what were deemed universalized "Western" views regarding aging reflected the tense relationship between the role and duties of the welfare state and its social responsibilities to citizens, but they masked the sharp differences among Western social policy experts in how they understood the characterization of old age in society, its ideological grounds, and its economic imperatives. The ICSW's view that Western approaches predominated reflected a separate tension in these meetings, raising the question whether the views of UN experts and its NGO advisers (who were predominantly from North America, such as the IFA), whose experiences stemmed from work with aging populations in the West, were an "international" vision at all.

However, it was not entirely accurate to claim the WAA organizers arrived at these views based on their Western partners alone, although Gelinek's claim that "people in the field" had not been involved in the UN's preparatory meetings was on the mark.[62] Based on the UN secretary general's directives, the secretariat for the WAA office in Vienna had initiated a series of regional consultations, through the support of UN regional offices, all over the developed and developing world.[63] Some of these engagements also tried to build interagency coordination between the WAA office, which represented the social development branch in the UN's Department of Social and Economic Affairs, and other UN agencies, in particular the WHO offices.[64]

UN Consultations and Their Results

What significance did these consultations spread through an entire year (1980–1981) have, and what did they yield? Advice and feedback on the needs of aging populations in regions such as Latin America and Africa emanating from meetings held in Costa Rica and Nigeria were dense, but the problem was that the WAA already set the parameters for discussion.[65] At these meetings, the organizers circulated demographically pessimistic documents on the implications of aging in the respective regions. These documents outlined the humanitarian and developmental aspects and issues of the aging "problem" and traced the unfavorable conditions challenging older persons in the present and likely to have more serious impacts in the near future.[66] What was said in regional meetings and what was refracted and heard by UN experts and international NGOs in turn also differed. The latter mostly emphasized a worsening situation for older persons caused by the "present" or the current economic, social, and cultural world situation.[67] The interdisciplinary experts invited to these meetings were expected to "assess" these documents and offer perspectives from the situation in their regions.

The Circulation of Experiences from the South to the North

The views from the South emphasized different perspectives. Experts who had been summoned by the WAA organizers and UN bodies to meet in developing regions emphasized the importance of social welfare services within a family framework, and therefore emphasized the needs to invest in rural areas to keep families and the young and old together, to strengthen the extended family and its role, and to enhance the participation of the old.[68] In contrast to the UN's perspectives on aging as a distinct issue and problem of dependence, nonproductivity, and marginalization, intergenerational support and solidarity was highlighted in this feedback, integrating aging as a wider agenda with concerns about families and communities in flux and experiencing social and health challenges was recommended.

In Costa Rica, delegates from across twenty countries made a statement that showed concern for the rapid demographic transition Latin America was undergoing; aging was seen as potentially affecting every aspect of social change and development to a lesser or greater extent across the region.[69] However, there was some criticism of the UN's lack of thought about who comprised the aged (beyond simply those aged "sixty and over"). In a reflexivity rare in official reports, it became clear that local participants and political leaders saw the aging agenda not as a new program the UN was offering them but as an initiative they were shaping based on their prior experience.[70] Aging represented issues they had already deliberated and acted on, as the Costa Rican President Rodrigo Carazo Odio noted. Odio discussed the establishment of a gerontological commission (1979) in Costa Rica, founded within the Family Care Council. These initiatives also implicitly represented a distinct opportunity for "developing" societies to advise Western societies on coping with social change. Local representatives also clearly stated that the challenges posed by aging were intimately linked to the wider social and economic inequities of the international economic order and the unchecked economic instability and dependency these had generated.[71] At any rate, these overtures demonstrated that new allies and networks were emerging in the 1980s, even before the WAA was held. There were meetings convened with other UN agencies, some of which agreed to sponsor forums or prepare technical papers for the upcoming Assembly. Most, however, still demurred about adapting aging-related policies into their mandate and activities, as we have seen with international population and development policies.

Some agencies, such as the WHO, were open to future discussions, but one WHO representative also admitted that the organization had so far not focused on aging programs, although they had some useful expertise with programs on aging in Europe.[72] He pointed out that their agency brought lessons to the table drawn from a new approach toward strengthening comprehensive primary health care (PHC) articulated a few years earlier in Alma Ata (1978), implying that aging could be more easily integrated into preventive approaches at the community level in its programs.[73] But observers of the WHO's growing challenges with defunding during the economic downturn of the 1980s knew that severe economic constraints were deepening in developing countries and that the PHC agenda already showed signs of a gradual erosion. In its place, the proposal was to establish a far more limited, vertically programmed strategy for child survival supported by UNICEF (1982).[74] UN experts organizing the WAA were therefore aware that the approaches laid out in consultations were not likely to be followed up in the immediate future. Even if there were interest in aging from a public health perspective, the WHO's resources and partnerships were in flux and needed rebuilding.

The Path to Vienna: Domestic Pressures in the United States and International Politics

What pressures led to the holding of a World Assembly on Aging if not mobilization led by NGOs and advocacy from the developing world? A decade earlier, in 1971, a motion in the UN General Assembly asked for further research on the condition of the old and elderly in developing countries. At this time, the director of the United Nations' Social Development division conceded "that the situation of the elderly and the aged varied among countries at different levels of development and in varied social systems," and that further study was needed to understand aging in countries at different levels of development.[75] Demographically, the "social problems relating to the old and elderly *in industrialized nations*," he concluded, were more "pronounced inasmuch as they constituted a significant percentage of the population."[76] Accordingly, the survey of policies and guidelines for programs that resulted from this motion was aimed at "countries where the socioeconomic problems of the aged are marked." The former statement gives us a hint as to how and why experts, mostly middle-level bureaucrats in the United Nations' Social Affairs division, mobilized wider support for a World Assembly on Aging.

Unexpectedly, the United States advocated to hold the World Assembly on Aging in 1982 under the aegis of the UN. It surprised contemporaries, and historians of international relations and population health continue to note it, for the 1980s are widely credited with having witnessed a crisis in multilateralism, with having been a time when the UN's role and influence was threatened and at a low ebb, as leaders and countries in both the industrialized and the newly decolonized world attacked its agencies.[77] The United States in particular demonstrated a strong distrust of UN international initiatives such as the World Population Conference and the negotiations over a New International Economic Order (NIEO).[78] Discussions over the NIEO had also created a growing rift between key developed and developing countries, with growing pressure from the latter to be allowed greater access to world economic resources and power.[79]

Domestic events were, however, precipitating a different course, and the inroads of neoliberal thinking regarding state welfare responsibilities influenced some political leaders and aging experts to initiate new strategies to mobilize pressure on the U.S. government. Frank Church, the Idaho congressman who headed the Special Committee on Aging, and Claude

Pepper, who headed the House Select Committee on Aging—the key figures advocating for U.S. support for the WAA—argued that the lack of purchase at the domestic level could be remedied by highlighting the international ramifications of population aging.[80] Church noted in an interview, "For one thing, the World Assembly on Aging would be an additional prod for development of policy on aging—something we had hoped the White [House] Conference [of Aging in 1971] would do." Church emphasized that a "retirement revolution" was likely to sweep the developing world as it had already swept the industrialized world, and added that "A WAA on aging could help them think and . . . prepare for the socioeconomic changes produced by longer life expectancy."[81]

Other experts, such as those from the National Council on Aging, voiced their disappointment with the Reagan administration's neoliberal leanings, its continuing failure to respond to the need for all but minimal state support and intervention for older persons, and its overt intention to study and make models of those elderly who did not need federal support.[82] They criticized the statement Dorcas R. Hardy, assistant secretary for Human Development Services, made to the 200 U.S. and Canadian aging experts gathered to draft recommendations for the WAA that "The vast majority of older persons is doing fine in our country because they are self-reliant. We have outgrown the myth that most older persons consistently require active intervention by society on their behalf."[83] They also challenged reports from a survey of 3,400 Americans, mostly supported by corporate foundations, that had been conducted before the White Conference on Aging. It stated that "the widely held view that people over the age of 65 have serious problems with poverty, loneliness and fear of crime is 'a myth." Its author, Louis Harris, observed, "On every single issue tested . . . the elderly are perceived as being in much more desperate shape than they actually are . . . 68 percent of those under 65 thought lack of money was a 'very serious problem' for 'most people over 65,' but only 17 percent of the older group found it a personal problem." Many members of the National Council on Aging challenged this, arguing with the view that "the majority of older persons are doing fine in our country because they are self-reliant. . . . More of us . . . are apt to conclude that more older people are today self-reliant than ever before because our people had the foresight to create public institutions to anticipate and prevent personal calamity. The development and expansion of social insurance programs to provide income supports, to meet medical cost, and to stimulate private pensions, to build housing and in recent years, to add indexed increases, have raised vast millions of older persons out of poverty."[84]

The impulses for the Assembly on Aging were partly prompted by a dead-end in domestic policies for aging where the battle lines were drawn sharply. Policymakers like Church and Pepper were responding to their disappointment regarding the White House Conference on Aging in 1971, the Nixon administration's continuing resistance to support the founding of a National Institute on Aging, and the limited increases in social security. The UN papers make little overt reference to the initiatives and pressures from the U.S. end, but correspondence between Ethel Shanas and Walter Beattie, who were invited along with other U.S. experts to participate in advisory meetings that shaped the draft report for the WAA, shows close engagement between U.S. political leaders and social gerontological experts in shaping the agenda for a World Assembly.[85] In 1974, even as U.S. experts began urging the UN secretariat to consider organizing a World Assembly, Shanas and Beattie were working closely with experts from the USSR, France, and other countries, such as Paul Paillat from France and D. F. Chebotarev of the USSR, whom they knew well from their common networks through the International Association of Gerontology (IAG).[86] Shanas wrote to a colleague from the American Gerontological Society, musing about the prospect of convincing the UN to hold a World Assembly, "As you know the Social Development Commission of the United Nations meets in January. I would hope that the recent efforts of Senator Church and the group on the World Assembly on Aging of which you are a member will have some impact on the United Nation['s] thinking about the aged."[87]

Shanas's and Beattie's influence in shaping the UN vision on world aging implied that a dominant strain of gerontology, focused on the social problems of aging, permeated their report advising on the WAA to the UN secretary general. In this line of thought, the social dependency of the aged should be addressed through a range of approaches such as postponing retirement, enforcing the right to work, resisting age discrimination, promoting adjustment and integration, and offering income security. These perspectives were the subject of IAG debates in previous years, and American experts' advisory role in preparing a plan to advise the UN secretary general (along with officers of the social development division) gave them the opportunity to insert these perspectives into an emerging and mainstream "world" vision. The repeated statements in several reports, asserting that all knowledge about aging was "new" based on the growth of "modern" gerontological knowledge in the postwar decades, are also interesting, for they allowed these experts the leverage to assert their unique experiences. The implication was that scientific knowledge about aging originated from Europe and the United States, where population aging and modernization had first been experienced.[88]

Ethel Shanas recognized in her notes on the UN expert committee's discussions that a lifespan approach and preventive approaches were important to maintaining health in old age. However, the group's report finally focused on addressing the "problems" of the old rather than taking a broader approach. The committee specified the need to articulate short- and long-term goals for policy change that they set for developed and developing nations.[89] In their discussions, expert committee members conceded that there was still a lack of data on who the old were and how they lived in many countries, and that these societies had not even framed basic policies related to aging and were unlikely to be able to accept and implement the goals set by the Assembly that they would need to meet. Their reports' recommendations reflected fears of dependency that were a significant and widely debated theme in social gerontology regarding aging populations in Europe and America. In the context of the developing world, their views addressed dependency by relating it to a few "basic" issues: the "problem" of aging in urban slums, the need of the aged for social security, and the role of the extended family.[90]

Shanas observed that the problems of developing countries still needed to be clarified, and that the committee was struggling to define and understand "who are the aged and what are the aged?" She noted that the meeting on policy and program development "recognized the limited resources and the often rudimentary nature of existing programmes for the aging in developing areas," and that "many of its recommendations, while constituting short-term objectives for the developed countries, should be considered long-term goals for the developing countries."[91]

A Meeting of Worlds

The WAA held in Vienna was attended by delegates from 123 countries and resulted in the passing of a detailed plan of action. William Kerrigan, secretary of the IFA, became the first American to head a UN conference when he was nominated Secretary General of the Assembly.[92] At the inauguration of the WAA, Kerrigan went to great lengths to assert that the

Assembly was hailing a new world agenda, one that would address a subject "basic to common humanity" and that aimed to look beyond the divide between developed and developing countries. He observed that although in absolute numbers there were more old people in developed than in developing countries, the number of the old was growing in all societies and continents; it would therefore "be a mistake to argue that the aging of societies was a matter of concern only to rich and developed countries."

Kerrigan's dilemma and indeed the challenge facing experts was to reconcile the differential demographic pace of aging in different societies, especially between developed and developing countries. The assembly proceedings were also complicated by the fact that many developing nations felt that the tensions, anger, and anxieties caused by the inequitable conditions in their societies were being aggravated by the world economic order and security concerns. In response, the Assembly's plan of action was lengthy, with a broad wish list of targets, and aimed to tackle the "developmental and humanitarian problems of the aging," but it lacked any specific allocations or assigned means to assist nations in implementing this programmatic focus. In an interview weeks before the WAA, Kerrigan revealed that the briefing materials (including twenty-seven background documents) prepared and circulated for the assembly were dense and that he had visited numerous countries to stimulate interest and solidarity in the common goals of the WAA. He observed that a Vienna Action Plan on Aging emerging from the Assembly would "provide an excellent blueprint for future activities. However, given the concept of zero-growth budgeting currently in effect at the United Nations, the implementation of the plan depends in a viable trust fund to carry on the Assembly's work."[93]

WAA officials tried to steer the debates at the Assembly toward the mobilization of national-level commitment and resources from member states. Underlying all UN rhetoric and ideals was a focus on the intersecting axes of aging, dependency, and development. The vulnerabilities of the "old and elderly" were characterized as posing a challenge to balanced development and as an impediment to achieving the full and final goals of modernization in the developing world. Unlike these trajectories, a "normal," measured historical trajectory of modernization in the West had resulted in industrialization, high standards of living, and longevity, with the state able to address the needs of dependency. Conversely, aging populations in developing nations reflected a distorted and imbalanced trajectory of modernization being experienced, with people living longer due to public health and technological innovations but still remaining dependent on their errant and migrant families for support, especially in the case of old people in rural areas.[94] The solution lay in advancing a modicum of humanitarian support for the old in terms of health, housing, and income security in particular, but also in ensuring that these interventions "do not result in the maintenance of a growing, relatively passive and disenchanted sector of the population." Therefore the old also needed to be supported in being "positive, active and developmentally oriented."[95]

These ideas received a mixed response from delegates, and were often the focus of criticism. In some of the statements and speeches delegations from developing nations made, ideological and even political differences in interpreting the implications of aging were clearly present. Most of these views did not outright reject modernization and Eurocentric models of development, but rather saw older populations both as representing the pain and suffering of economic and social transitions in their societies and often as inextricably linked to the lives of youth and families. Kenya's minister of culture and social services observed that the social, political, and even religious roles of the elderly were eroding and that that was an inestimable loss:

> It has become very difficult to believe that in the past, the aged were held in high esteem and they had significant roles to play. In Kenya society, the aged people gave advice to traditional leaders in passing out judgement on local cases. . . . They participated in the counseling of marital conflicts or family disputes and . . . they directed the behavior of youth so that they could adhere to norms, values and culture of society. The aged also prepared mature members of the society to become leaders after them. But due to the advent of modern changes, these roles are no longer being played by the aged. . . . These changes are due to developmental issues. One of the most glaring institutional changes that occurred in Kenya pertains to economy. The traditional economy, which was largely agrarian kept the family in a state of cohesiveness and stability. . . . But with the ravages and the demands of modern production and attendant economic demands together with the population explosion, family members who cater for the needs of the elderly often have to work in the urban areas away from their families and this leads to disruption.[96]

He added that apart from the economic sphere and its deprivation, the most devastating change for the elderly was their loss of place in religious leadership and as repositories of wisdom and information; further, because they lacked education, they lacked the political skills necessary in modern political settings.[97] Other leaders, such as the representative from Malawi, related similar experiences, emphasizing extended kinships that went as far back as three or four generations. Old people had served as moral custodians of the community, and these roles, he observed, were threatened by urbanization, industrialization, and migration, although Malawi still relied on the strong interrelationships that persisted between the young and the old.[98]

In response to the institutional structures suggested and discussed at the WAA, many developing countries that were already coping with the uncertainties of a worldwide recession responded by stating that their solution to the provision of social security and care for the old was the family. The institution of the family was no doubt under pressure due to urbanization and industrialization, but the focus remained on reordering and safeguarding family values.[99] A delegate from Nigeria at the WAA stated that the importance of traditional family values as well as the dilemma of finding the means for state social welfare schemes left no recourse but to invoke African values and support: "Nigeria is a developing country and suffers from all the problems and disabilities of underdevelopment. She is anxious to develop in her own way. The European models of welfarism are doubtful models for solving our problems including those of aging. We have not got the resources to cope with the already worldwide now innumerable problems of aging and the elderly, but we have our African culture, tradition, practices, and institutions to fall on."[100]

For many others, their political ideologies and social structures had thrown up solutions, and often both the changes they experienced and their solutions were different from the normative assumptions about aging offered in discussions at the WAA. Some delegates offered examples of ways families and the state had worked together to reinforce and retain "their traditional sense of values towards their old parents in spite of recent economic and social changes caused by industrialization" or ways they had initiated the integration of older persons into a strong network of primary health care, with services provided by social welfare officers.[101] These responses implied that the provisions offered in countries such as Japan and Korea were already addressing the problems of loneliness and alienation faced by the aged. Long-term measures had been introduced in Korea, such as a Charter for Older People (1982) and Welfare Laws, including a medical insurance system (1979).[102]

In other cases, the phenomenon of an aging population was seen positively, as representing the success of the countries in implementing family planning policies and public health programs, and the political ideology of these nations offered a place and role for older persons to contribute to both "material and cultural development" in society.[103] These countries did not see the end of working life being defined by retirement but argued that older persons continued to be engaged in work lives of a formal and informal nature, especially in the rural areas. An "active" old age did not have to be introduced as a novel pedagogy and lifestyle in these societies as it had to be in the West, since the old had already contributed to their families and communities as long as they possibly could. The delegates from China and the socialist countries pointed out that their political systems had been able to mitigate the negative implications of modernization and aging. The head of the Chinese delegation, Yu Guanghan, emphasized that "China is a developing country. [Al]though our economy and technology are still relatively backward and our people's average living standard not high, we have ensured the life and health care of the aged. . . . In the rural areas, old commune members normally do what they can for the communes and production brigades and their own families."[104] The founding of New China, he said, had moved forward the Chinese nation's fine tradition of respecting, taking care of, and providing for the aged, and the communist system had in particular ensured retirement benefits and free medical care.

These views reflected a tendency to avoid acknowledging the need for a distinct agenda to tackle the issues of aging, as countries listed many state schemes and programs, or family solidarities as a means to assert that aging populations did not yet warrant a special position in their developmental and welfare priorities. In the case of China, despite Wu Cangping's protracted struggles to raise interest in gerontological thinking, the Chinese delegation's assertions that its existing welfare provisions for all laboring classes, including the most vulnerable, together with intergenerational family support created the appropriate conditions for its aging population implied that China was committing to very little investment in policy changes.[105]

Writing a few years after the WAA, Kenneth Tout, a senior functionary in the international NGO Help the Aged (later HelpAge International) and a keen observer of aging projects in the global South, reported that of the sixty-two recommendations made at the WAA, there was little of interest that met the needs and requirements of developing countries. "From the point of view of developing countries," he observed, the Plan of Action formulated by the WAA, "although detailed and exhaustive is bewildering, and lacking in certain important aspects. It tends to assume always the existence of structures similar to those existing in Europe or North America and aims at detailed targets which have generally not been attained even in the most advanced countries, after decades of planning and organization, or only in a way that they are not easily accessible to the totality of the aged population of the country."[106] The WAA discussions, with country papers submitted by more than a hundred member states, had already suggested these deep differences in perspectives and resources. Though well intentioned, the WAA recommendations lacked "significant and realistic financial recommendations and projections," and the Assembly's priorities and understanding of the place and needs of aging populations were not easily shared by many countries in the developing world.

Seeing Beyond the State

The World Assembly on Aging was planned and held at a historical conjuncture dubbed by some international politics scholars the "decade of conferences." These years were emblematic of the emergence of a global "nervous system" marked by the rise of international NGOs involved in humanitarian and development work.[107] The growing power of international NGOs—so visible in the making of environmental activism, in population programs, and in scores of other development issues that jostled for space in the international arena—was missing during the Vienna discussions.[108] They were consulted and gave their opinions in the preconference meetings, and attended the WAA in large numbers, but were not official representatives at the table. However, although they did not directly build the networks and discourse that made up the concerns voiced at the Assembly, activists and experts who worked for international NGOs and social workers at the local level began to shape the afterlives of the Vienna Plan. Regional meetings in Asia and Africa helped to dispel the notion of aging as a uniform universal problem, as it was represented in Vienna. Even as activists used the same gerontological terminology, it often masked a separate set of concerns, which had a local and regional genealogy rather than a global one. International NGOs such as Help the Aged (1961) were part of these national collaborations, funded increasingly in the 1980s by a growing sentiment and support for the Third World voiced, as Didier Fassin has termed it, in the vocabulary of humanitarian reason.[109]

In the mid-1980s, developing countries began to mobilize themselves, in complex social and political ways through new associations of regional trading and economic zones; the social agenda for specific regions began to be voiced collectively, and thus began to seem more coherent. This had an impact on aging issues as well. For instance, in an Asian Regional Conference on Active Ageing in Manila, a leading social activist from India, Walter Fernandes, noted that in the case of some South Asian countries, the "similarities of their neo-colonial economy" and their history and social structures brought them together. He admitted that all of them could not be treated as a "unit" in every respect—that their differences were prominent—but added that they shared a quest for a new identity to keep them united.[110]

"The Aging of Africa" in Dakar

The birth of world aging at the UN-led Assembly was followed by rebirths in various regional settings. In 1984, the first African Conference on Gerontology, mentioned at the beginning of this narrative, was held in Dakar. The conference began with delegates from Francophone and Anglophone Africa invoking the Assembly, with their references to the African Conference following in the footsteps of the WAA. However, since the WAA's Plan was not relevant to developing countries, it seems likely that referring to the Vienna Plan as the meeting was inaugurated was a means to mobilize and assert a distinct agenda about "the aging of Africa." Even as the meeting began, delegates noted that aging was a new field of expertise. They underscored 1984 as a starting point in this process, when aging as a category and object of study, analysis, and policymaking was gaining visibility across the entire continent. They observed that Africa "does not escape general historical movements," and that the problems of aging in Africa were also exhibiting the effects of rapid urbanization and industrialization.

These observations echoed concerns dating back to the late colonial decades, voiced by colonial administrators, missionaries, and anthropologists, about fast-paced social change in traditional societies in Africa, as well as concerns more recently expressed by many present in Vienna. The

Dakar meeting report noted that the migration of young populations from rural to urban areas threatened "traditional structures" and the status enjoyed by the old, and it destabilized social relations—assertions along similar lines as some made in the Rhodes Livingston Institute studies tracing migration and urbanization in the 1940s and 1950s Copperbelt.[111]

In asserting that social gerontology was a new subject of study, the participants at the Dakar meeting may not have acknowledged these past links with older research concerned with families, migration, and aging, as these studies had focused mainly on parts of Anglophone Africa and the sub-Saharan region. The participants in Dakar were overwhelmingly from Francophone Africa, representing Algeria, Tunisia, Rwanda, Lesotho, and parts of northern Africa, and this may have represented a divide, alluded to at the beginning of the conference, of language and familiarity between English- and French-speaking Africa that remained a challenge. A decade later, an African Union-led meeting held to translate the recommendations of the Madrid Plan of Action on Ageing (April 2002) following the Vienna meeting resulted in tense exchanges between representatives from states with Francophone and Anglophone histories and saw the articulation of multiple competing local interests.[112]

The meeting in Dakar was not only rooted in the events in Vienna. Its sponsors were French experts who ran the International Center for Social Gerontology (ICSG) in Paris and drew resources from French pension funds that supported the ICSG network and its conferences and workshops.[113] Father Hampson, who had attended the Dakar meeting, said that the sponsors of this meeting were "like a new comet that flew across the skies of Africa and then disappeared"; however, he said, this meeting encouraged him to hold a meeting in Zimbabwe with some support from a local International Labour Organization (ILO) officer and from the social work department at the University of Zimbabwe in Harare.[114]

This also helps us uncover the wide-ranging networks that experts on aging in various sites across Europe and the United States, as well as in Asia and Africa, had fostered with different UN agencies separate from their recent engagements with the Social Development Office at the ECOSOC that led the charge in Vienna. Experts from the ICSG in Paris, such as Georges Lambert and Joseph Flesch, repeatedly courted ILO officials who were invited to the gerontological meetings they organized over time; the ILO officials, in turn, engaged with them closely. ILO correspondence housed in the Geneva archives documents these contacts in the 1980s with the ICSG, but, interestingly, it makes little or no reference to the Vienna Plan of Action, except for responding to a letter to send an update for the Vienna meeting.

Responding to an invitation to attend a meeting of experts to discuss aging in Africa that the ICSG was holding in Versailles, ILO officials observed, "We have entertained excellent relations for many years with the International Institute [Center] for Social Gerontology that organizes high level meetings. This meeting in question discusses a current subject that will be discussed by experts directly concerned [with aging]. . . . ILO presence at this meeting seems opportune. It will allow us to sensitize participants to recommendation no. 162 and our politics in the field of social security and to contribute to directly shaping recommendations."[115] The recommendations referred to, relating to older workers, had been passed a few years earlier (1980) and regarded discrimination at work, protection in employment, and access to retirement benefits.

The meeting in Dakar also included members of the International Social Security Association and policymakers from the labor and social welfare departments of Senegal.[116] Their attendance in Dakar suggests a range of other interests in social security-related advocacy that intersected on and off with the agenda and plan passed at the WAA, but in effect demonstrated that agencies with long-standing networks, credibility, and connections in Asia and Africa, such as the ILO, were not consistently involved in advocating the goals articulated in Vienna or in the field; rather, they worked separately and often alone rather than in packs. The experts at the Assembly and the experts who had worked on and prepared its agenda understood aging in historically specific ways, as a fallout of rapid development and lack of humanitarian empathy; but these ideas did not engage sufficiently or consistently with other influential international networks that stemmed from rights-based views of old age and labor or social security in the 1980s, as the UN sought to project a world agenda for aging.

Yet those attending the Dakar meeting overwhelmingly emphasized the family in Africa and African realities. This was given primacy over importing large-scale social security provisions, though changes in needs were recognized and setting up retirement programs and social benefits was recommended.[117] The lessons of importing Western models of development in the previous decades hung over the conference's cautious recommendations. The Dakar report advised, for instance, that "the following pitfalls should be avoided: Undigested imitation of European and American models, lack of information on and research into the situation of the elderly . . . political instability, inability to use the Western experience objectively." Although it was not clear how political uncertainty could be an avoidable pitfall, it was evident that delegates in Dakar were emphasizing an intrinsic African identity as well as reversing Western prejudices and assumptions about Africa by implying that Western models had inadequacies when blindly applied in other settings.

Even as scholars have debated the notion of and claims to an essentialized "African identity," the statements made in Dakar served an important purpose: to see gerontology in Africa as deriving or originating from Western models of aging and care, but also as representing a distinct mutation from the West. This meant that statements at the conference could often seem contradictory.[118] Although there seemed to be fissures between perspectives about aging and its problems within Africa, there were continuous references to a homogeneous traditional society and its values, intrinsic to all of Africa, that was being overtaken by urbanization and modernization. Much like the call Walter Fernandes made for a regional identity regarding South Asia, African gerontology's reference to a common history and past of traditional societies under threat was a useful device meant to invoke Africa, as Frederick Cooper terms it, as a "category of practice" rather than a social or political reality. It acted mainly as a foil to all that was European or American, and a way to free themselves from all that was European or American, and as a starting point for making new contentions.[119]

The Rebirth of Vienna in Zimbabwe

In the 1980s, experts at conferences on aging often produced long wish lists of what they wanted governments to pursue. Their expectations were usually inversely proportional to the resources that they mobilized or that governments would set aside for aging. The first African Conference on Gerontology produced the Dakar Recommendations for Action on Aging, which called on concerned governments to address questions about aging in their development plans, advised the establishment of an African Institute on Aging, suggested holding an African Elders' Day, and urged contributions by governments to the UN Trust Fund for Aging to assist African states. There is little follow-up in their reports and records to tell us whether any of these recommendations materialized or if they remained, like the sixty-two "specific recommendations" passed at the WAA, largely recommendations.

The Institute for Social Gerontology (ISG) hosted several other international meetings that were partly successful in mobilizing some political will, but as Kenneth Tout, who was involved with the ISG's meetings in Dakar and later Bogota, recalled, they were not successful in raising large resources for programs. Their main contribution—and this was not to be underestimated—was adding "relevant detail" based on local interests and laying the groundwork for debates about aging policies.[120]

There were also less visible fallouts from Dakar. Father Joseph (Joe) Hampson, a missionary and social worker who had worked for decades in setting up social work programs at the University of Zimbabwe, left the Dakar meeting with ideas of his own, to relate the legacies of the Vienna conference (1982) to a "national" plan that would address a vision for aging "from below."[121] He also realized that the agenda of the Dakar Conference, with its focus on a regional mission and policies and its aim of building institutional and training networks across Africa, did not address the pressing needs of an aging population in Zimbabwe, though the meeting he would organize in Harare would refer to continuities with the Dakar meeting, where African governments had been encouraged to include aging in their development plans.[122] Hampson was principal of the School of Social Work in Harare and, working closely with a local ILO official, organized a workshop to formulate a national plan for the needs of the elderly in Zimbabwe. Hampson found some support from the UN office for Social Development in Vienna through some local UN connections, and got in touch with a WHO officer and two HelpAge staff members to organize the meeting, which government ministries in Zimbabwe and the School of Social Work would also support.[123] The workshop held in Harare drew an impressive range of national figures and international experts as participants. Even though Zimbabwe was not among the 32 African countries that participated in the Vienna Assembly, it declared the WAA a benchmark.

Conscious of the new political leadership in their midst, including the violence-based totalitarian power assumed by Comrade R. G. Mugabe (even as his party promised a socialist transformation), the WHO official speaking at the meeting offered circumspect praise for the revolutionary and "progressive" spirit pervading the "entire National leadership in Zimbabwe," which had led it to take up the aging agenda, "long before the expected explosion"—a metaphor regularly applied to aging, the population bomb, and its urgency in those years.[124] The WHO official addressed the seeming conflict between the problems of population growth and aging by clarifying that both the structure and the geographic distribution of population affect aging.[125] He must have been aware that such an argument was crucial and locally relevant, because Mugabe and others had also brought up the issue of aging in Zimbabwe as an imbalanced distribution of the young and the old rather than a changed population structure with an increasing proportion of older persons, as in the West.

The speech given by the UN-WHO official in Harare implied that the growing gerontocracy in the world held critical new challenges, and that society needed to be protected from the fallout of these challenges. In Harare, however, the emphasis was on both the humanitarian aspect of the needs of the old and the need to save and secure the old through recourse to the family, resettlement of young persons, or some minimal benefits from the community. Ultimately, the conference's objective was "to plan for a comprehensive and coordinated approach to meeting the needs of the elderly in Zimbabwe."[126] The UN approach to saving the world from the challenges of aging was reflected more widely in its later reports and was part of its larger vision of development and its feared setbacks. In a report by the United Nations Development Programme (UNDP; 1999), the section on population aging noted that "Population ageing will result in the continent's inhabitants aged 60 years and over to increase from 38 million in 2000 to 212 million by 2050 (UNDP, 1999). . . . Yet, African country governments have for the main part not started to visualize the scope of the challenges ahead."[127]

Mugabe, in his address, spoke of the old in the context of an Africa where custom and tradition offered them "a special place of honor in society. Traditionally, our society granted people in their old age both security, honour and respect."[128] However, the demographic impact of aging would be uneven, he said: the urban drift of younger persons would become compounded as agriculture was "left behind" for old people to manage and rural areas became the reserve of the old. In the context of Zimbabwe, he noted, the Socialist government would look to protect older persons from these insecurities by providing the young with gainful employment in rural areas and strengthening the family—the first natural institution to look after the old. Social welfare, however, was a part of his government's socialist ideals, and he offered to provide a share of care and protection where required.

This tendency to view the elderly as needing support from the society around them is voiced more clearly in Hampson's work and some of the research and programs that came out of the School of Social Work in Zimbabwe. In a book on old age in Zimbabwe, Hampson stated that his efforts to work with old people originated with finding them bereft and abandoned amidst the destruction caused by the war in Rhodesia in 1979. He described the failing Muzorewa regime and the violence perpetrated by Zimbabwe African National Union (ZANU) rebels, and contrasted them with the sterile inauguration of the Commonwealth Summit in Zambia, led by Kenneth Kaunda, the first president of Zambia, with Queen Elizabeth "listening impassively." He discussed the implications of this escalating war and political indifference toward a group of old persons, whose stories of suffering, neglect, and oppression made them representative of "the whole of South Africa" and not merely Zimbabwe.[129] "All the group are destitute aged," he wrote, "and as I look at their wrinkled faces, some squinting in the sun, others sightless and impassive, I begin to realize that I am looking at the cast-offs of society. . . . In the garden lies the debris of city life—cans, rusted wire, paper, bits of wood and the saddest debris of all are the old people themselves."[130]

Hampson saw his research and the work on aging in Zimbabwe as representing a first, because the experience of the elderly and the process of aging in Africa, he argues, had not been studied, and Western categories of aging and adjustment offered few insights in the African context.[131] However, this research and perspective were not completely new, for they represented an older current involving social workers and their interests during the 1940s and 1950s in marginalized urban groups, such as destitute old people, beggars, juvenile delinquents, and hawkers, who were part of an unstable and unregulated urban population in working-class towns and cities.[132] The aged in this case were defined not by chronological age but by the conditions of vulnerability and abandonment by family and society, which resulted from the racial tensions and political instability that characterized southern African societies.

The workshop to discuss a National Plan for the Elderly in Zimbabwe saw old age primarily in terms of poverty, deprivation, and destitution. It was voiced in the propagandist vocabulary of Mugabe's early years, promising the old the help and protection of the state "as a right" for citizens. But these promised rights were chimeric in the following years of unabated political violence and suppression of liberties.[133]

A "Rosy" View of Families and Elders

In other sites, such as India and China, the circulation of the Vienna Plan or the fallout of the WAA took unexpected turns. In India, a group of activists at the Indian Social Institute (ISI) and HelpAge, India cited and criticized the Indian government's official statement at the Vienna Assembly that "in India there is no problem of the aged, that there is joint family system in which old people are looked after by kith and kin; that we have a state apparatus of medical care for all, and the aged can participate in that as much as any other sections of the people and so on. This is, if I may say so [noted an Indian activist], rather a rosy presentation of things and it does not behoove thinking people to almost overlook the problem."[134] The Indian representative at the WAA, M. C. Narasimhan, admitted that his government recognized new challenges but had termed aging an "emerging problem." He observed that government protection of the old and their tendency to work in large numbers throughout their lives in the unorganized sector—"there is no retirement except on a voluntary basis"— made them economically active.[135] This, of course, avoided addressing whether the minimum public assistance offered those working in this unorganized sector was sufficient to their needs. It was clear that in the absence of political will, the state would not meet the Vienna plan goals in a comprehensive way, and it would fall to national-level and local NGOs to put pressure on the Indian state.

The Indian Director of HelpAge argued that India's traditions of caring for the aged were similar to Africa's, but the disintegration of the family posed new challenges. These discussions elicited different visions of aging and its constituency from those who addressed the needs of retired senior citizens to those from the ISI who spoke of the old as comprising the most disenfranchised ranks of Indian society. The afterlives of Vienna thus demonstrated a recasting of the WAA and brought out a global agenda that was largely ineffectual and divided in its reception within the UN and its member states, but was far more dynamic as it circulated because it was coopted by a range of ideologies and activists, whose work pre-dated Vienna and would only deepen in the coming years.

6

❧

International NGOs and the Aged in the Developing World

THE ECONOMIC CRISIS of the 1970s and the failures of the development decades that promised and failed to uplift all developing nations cast a shadow over the World Assembly on Aging (WAA) in Vienna (1982). Even in the early sessions of the Vienna meetings, delegates from developing nations voiced a moral parable of development and its discontents. Aging populations of the world were seen as victims of the disease, poverty, rapid social changes, and insecure habitats that grew out of failed and unequal development initiatives. Children, women, disabled persons, and the aged shared in the misery of development's social and economic fallout, and many at the WAA expressed the view that this negative fallout needed to be addressed.[1] It is not surprising that in the UN WAA leaders' inaugural declarations, humanitarian sentiments predominated. The delegates asked policymakers, social activists, media, and citizens across the world to see aging as a worldwide moral and social responsibility and urged, "The Assembly should arouse the consciousness of the world for the benefit of the aging."[2] This human aspect of development increasingly took on a new focus in the 1980s and 1990s, as new international emergencies in the areas of human, health, and ecological disasters deepened.

In the eyes of a transnational public, aging became increasing visible as a humanitarian issue through its association with a few crisis-centered campaigns and with NGO and UN efforts on relief projects and refugee problems. Many such efforts echoed a colonial past of rescuing backward subjects, but focusing now on the postcolony and its needy populations instead. These were short-term, emergency approaches for times of crises rather than longer-term policy investments focusing on social justice and security for old populations, but they allowed certain international and national networks to deepen. But even as aging became internationally visible, activities and services for the old in need and crisis underscored their "difference" and aberration from the rest of the population. Thus aging became associated with the most marginalized and, particularly, those in emergency situations, including those experiencing acute health crises such as HIV/AIDS, which caused devastation in developing nations.

At the level of the everyday lives of the aged, these NGO campaigns and interventions addressed acute care needs and services such as disability and other physical vulnerabilities. However, international campaigns centering on the old's precarity and on catastrophic events obscured the experiences of aging in families and communities over time, as well as the changing life course older persons experienced due to social and economic changes. Local activism and national policy statements were also increasingly vocal in their views about aging, propounding a discourse that set ideals such as older persons needing to contribute to the social development of their developing societies. Yet most countries were still unwilling to commit substantial resources to supporting the needs of older populations.

The need to look elsewhere, at campaigns that did not strictly align with the long-term, policy-focused plan of action the WAA outlined—at campaigns that emphasized integrating aging with developmental goals and providing relief to the aged in the health, housing, and social sectors—had immensely pragmatic roots. In September 1989, at a high-level meeting on aging, UN officials and international NGOs all readily agreed that funding for policies supported by the WAA's plan of action "was not being adequately pursued and that there was a gap between the needs of the elderly and the resources available to meet them." Furthermore, this "funding gap" needed more flexible financing: private sector support should be pursued, and public awareness of the elderly's productive potential should be increased.[3] The international profile of aging, participants at this meeting argued, needed to be assigned "a higher priority on global and national agenda[s]," and aging needed to be on global developmental agendas such as the strategy for a fourth development decade.[4]

The United Nations Trust Fund, founded at the time of the WAA, had been involved in raising funds to increase developing countries' capacities to respond effectively to issues of aging, but its efforts were limited and mostly small scale due to the limited grants it received from various governments. It could not adequately support intergovernmental programs and large-scale regional cooperation. In 1988, for instance, the gerontology meeting in Dakar received support from the UN Fund, as did some small income-generating projects for the aged in Kenya, relief and rehabilitation projects in Uganda and Thailand, and a few small training courses for care of the elderly.[5] A few more activities, such as travel for scientists to the Fourteenth Gerontological Congress in Acapulco, and some other seminars were also funded, but the scale of UN funding for implementing the Vienna Plan of Action remained limited to seed grants.[6]

Because of the funding gaps and lack of large-scale projects and programs drawn from the UN's Vienna Plan of Action, international NGOs and national level activists began to undertake campaigns that aligned with and inserted aging into areas that evoked public empathy. At a national level, this often consisted of a small but steadily increasing number of projects focused on aging and its implications for society from a "disability" perspective. In the 1980s, the UN's *Bulletin on Aging* regularly reported on such projects as those for the hearing- or vision-impaired in India and Belize, or hospice care in the Dominican Republic, and so on.[7] This focus on the needs and vulnerabilities of the aging deepened, since it coincided with international crises over the situation of "dependents" and vulnerable groups like refugees.[8]

A Climate of Empathy for the Old

Interestingly, in the years following the Vienna Assembly, even as aging in the West became an increasingly politically charged issue and subject of debate, and even as older persons were viewed as independent and vocal, efforts led by international NGOs still represented the old in the Third World as a disenfranchised, silent, needy group, isolated and alone as refugees and later as survivor grandparents during the African HIV crisis.

Moral claims about the aged and the urgency of rescuing them in times of distress were the compelling arguments behind these campaigns; they formed an effort to reconfigure the distinct needs of older persons in developing countries. By contrast, these debates in the United States in the 1980s shifted dramatically as vast resources for research on aging became available to the National Institute on Aging and to aging programs. American politicians acknowledged the power of the Gray Panthers advocating for intergenerational solidarity by campaigning against retirement age and ageism (as well as opposing the Vietnam War and nuclear weapons).[9]

In the 1980s, in the corridors of the UN, attention increasingly shifted from debates about aging to more dramatic sites, in particular the effects of war, famine, and disasters on population displacement and the mounting numbers of refugees across developing countries. Human emergencies, disasters, and migration caused by wars, famine, and apartheid, stretched from the Horn of Africa, El Salvador, and Khmer camps to internal displacement across sub-Saharan Africa and were growing international concerns.[10] These refugees, concentrated in the largest numbers in Africa, mostly fled to other low-income countries, leaving agencies like the United Nations High Commissioner for Refugees (UNHCR) with few "durable solutions."[11] The upsurge among the public and politicians of what Didier Fassin has termed "humanitarian reason" in response to these crises also created opportunities for founding new international NGOs in the aging field and redeploying these sentiments and resources.[12]

Elderly refugees became a growing focus of funding campaigns and calls to political action in the Third World, originating from a growing network of NGOs that emphasized the vulnerability and immaturity of the countries in distress as well as the neglect caused by aid administrators. As they competed for support and compassion, their appeals and writings pressed for the "friendly, enlightened world" to save these refugees, who had been spurned and abandoned by their own societies.[13] This shift was significant in bringing to light the human rights of older refugees and in reshaping the Western public's understanding of the vulnerabilities of the aged in Asia and Africa. Paradoxically, while designing relief programs, some development experts would associate even old and abandoned refugees with productivity and emphasize their need to contribute to society, thereby resurrecting an older, persistent view of aging as a form of dependency solvable with income and work.

Making the Invisible Visible in the Horn of Africa

The new ideas and movements, and some recurring stereotypes, can be traced through the institutional trajectory and campaigns of HelpAge International, an international NGO that emerged from the overseas work initiated by Help the Aged, UK.[14] In its early years, in order to represent the old refugee as a morally vulnerable category marginalized by family and communities, HelpAge International's founders obscured the complexity of both the conditions surrounding refugees and the identity of the old among them. They also engaged with the politics of humanitarian relief and its priorities in identifying vulnerable refugees.

In 1990, HelpAge International reviewed an aging dimension to refugee policy, a new focus area introduced to its international agenda in the preceding years. Its reports from the field described how aged persons had been "uncovered" in refugee camps and the intensified work toward their rehabilitation that had followed.[15] Ken Tout, a senior employee, described one memorable early encounter that eventually led to HelpAge International's founding. One characteristic of refugee migration into Somalia, he observed, was the "invisibility" of older refugees. Tout spoke of how, while his colleague Dr. Christopher Beer was visiting camps in Somalia, members of other relief agencies informed him there were very few refugees at the camps and reception centers who could be termed elderly. Undeterred, Beer persisted in visiting refugee shelters to find out for himself. There he found "many older persons who had secreted themselves in the darkest corners of the shelters. In some cases the elders were too weak to venture out into the rough desert conditions. . . . In the majority of cases, the older people were deliberately denying themselves supplies so that children and nursing mothers might be fed."[16]

There are several interesting features in Ken Tout's account of how Christopher Beer, the chief executive officer of HelpAge International, made the old refugee "visible." This description of a specific episode in a camp in Somalia hints at the assumed authority of the visiting refugee experts like Tout and Beers who interpreted behaviors and spoke on behalf of the old regarding their priorities. Tout observed that the old were passive and tried not to draw attention to their needs, and that their noble efforts at self-denial were often in favor of other generations—until HelpAge interceded and assisted them by making a case that they needed separate relief efforts. Tout's narrative described the situation in Somalia but shared much in common with later narratives on the same subject HelpAge International published, even a decade or so later.[17] It marked the beginning of an effort to refashion the aged among refugees as a distinct category evoking neediness, wherever they were to be found during displacement and relief operations in developing countries.

Part of the barrier in "seeing" the old, Tout wrote, stemmed from the lack of local expertise in the matter, because both aid agencies and their workers, mostly trained to support children and mothers, lacked the ability to identify older persons and provide them special relief. Tout noted that pediatricians were encountered often in relief camps, but geriatricians were encountered "very rarely." But what distinguished the old among refugees was that their fate differed from those "engaged in the full labors of everyday life."[18] Oxfam calculated that, in the movement of refugees from Central Tigray in Ethiopia into Sudan, up to 40,000 elderly people may have been left behind in deserted villages. Oxfam also reported that, at times, older people's attachments to their cultural roots discouraged them from leaving, and they continued to live in precarious ways in war-torn cities such as El Salvador.[19] Others who did venture out often went missing in the course of arduous treks, and lost contact with their families due to their illiteracy, frailty, and disabilities. Arrival at the relief point was no better, as funding sources "unashamedly left them out of priority lists as they were considered to have had 'had their day.'" Tout explained that as "non-producers" in a refugee community situated in a resource-stricken developing country, elderly refugees found little support and were often abandoned to beg on the streets or become outcasts, as they did not adapt to skill-building rehabilitation programs. All of these physical and psychological complexities relating to elderly refugees required specialists "both within UNHCR and in NGOs, who can render this essential initial service," guide policy, and rectify myths about elderly refugees.[20]

When Tout wrote this account in the 1980s, he was a senior officer in HelpAge International, in a period when there were recurring disasters, refugee movements, and conflicts across the developing world, as well as violence in new postcolonial states, some compounded by Cold War rivalries and environmental disasters such as famines.[21] These events stimulated large-scale humanitarian interventions from UN agencies such as the UNHCR and the Food and Agriculture Organization, when the UNHCR transformed from a refugee organization into a more broad-based humanitarian agency.[22] In these years, a growing number of foundations in the West, particularly in the United States, were supporting grants to human-rights programs in developing countries, and many international NGOs were working with and pressuring UN agencies and states regarding their humanitarian policies.[23]

Mobilizing Compassion in the Metropolis

HelpAge International itself had an indirect history in refugee work: its founding director, Leslie Kirkley, worked for the Oxford Committee for Famine Relief, transforming it later into a leading international organization. Help the Aged, its parent organization in the United Kingdom, had been founded a few decades earlier (1964) by Cecil Jackson Cole, also a founding member of Oxfam and a pioneer in modernizing the charity movement by reaching out to people rather than large foundations, an approach that suited the international aging agenda since it had little support from large foundations.[24] We have seen that the beginnings of gerontological research received support from the Nuffield Foundation at the University of Oxford and from institutions in the United States such as the Josiah Macy Jr. Foundation, and that U.S. federal agencies supported international meetings and travel for experts, but not international programs.[25] International development agencies were still largely invested in population control in developing countries, and the international trust fund established after the WAA (1982) to implement the Vienna Plan of Action had the capacity to fund only limited programs.[26]

HelpAge International, with its roots firmly in the traditions of UK public charity campaigns, resorted to publicity and to raising funds largely from the British public. The constituency addressed by agencies such as Oxfam and HelpAge International was broadly similar. HelpAge's search to mobilize volunteers among liberal members of the public committed to improving the lives of the poor abroad was similar to Oxfam's, too. As an Oxfam volunteer admitted, this was often due to "the guilt of a former colonial super-power" and, as a news item bluntly summed it up, wanting "to improve the lives of the blacks out there so they don't want to come over here."[27]

From HelpAge's launch after a high-profile service at Westminster Abbey (1974), Christian sentiments about rescuing the poor and suffering as well as newer concerns colored the campaigns and support it received.[28]

Hudson, who mapped HelpAge's institutional history a decade later, wrote about the motivating philosophy behind the organization that

> The desire to convert the heathen is not the main motivation now. . . . A high proportion, possibly the majority of those who support campaigns aimed at mitigating effects of disasters in poor countries, have no markedly Christian beliefs, but they certainly have strong feelings of guilt about being so much better off than their fellow human beings in Uganda or Uruguay, or wherever disaster has struck more recently. It is possible that some part of this guilt derives from a feeling of shame, conscious or subconscious, that Britain once controlled an enormous empire, but it seems more likely to be due to the fact that the British are fundamentally a kind people, with an above average wish to be helpful to others.[29]

These comments are significant. They explain the strengths of a committed army of what were termed low-paid "god's agents" who mounted the early Help-the-Aged campaigns to raise money for the victims of the Rwandan civil war (1964), famine in India (1966), the Tibetan cause, and the Biafra wars (1968). They also explain why it was harder to forge institutional ties and raise funds in other developed countries through the same methods and campaign. For instance, close personal relations marked HelpAge International's early years, and strong individual networks were cultivated with U.S.-based gerontological research bodies and the American Association for Retired Persons (AARP). However, these efforts did not immediately result in a larger network of collaboration around this agenda. Mark Gorman of HelpAge International recalls frequent visits abroad to attend meetings of the AARP and participate in networks where U.S. delegates had a strong presence, such as the International Gerontological Congress, but no real institutional collaborations to advocate for refugees emerged except when pressures to mobilize for a second Aging Assembly in Madrid (2002) began to build in the 1990s.[30]

Even in the late 1950s, with campaigns such as the first International Refugee Year launched to address the cause of Second World War European refugees, many NGOs in Britain had begun working closely with UN agencies in international humanitarian work, and Kirkley and others had coordinated efforts such as relief work after the famine in Greece.[31] In 1967, Kirkley, then director of Oxfam, observed that these NGOs had begun reappraising their role after these experiences, and now aimed not only to meet urgent needs but also to shape rehabilitation policies.[32] For instance, when bodies such as Interchurch Aid (later named Christian Aid) had assisted during the earthquake in Yugoslavia, Christian charities began drawing attention to the condition of aged refugees in the UK, and Kirkley and Christopher Beer had worked closely with Christian aid agencies in some of these early relief efforts. The networks among many of these NGOs were already well established in the 1960s, when the British Council for Aid to Refugees was working to help old Hungarian refugees settle in the UK.[33] By the 1980s, the sites and strategies had shifted, but the experience of working on these campaigns could be revived.

The 1980s, however, marked a shift in this thinking, and the arena shifted from parts of Eastern and Southern Europe to the developing world. The category of the "old refugee" that emerged from the initial years of HelpAge International's developmental vision and vocabulary would be used more often, to designate a group with distinct needs and vulnerabilities. Chris Beer had reported on the neglect of old refugees while he was undertaking a consultancy project in Africa Leslie Kirkley, then chair of the Help the Aged Overseas Committee, assigned to him in 1980, and he and others conceived of the need to support the cause of aged refugees in developing countries. He said, "It was the time of the Ethiopia and Somalia wars. . . . It became clear that older refugees were not being looked after by other agencies. The idea was to become a lobby for older people and develop programmes such as . . . community care."[34]

Narratives of Abandonment

Studies of the politics of compassion and humanitarian relief that emerged in the 1980s and 1990s have pointed out that activists represented refugees displaced by disasters and emergencies as passive, traumatized recipients of aid and support and that, in stark contrast, they represented refugee agencies and their experts as offering ready solutions to a complex humanitarian problem.[35] However, voices from affected areas such as Darfur, as captured by filmmakers and journalists, often did not corroborate this emerging narrative of elder refugees; neither did many of the contemporary refugee studies and surveys. Older persons were undeniably affected and marginalized in refugee reception centers and camps, and they were in dire need of support. However, I argue that in the 1980s, in the process of

representing their cause in the language of social and political abandonment as distinctly moral, activists did not adequately define who the "old"
were, nor did they attempt to understand how their location, their family
histories, and their social histories before migration continued to affect
their condition.

In *Darfur Diaries*, an account consisting of travel and filmed interviews
with locals regarding the violent conflict in Sudan, the narrative was pep-
pered with old people who served as informed, politically astute narrators
who often participated in training young boys to join the armed resistance.
Often, older persons in these camps and outside of them saw the condition of women, children, and elders as a common, shared plight, with all
of them extending mutual care to each other because the young men had
left to join the anti-Arab Sudan Liberation Army leading the resistance
against the state and the Janjaweed.[36] Other documentaries in sites of conflict, such as between Ethiopia and Eritrea (1998), described conflicts
in which entire cities, such Asmara, were populated only by "women,
children and the elderly. Every fit man is, in fact, at the front."[37]

Part of the problem in trying to identify the distinct needs, claims, and
rights of the old lay in the spaces they occupied. As studies have shown,
refugee camps, with their frightening historical legacies from the war in
Europe, could both protect and persecute; therefore contemporary sites
were more often than not termed "reception centers" instead. However, in
most developing countries, the camps were often porous rather than
demarcated and closed as those in Darfur and Zimbabwe were.[38] Contemporary migration histories that featured the elderly also suggested that
older people were not in these camps in large numbers. In a study Beer
commissioned at Help the Aged on the health of elderly refugees in camps
in Sufawa in East Sudan (1985), Nancy Godfrey reported that "over half of
the old elderly had already been left behind in Tigray. Severely disabled,
old elderly especially women were not found in Sufawa and were likely
to have been left behind. . . . The migration of entire villages and families to
Sudan removed many (possibly all) support systems normally available to
the elderly who remained in Tigray."[39] Godfrey noted that in terms of
health indicators, "the medical problems identified were similar to the
problems of the elderly elsewhere in the world. . . . These problems are as
significant in Sufawa as in stable communities; the elderly should be recognized as a physically vulnerable group."

Ordinarily, refugee camps were sites of enumeration and classification to distinguish the able from the dependent. In this case, camp officials and local Sudanese administrators lacked data on age in camps and, in Tigray, on places of origin. As a result, studies such as Godfrey's only reinforced the inability of those delivering humanitarian aid to establish the problem of the elderly in refugee camps as a priority. A more familiar problem also raised its head: studies of old refugees pointed out that, due to disabilities, poor women in Africa experienced old age earlier, and Tout's report conceded that, while distinguishing medical services provided for children below five years from others was easy, all other age groups often drifted to the HelpAge facilities. In some villages, life was already characterized by migration patterns that left only the "old" behind. A study by the International Federation of Aging on the changing structure of villages in Zaire showed that in 1978, "there were no persons between the ages of 20 and 34, the most economically active age group, in the village. This group has left for urban areas in search of employment and education. Almost . . . 44% of the village population was between the ages of 35 and 60, and 7% were between ages 61 and 85. Since many persons in their 40s in Zaire, as in many developing nations, are considered elderly, these statistics underscore the deteriorating dependency ratio in the village and the vulnerability of the elderly."[40]

Even as other studies corroborated this narrative of migration, some researchers argued that, in times of rapid change and social pressures, communities of older people, such as in Botswana, both assumed new roles and continued to fulfill previous responsibilities in the village. The departure of the young and the return of aging urban migrants implied that many rural areas may have already devised strategies for coping with the loss of manpower or that emergencies and refugee migrations only compounded already-present poverty and dependence. According to a study of Darfur, not only the aged, but also the already poor and destitute had higher mortality, and the locations of both refugee camps and villages were critical in determining the survival of vulnerable groups.[41]

International NGOs' efforts to represent old refugees' needs as a distinct, humanitarian cause and to underscore the conditions abandoned elders faced were also challenging because the vulnerability of children and mothers and, to a lesser extent, women during crises was already recognized and prioritized. Childhood as a moral and social category in international humanitarian causes had drawn increasingly more attention after the Second World War, the creation of UNICEF (1946), and UN declarations such as the Declaration on the Rights of the Child (1959), which initially highlighted issues of child abuse and later highlighted children's purity and innocence as victims of adult vice with the spread of HIV/AIDS.[42] In the case of older persons who were refugees, some studies tried to allege that elders' disrespect of the young, cruelty, and tendency to monopolize scarce resources were responsible for their marginalization. However, there were significant contradictions to this perception, since the old were also portrayed as playing an important role in caring for their grandchildren in camps.[43]

Behind God's Back: Abandoned by Families and the First World[44]

I would like to situate the continuities and changes in these narratives of abandoned and bereft old refugees, which formed the focus of HelpAge International reports in these years. Many of these founding activists had Christian fund-raising background, which gave them a missionary zeal for relief and rescue that had some continuities with missionary efforts under colonialism (see Chapter 1) in terms of drawing attention to the vulnerabilities of the old and frail, who had been left behind due to local "custom." Notions of abandonment have a long history in missionary thought. In the case of Christian missionaries such as Robert Moffat, encounters with the Xhosa tradition of abandoning elders in the wild represented a deeper encounter between cruel heathens and civilized Christians.[45] In postcolonial contexts, a more specific responsibility for the abandonment of aged refugees in villages, during a family's migration, and in refugee camps was difficult to fix, since generalizations regarding civilizational difference and racial inferiority were no longer relevant. However, accounts of refugee distress, especially in the media, still centered on Africa's "inherent" and changeless pathologies of moral and material distress.[46]

Neglect and abandonment were therefore attributed to the "First World" by international NGOs working for the aged. In the 1980s, international charities such as Oxfam and Christian Aid ran powerful and emotive campaigns focused on the plight of refugees that emphasized the developed world's responsibility to contribute aid to mitigate human suffering overseas, appealing especially to liberal middle classes to support and remedy this suffering-at-a-distance. Appeals regarding the neglect of old refugees were voiced in similar registers. Tout described a family group in Hong Kong who arrived from Vietnam by boat in 1982: "In due course the younger family members with their small children were offered retraining and settlement in North America, which they felt constrained to accept. However, it meant leaving two 80 year old women . . . in the refugee cages in Hong Kong with very little hope of ever being reunited with their family again."[47] The suffering of older refugees now took on an aspect of abandonment both by their Third World families and by powerful states and their immigrant regimes that selected the young and productive over the old and encouraged only the former to migrate. Missionary narratives of the Xhosa had described the "tribe" going forward in search of food and shelter, leaving behind the aged and sick in the wilderness. Tout's description underscores a similar migration to the developed world. In this case, both family and industrialized societies were responsible for this humanitarian neglect.

Inserting aged and abandoned refugees' needs into a hierarchy of international humanitarian empathy and support for the displaced and homeless required ideas, images, and oppositions to persuade those who influenced resources, policies, and public opinion. The founding members of HelpAge International, such as Kirkley, Beer, and its public relations advisers such as Harold Sumption were closely associated with campaigns to build international charities' profiles in the UK. New rules and strategies of charity publicity were being established in the 1960s and onward, and powerful direct marketing and advertisements depicted need in the developing world that shocked and provoked, attracting volunteers and funding even though the 1980s were dogged by world economic crisis and recession.[48]

HelpAge International benefitted from these campaigns and experience, and Kirkley's efforts to found the Standing Conference of Refugees, an assembly of voluntary agencies in the UK, allowed HelpAge International to participate in a wider network and be eligible for government funds for disaster relief work.[49] Even though refugee campaigns were hard-hitting and sought funds equally aggressively from the public elsewhere, such as in the US, in these years the condition of the aged refugee was not highlighted in publications of the US Committee for Refugees, and HelpAge International continued to center its campaigns in the UK. Other international NGOs set up in the 1970s, such as the International Federation on Aging (IFA; 1973), became platforms for a range of national NGOs to find a collective voice with which to advocate in the UN for the aging, but they were not shaping a new humanitarian paradigm as HelpAge International was venturing to do in these years.[50]

Social Development in Camps

Even as these networks and campaigns spoke about aged refugees and their vulnerability, many in the field were asking how work and resources were being mobilized in refugee camps and whether these international NGOs' approach was actually solving local problems concerning aged refugees. The humanitarian campaigns HelpAge International supported worked with the support of local social-work schools and workers experienced in other development projects. Zimbabwe, where following the Vienna Assembly on Aging, a leadership trained in social work was taking interest in national programs for the elderly, emerged as a site where these collaborations between HelpAge International and local social workers could be examined.

Field reports and reviews submitted to the HelpAge Zimbabwe office described the hiring of six social workers, who first collected population statistics in three refugee camps, carried out needs assessment surveys, and began working with older persons to identify training programs for them as well as to ensure a more equitable share of goods, medical services, and shelter. Elderly refugees, it was reported, were now under less stress as they were productive and participating in camp activities.[51] The report concluded: "Through these activities their confidence has been built up and enhanced. They are beginning to experience less stress because they can now approach our social workers for advice or counselling. Previously they felt themselves to be in a position of helplessness. Elderly refugees now identify with each other. They hold meetings, have discussions, and organise social functions. They recently organised activities to celebrate Mozambique's anniversary of independence, when they performed dances, sang songs and told stories. . . . *The old attitude that there is little point in doing anything to help elderly refugees has gone.*"[52]

The field report was clear in its statement that in the five months the HelpAge officers worked in the camp for Mozambican refugees, they had solved the problems of old refugees. The main competition for authority they faced was not only from camp administrators but from researchers and experts who visited the elderly and offered little to them, unlike the

HelpAge workers. The HelpAge staff noted that, once they had won over the older refugees and offered them services and training, they had been successful.[53] Reports and studies conducted in the years that followed, however, challenged these claims. R. Mupedziswa, the director of the School of Social Work in Harare observed in a presentation that of about 70,000 Mozambican refugees in Zimbabwe who fled famine and war, 8–10 percent were elderly men and women. He noted that the developmental approach toward old refugees could not be the sole approach, as it emphasized their participation and productivity through self-help projects, but neglected to find ways to restore their social status through new means. Mupedziswa observed that now, dealing with old refugees emphasized a social development perspective rather than the earlier remedial approach that treated them as a "problem," but the new perspective still did not respect their role and place outside of their physical contribution as individuals, and tended to see old age as a disability. "A cursory glance at the activities that elderly refugees are involved in, within the camps," he observed, "will show that while the economic facet has been promoted with gusto and energy, the same cannot be said with regard to the social status dimension."[54]

Mupedziswa admitted that longer-term factors involving colonization, urban growth, loss of resources, and poverty were also at play, but his account emphasized that the developmental approach, with its focus on productivity and activity, neglected other aspects of old refugees' roles in camps where resources, such as command over rituals, livestock, and land, were missing.[55] Later studies among the refugee camps also emphasized that elderly refugees, especially poor older women with little experience of markets, were more marginal to schemes to adapt them to livelihoods and often continued to feel isolated both by younger persons and by camp officials.[56] Due to the demographic imbalance in camps, the status of women—older women in particular—was adversely affected because male labor was more in demand and old refugee women were not able to rebuild their social networks easily.[57]

The campaigns HelpAge International and its national allies led to raise awareness of abandoned and marginalized old refugees were a significant new means to garner international attention and mobilize funds for running programs benefitting from a build-up of humanitarian concern for the developing world's suffering. However, at both the international and local levels, the efforts to represent the "older refugee" as an individual with an autonomous occupation who shunned economic and social dependency tended to undermine social complexities on the ground, such as the interdependence of old and young across the life-course, and tended to compartmentalize these identities. As Mupedziswa perceptively voiced in his critique, even in refugee camps, the place of the old was anchored in their social status and their family and community roles, and was drawn from unpaid social functions. Restoring their status required bringing old and young refugees together. More often than not, even as the old were projected as a separate humanitarian cause, distinguishing the differences between approaches to aging and to other development projects and workers was easier said than done. At the field level, a shortage of trained labor for humanitarian work more generally made identifying a separately trained workforce oriented to older persons and their resources difficult.[58]

HelpAge-supported programs suffered from the same problems as other development initiatives for refugees—and also shared the optimism of other development interventions and donor rhetoric that concluded, based on a few surveys and interviews, that they had affected the complex social realities older refugees faced.[59] Workers with a few years of social-work training and a few weeks in the refugee camp were projected as having solved a whole gamut of problems faced by old refugees, and their accounts emphasized the use of ubiquitous development tools, participatory evaluations, and need surveys to develop targeted programs for old refugees. However, the old were a differentiated group even in refugee camps, leading to the neglect of the more vulnerable among them, such as poor women (who noted that they did not understand the livelihood generation plans) and other elders who were frail and disabled. In the case of assistance to women refugees, for instance, the UNHCR, reflecting idealized notions of good and bad practices and behaviors among displaced populations, pointed out that not all women needed to be considered vulnerable;[60] rather, specific characteristics had to be determined, and adding women to the arena was not by itself a means to generating a gender perspective.[61] Finally, targeting the poor and vulnerable among these groups held its own challenges, such as identifying them from among the mobile population of a refugee camp. Studies such as Godfrey's and Kalache's tried to document the health needs of older adults in Sudan, but even in the 1990s, there was a dearth of information, including demographic data, nutritional information, and data on social, ethnic, and gender divisions in societies with large displaced populations, such as those in the Horn of Africa.[62]

Refugees, Social Justice, and Rights

What impact did campaigns by international NGOs such as HelpAge International in the 1980s have? In terms of sensitizing humanitarian experts and building on a growing public arena of humanitarian support, they made definite inroads. By representing aging as a humanitarian agenda linked with poverty and vulnerability, NGOs secured recognition for these campaigns, since the image of aging associated with debates over the age of retirement and social security more relevant to industrialized nations had little or no purchase among a wider community of social and development activists or policymakers. These campaigns allowed HelpAge International to build a substantial presence in international aging programs, and by the time the Second World Assembly on Aging was held in Madrid (2002), its director, Todd Petersen, noted they were active in over eighty countries.[63] The focus on support for older refugees has persisted with support from the UK Disasters Emergency Committee (DEC), which comprises the UK's leading charities and allows HelpAge International access to resources for disaster-relief funding. Due to a need, prompted by its grants from the DEC, to demonstrate its efforts and spending in this area of refugee relief, HelpAge continues to highlight the condition of old refugees, and references to old refugees as "hidden victims" and forgotten casualties continue in their recent campaigns in Syria.[64] The rhetoric of missionary zeal and "First World" rescue has, however, dissipated, since replaced by a tempered emphasis on "well-being." Additionally, these programs now emphasize the need for trauma counseling for old refugees ("the neglected generation") in conflict zones.[65]

Inroads were also made in the arena of older refugees' human rights through advocacy within the UN, since HelpAge International activists were in close contact with UN relief agencies and local policymakers. To step back briefly to make a comparison, in 1967, at one of the first conferences to coordinate refugee relief efforts in Addis Ababa, Lars-Gunnar Eriksson, the representative of the Group of Voluntary Agencies, summed up the profile of refugees in Africa in a somewhat undifferentiated manner: "More than 50% of Africa's population consists of children and adolescents, and of course, the refugee population reflects the same demographic trend. There even tends to be a higher percentage of children and women among the refugee population, for obvious reasons. We therefore feel that special efforts to provide for the many children, and, in particular, to develop further educational programmes for their benefit is a high priority."[66]

In the decades and humanitarian campaigns that followed, children were still the highest priority for relief, but a somewhat more complex understanding of who were refugees and their distinct vulnerabilities had emerged. In 1983, for instance, a landmark meeting held in Arusha, inaugurated by Tanzanian president Julius Nyerere, emphasized the urgency of refugee relief as a path to human and political recovery in Africa. Among the priorities highlighted at the meeting were "the elderly," formally listed as a separate category of concern among marginalized groups.[67] These were still small steps as far as human rights laws and conventions were concerned. As compared to other groups recognized in the core international human rights conventions, aging persons were still not considered a core human rights issue. It would take a deepening awareness of aging and of elder rights abuses in the next decade, especially in the developing world, to begin building a wider consensus.[68]

In the 1990s, efforts to campaign for the rights of older persons began, with the IFA and HAI at the forefront in the United Nations. These NGOs had built a network of local partnerships on the ground that gave them a stronger voice in these campaigns as they sought to link aging with humanitarian crises and displacement.[69] The UN Principles for Older Persons (1991) were passed, but the larger question of whether the rights of older persons merited a separate human rights instrument, which would allow the situations in individual countries to be monitored and reported on and would safeguard their rights, continued to be a focus of intense debate.

Elders as Abused Survivors in the Time of HIV

By the end of the 1980s, as the state of emergency associated with the refugee crisis became normalized and HelpAge International consolidated its relief programs, another humanitarian crisis was looming. Many national NGOs and affiliates of HelpAge International were already involved in campaigns against elder abuse, in particular abuse in long-term care institutions and by healthcare professionals in the West, but the integration of newer issues, such as the challenge to elders from HIV deaths, was slow to gain acceptance. In an interview, Ken Tout from HelpAge International noted that, even though national affiliates such as their partners in South Africa were beginning to highlight the condition of older persons, in particular grandparents who were caregivers of HIV-afflicted children and grandchildren, international partners in the developed world had not recognized this humanitarian issue until it assumed very serious proportions.[70]

Tout and Chris Beer from HelpAge International attended the First International Conference on the Global Impact of AIDS (1988) and raised the issue of what they termed "The Grandmother's Burden." They warned that the phenomenon of the abandoned grandmother, left to care for the children when youth from the village migrated, was now compounded by the role of grandmothers as survivors.[71] These remarks were made in passing at the AIDS conference, but they have an important historical resonance if we try to understand how perceptions of the older persons' vulnerability in the Third World was constantly changing. In the 1950s to1970s, the abiding concern was grandparents being left behind due to rapid urbanization. As we have seen, anthropologists at the Rhodes Livingston Institute such as Godfrey Wilson, Isaac Schapera, and others were already examining the social aspects of these changes as far back as the 1940s, paying special attention to the exodus of young men drawn by jobs and capital in the Copperbelt, and the women and elders left behind in this exodus. Later scholars such as James Ferguson have also traced old retirees' return to rural areas in their research.[72]

During the 1980s and 1990s, this history would be recast as one that intensified "an already desperate situation for old women with young orphans."[73] For the majority of older persons in developing countries who looked after children and homes, the earlier situation was characterized by reciprocity, with almost half of those interviewed in one study in Zimbabwe reporting that they received support in small cash or noncash contributions from their children.[74] The loss and disruption of these intergenerational ties due to HIV-caused mortality had devastating implications across generations. In a HelpAge-supported study with local partners in Tanzania conducted among 1,500 older persons, frail old persons with young orphans were reported to be caught in a vicious cycle of poverty: in which they scrimped to send these orphans to school, but the children missed school, had a poor diet, and were "severely disadvantaged."[75] Further, with their adult children sick or unemployed, older persons were not only overburdened but often ill-treated at home.

South African activists who took up this issue and were invested closely in these questions would point out in a later critique that the tendency to define human rights issues concerning the elderly according to Western terms of reference was a barrier to recognizing elder abuse in developing countries. Categories of elder abuse originating in the West impeded the recognition of abuse and cruel practices that were culturally specific.[76]

International NGOs, often with roots in Church-centered charity, had pursued the agenda relating to abandoned old refugees with zeal, as their concerns reflected both a sense of Christian rescue and medical and moral concern for the poor and their souls. Their agenda also overlapped with funds and resources offered by the UN and development programs in the UK for disaster relief. But older persons who took on the role of caregivers for HIV orphans and whose kin abused them for their social security payments continued to be isolated figures drawing limited support. Their cause could not be aligned easily with UN campaigns, nor did they match descriptions, centered in institutional settings and around caregivers rather than in homes and families, of elder abuse in developed countries.

Maturing Networks in Developing Nations

In 1986, an IFA-supported journal reported that the government of Belize had drafted "a strategic plan for the aged." The report noted that, "In an unprecedented move, the government brought in an international organization, HelpAge International, with multinational funding to survey the national scene and consult on the problems of the older population. . . . Finally to implement the study, the public and voluntary sectors joined together in a representative and effective national committee on aging to provide the credibility needed to obtain international funding."[77] Countries such as Belize, the Dominican Republic, Ghana, and others were important examples in these years of how international campaigns to support aging rights or effect development programs for the aged were implemented, often by the mediation of international NGOs who worked with national governments in planning aging policies.[78] HelpAge's significant contribution was to offer validation or credibility for these plans; HAI would then work closely with governments in advocating for mostly international funds to roll out the programs envisaged as national-level strategic plans for the aged.

International funds especially were still scarce. They continued to be restricted to more generally allocated development aid, such as food aid and funds for rehabilitation and health that were also available for aged persons. The lack of large donor support was starkly shown in a 1998 HelpAge study that surveyed the "Status of Ageing in Development Cooperation," which concluded that both multilateral agencies, such as USAID, and bilateral agencies in Denmark, Germany, France, Norway, Sweden, and other West European countries were not supporting development activities that targeted aging populations.[79] The PanAmerican Health Organization supported some programs, mainly aimed at developing infrastructure within countries; however, other powerful agencies such as the Organization for Economic Co-operation and Development and even the United Nations Population Fund (UNFPA) had yet to make aging a stated priority in their development strategies. Even the World Health Organization (WHO), which had established a new program on "Ageing and Health" (1995), did not set aside a sufficient budget to pursue some of the aims voiced in this program.[80] The campaigns to draw attention to the vulnerability of old refugees did pay off, most immediately in the UK and, to a limited extent, in garnering support from the European Community's Humanitarian Office programs, and some emergency relief and development support from the UK government's Department for International Development became available. But by and large, the message for leaders of aging-related NGOs was clear: mobilizing support for national or international programs meant raising funds from the public and from individual states.

The effort that networks of experts made to cobble together aid and programs were quite widespread, however. These networks might be between visiting HelpAge International executives, leaders of local NGOs, and government officials, as well as local researchers who conducted initial development surveys and evaluations. The constituency of older persons whose interests these experts supported, however, was not always as diverse. Unlike in Belize, older affiliates to this international NGO network such as HelpAge India had begun to successfully raise funds domestically. HelpAge India had also worked closely with Help the Aged, UK in the early decades after the former was founded. As early as 1974, Samson Daniel, a local Indian philanthropist, had approached the enterprising Cecil Jackson, an influential founding member of Help the Aged in Britain, with the aim of founding an affiliated organization in Delhi.[81] In characteristic fashion, instead of offering funds, Jackson chose to train Daniel in England in fund-raising techniques. Based on these skills and the ties cultivated with corporate donors in urban areas, the newly founded affiliate found support among an urban middle-class constituency.

The founding of HelpAge in India was also seen as an experiment in relocating the original model of Help the Aged to developing countries, although an observer writing in the 1980s noted that not all ex-colonies were as amenable to this transfer of skills and training. He observed in a tone laden with colonial presumptions, "there have been disappointments, mostly due, one is sorry to say to have to say, to the fact that British institutions, however admirable in themselves, do not transplant satisfactorily overseas. One has to record, for instance that parliamentary democracy has for the most part been a dismal failure in those recently liberated African territories. . . . But British habits and traditions have, it is true, struck much deeper roots in certain other former dominions and colonies, and one of those is certainly India."[82]

The India "model," as officials have tended to refer to it, was clearly a postcolonial "jewel in the crown" for Help the Aged, UK, whose international operations would later be separated from Help the Aged, UK and taken over by HelpAge International. Predictably, this model had a limited public reach, and was limited in its perception of the aging population—as retired, middle-class, "senior citizens"—although it succeeded in building on a core group of volunteers and donors in Indian cities that included Indian "salesmen and school teachers."[83]

Its fund-raising campaigns and partnerships also remained conservative, aiming at a constituency with striking parallels to that of Help the Aged, which banked mostly on middle- and upper-class generosity even until the 1970s and 1980s.[84] Its understanding of aging and its needs was focused on disease and care. After three fund-raisers held soon after its founding in Delhi, Bombay, and Madras respectively, it established a series of institutions for the elderly and poor, including a Help the Aged Ward and other care-giving facilities.[85] Samson Daniel and his wife had raised funds for their early campaigns through walks, and more than a decade later, in the late 1980s, HelpAge India was still raising funds to partner with a local NGO, Kalyan Samiti, through mail appeals, walks, and—a first—an art auction.[86]

NGOs' role in pressing for national aging-related policies in developing countries was now well consolidated. Often, new partnerships and interests that were emerging from developing countries helped in this role, and HelpAge International's priorities had to adapt to pressures from potential affiliates in developing countries. In India, NGOs in the aging sector also spearheaded partnerships with members of the International Federation on Aging, another international NGO with links to the AARP in the United States. As the number of NGOs associated with various aging-relating causes increased in India, they also had a show of strength: in 1988, it was emphasized that NGOs working with older persons had become a crucial source of innovation in spreading the cause of aging to a broader public.[87]

However, these NGOs' coming together still did not spell a break from past approaches to aging, such as a middle-class worldview of social change and progress with inherent biases toward rescuing the old and destitute and providing retirement and family support for the resilient and middle class. Pronouncements by members of a national symposium of NGOs working on aging in India (1988) reflected this by noting that the elderly in India were of two kinds: the needy, who already received considerable attention through medical and housing aid or through small loans, and those who wanted "to continue contributing to society and to the development of India."[88] The Indian government's minister for welfare, who was invited to the meeting, reinforced these viewpoints, adding that while "nearly all Indian states had schemes to support the destitute elderly with low levels of assistance," it was "clear that support for the aged currently lies mainly with themselves and with their families."[89] These generalizations did not capture the interests of either group, and they left out a large heterogeneous group of older persons who did not fit into either category.

Prioritizing Development among Emerging Economies

In terms of international voices and networks, however, NGOs such as HelpAge India and others did not offer a sustained critique of the changing welfare priorities of states and international institutions; rather, they focused primarily on services and aid for the most vulnerable. Their humanitarian discourse was reserved for older persons deemed vulnerable and needy, and those caught in poverty traps. Older persons included in new ideas about productive and active aging were perceived as able to contribute to furthering their nation's developmental goals. In the 1990s, as neoliberal regimes spread across developing economies, ideas about active aging voiced by international and national NGOs, experts, and governments in many developing nations began redefining the terrain of aging

and development. The focus on productive aging aimed at fostering qualities of secular self-reliance and independence because these contributed
to national goals and rapid industrialization. This emphasis also included
roles for family, culture, and interdependence based on family rather than
state support.

These new paradigms of aging, in which the family rather than the state
provided support, and aging was not necessarily a distinct political and
policy category, underscored the ambitions of developing and emerging
economies. A 1999 survey of the status of national aging policies in forty-
six developing countries showed that most countries had limited social insurance (for former government employees only) and no plans for further
expansion. Their aging policies were either absent or underscored measures to maintain family support and prevent abuse of the most marginalized, to whom they offered social assistance or poverty pensions.[90] Very few
of them were as yet implementing policies focusing on better integrating
older persons into society, nor did they perceive aging as an agenda that
had synergies with other age groups and developmental programs.[91]

NGO reports reflected priorities such as older persons needing increasingly to find coping strategies to remedy their poverty and discussions
about whether aging could still be inserted in the UN's goals to alleviate
global poverty by 2015.[92] The dawn of neoliberal health priorities and the
privatization of health also made the search for new approaches to aging
urgent. In Tanzania, a report noted that individual self-reliance was key in
an age when health services were being withdrawn. Quoting from local
interviews, the report elaborated that, "Many older people say that nowa-
days they have to work harder in order to make ends meet, which adversely
affects their health. Older people insist that coping strategies have changed
over the years[;] in the past there was more community support, families
were less fragmented, and there was less necessity for money, particularly
because health services were free."[93]

In the case of China, at the first International Forum on Ageing, held in
Beijing (1986), a report of the Sino-US supported meeting stated that due
to its successful family planning policies, China would be "telescoping in
several decades a demographic transition that took a century to occur in
the West. . . . However, it is a price that Chinese policy-makers are willing
to pay in exchange for the more rapid economic development that may
result." The report observed that the Chinese foresaw their old people contributing toward social and economic development: "Even older persons

who remain at home today helping in household chores believe they are making a contribution to China's economic development by permitting the release of their children's time for productive work. . . . It is not surprising that Chinese planners are optimistic about harnessing more of older persons' energies in the future for economic growth."[94] In both the Indian and Chinese reports that followed the Vienna Assembly on Aging, and in later discussions of the Zimbabwe National Plan on Aging, we increasingly see a "new" old person emerging: a productive contributor to social development who is distinct from the poor, indigent elderly still supported through poverty programs.

Mainstreaming the Old

Interestingly, the grandmother's tale follows us here too. Recent studies of HIV and grandmothers, rather than tying their condition to older narratives of being left behind or being burdened survivors, have tried to represent older persons' ways of coping with HIV orphans as strategies of resilience. An article in *Ageing and Society* (2015) portrays South African grandmothers raising grandchildren as demonstrating a process of responsibility, fulfillment, and resilience rather than simply compromising their own health and personal security.[95] Such articles are often based on models of resilience studied and tested among custodial grandparents in the US; this implies that poverty and adversity among the old and marginalized is not restricted to developing countries, but exposes elders to the same challenges worldwide.[96]

In turn, the emphasis is on turning to limited state allowances and support and translating what were once considered vulnerabilities into strengths. At the same time, economic studies demonstrating the gendered nature of care by grandparents have tried to show that wider social development goals of child health and nutrition are met when grandmothers care for their granddaughters. This reinforces the shifts, in both research and policies in developing nations, to portraying aging as something to mainstream and connect with other development goals and to recasting the geographies of deprivation and marginalization as not confined to Third World spaces but including old people, in other parts of the world, making efforts to cope and thrive in globalized societies.[97]

By the 1990s, even the aged and helpless refugee who formed the early parts of this narrative had been taken "out of Africa," if only briefly, when attention among NGO experts shifted to the plight of older refugees in the "transition economies of Eastern and Central Europe," where failing social policies, inflation, and conflicts such as in Kosovo, Yugoslavia (1998–1999) brought up the need to extend emergency relief.[98] Reports estimated that more old people in countries *under* transition lived with their families. In Hungary, in 1984, almost one-third of those over sixty-five years lived with their children, compared with 6 percent in Sweden, and their physical and mental well-being were threatened.[99] The shifting focus of this relief work underscored that older refugees were vulnerable not only in the global South, but also in other parts of the world. These relief campaigns emphasized that social, political reversals and historical experiences made supporting aging populations a challenge in Eastern Europe as well, where demographic aging was not a new and uncertain process as in Asia and Africa.

These shifts in ideas about aging in developing nations also bore the marks of changes in thought within and among UN agencies. Prominent UN experts urged "mainstreaming" aging into development and national-level plans and integrating it into cross-cutting issues and policies across the social sector.[100] International NGOs and their national partners were critical in shaping this. However, many countries made clear that the economic status of the elderly differed in the developing world, as did their potential to offer universal social security benefits and institutional care. We increasingly see policymakers highlighting the family's responsibilities and even strengthening the family's role and increasing reliance on it. At the same time, in political declarations and policies, political leaders emphasized older persons' need to play a productive role in national development, although they offered limited support in public programs for healthy aging and work.

In a meeting the WHO held in Brazzaville (1988), where NGOs from across Africa were invited to participate, the WHO acknowledged the crucial role of NGOs in mediating health programs for the aged. It was also clear that African countries were choosing to appropriate population aging as a category so that they could imbue responses to it with multiple meanings. The delegate from Botswana reported that in Botswana, there were no programs "tailored specifically or exclusively to the elderly, but there are programmes for the elderly that are integrated."[101] In Tanzania, the response was similar, with the delegate from Tanzania noting that aging as a separate and distinct health agenda was not sustainable there, since the economy "was currently too weak to support a nation-wide plan for the elderly." Many countries emphasized the need to rely on existing primary healthcare services and to integrate eldercare with the infection management and other health campaigns.

The complexities of addressing the needs of aging populations among a still youthful majority, of coping with the burdens of infectious disease that were still prevalent when chronic diseases were rising, and of population control programs that had barely ended when longevity and a fall in fertility also needed policy support implied that the realities of aging populations in Asia and Africa were going to be complex and, often, contradictory. However, there were now new emerging worldviews of aging articulated during these humanitarian campaigns and in their wake: a focus on older persons' welfare needs and the emphasis on making them productive and self-reliant from a social development perspective, and also a focus on the international rights of older persons. The latter was drawn partly from campaigns in the United States and Europe relating to elder abuse, but the debates led by activists in South Africa working with older persons reinforced the need to understand elder abuse and rights based on the experiences of generations with HIV/AIDS and economic and social disparities rooted in the global South.

From Decolonization to Globalization

IN A SPEECH delivered at the Indian Parliament in 2007, Meira Kumar, the minister for social welfare, reflected on the country's coming of age: "Today sixty years have passed since the country became independent. We are going to adopt the modern culture."[1] Kumar was introducing legislation mandating that adult children maintain their aging parents.[2] The Parental Maintenance and Senior Citizens Act (2007), passed unanimously by India's legislators, decreed that adult children should support their old and dependent parents as a "statutory duty"; it declared that "the family is the most desired environment for the senior citizen or parent to lead a life of security, care and dignity" and aimed "to ensure that the progeny performs its moral obligation towards their parents who may otherwise be left . . . destitute in their old age."[3]

The minister elaborated on the demographic and historical implications of the momentous problem the Indian government faced. The growing numbers of an aging population, she said, partly reflected India's "national progress in areas like public health" but also represented the alarming social aspects of modernization, migration, and urbanization as well as a growing neglect of older persons in Indian society. Other voices, from civil-society groups and various political parties, spoke in the same registers; it was evident that the subject of care and family support for the aging was now part of a globalized narrative. As parliamentary debates on the legislation followed and were reflected in the public sphere, anguished speeches and letters dwelled on the decline of filial piety and narrated dramatic stories of parents abandoned by derelict children who had migrated abroad in search of jobs. Errant children, it was agreed, would be pursued not only along their migratory paths from rural to urban centers but also across the globe as they migrated to the West.

Notions of the family as welfare provider for older persons echoed concerns expressed in the 1940s and 1950s in Asia and Africa. Social experts in the context of late colonial developmental projects and, later, serving as advisers to newly independent and modernizing nations were anxious to understand the implications of rapid social change. They were concerned about problems of dependency, as in the case of children and the elderly left behind in rural areas as young adult workers migrated to towns and cities. The problem was now assuming a global dimension, with national policies such as the one in India recognizing the transnational nature of the social changes: labor migration was increasing, the endpoint destinations were changing from cities in neighboring states and countries to distant centers across the world, and the "abandonment" of children, wives, and elders in villages had correspondingly increased. New policies tried to address and pursue parental claims across borders.

When the Indian Minister introduced this legislation in India, similar perspectives were already entrenched in other parts of Asia and in Africa. In China, adult offspring had already signed more than 13 million family support agreements in rural areas that mandated the maintenance of parents and relied on family for caregiving.[4] Policies requiring informal support from families were also in place in Singapore and other states in Asia. Member countries of the Organization of African Unity also emphasized the importance of family support as a moral norm and responsibility, the need to sustain African traditions of family solidarities, and elders' roles. In a statement issued while preparing for the 1984 UN Assembly on aging, they also spoke of most African states' inability to provide formal and universal support for older persons.[5]

Not all care is seen as flowing from the young to the old. In the wake of the challenges posed by HIV/AIDs in Sub-Saharan Africa and the high rates of morbidity and mortality of young parents, the pressures of caring for orphaned children fell on grandparents, whose families relied on their old age pensions. This raised searching questions about the rights of these older persons and their care, since an entire generation of younger family members had gone missing. In a speech at the founding of the South African

Older Persons Forum (2005), Zola Skweyiya, South Africa's minister for social development, spoke of "mothers and fathers of the nation" who were forgotten and abused, lived in poverty, had contributed to saving the lives of AIDS orphans, and now needed support from the young.[6]

Modernization and Its New Normal

These political speeches and policy shifts bring out the contradictions many political leaders and the public in developing countries see in population aging. It not only represents aspirations to modernization, a better quality of life, improved health, and longevity but is also symbolic of a rapid, unanticipated turn. In these countries, the trajectory of industrialization, urban migration, and changes in standards of living has not taken the same historical course as in the West, where aging followed industrialization. Developing countries face the issue of aging populations alongside other challenges, such as large youth populations facing unemployment, the persistence of infectious and chronic disease burdens and co-morbidities, and the lack of improved standards of living among the weaker sections of society.

In many areas of the world, the emerging optimism of industrialization "slipped off the tracks" as James Ferguson describes it, and reversals of industrialization and urbanization have occurred.[7] As a 2013 UN report on aging reveals, many countries in the developing world rely on private transfers from earning family members to support older persons, and they fear a decline in these. Several have social security for older persons, but countries like Brazil, where most of the needs of older persons can be met from such public transfers, are the exception. Many express these anxieties as a narrative about modernization resulting in a dramatic decline in family relations and solidarities, including the ills of individualism among offspring; having made this case, policymakers have asserted that the state needs to intervene and regulate the conduct of the young and the dependence of the old.

Attitudes to aging centered on the role and reciprocity of families are likely to determine future debates around global aging, especially with the growing focus on long-term care in countries where the state is unwilling or unable to provide substantial welfare provisions. This may also change the focus of the politics and priorities of aging, which have so far reflected the same concerns about aging prevalent in Europe and in North America—

that is, retirement, social security, and worries about keeping up a large and productive workforce—and have therefore focused on debates about chronological age thresholds. The perspective of family responsibility offers a fresh set of reductionist assumptions and arguments about aging and social change. It characterizes aging as a family peril and signals a loss of moral compass and values in a society that needs older people to be supported for the sake of past legacies rather than as a matter of right. New "global" campaigns and stigmas, such as those against the abuse of elders, accompany this thinking. We have discussed earlier that, in colonial India, the abandonment of the old was criticized by missionaries and its stigma was associated with native practices of leaving older family members to die in the wild or on the banks of the Ganga; now, its sites and spaces have shifted to old age shelters and even domestic spaces, where the errant can be regulated by the state and global regimes, such as international NGOs and the UN. At a national level, the younger generation in society and the forces of modernization are viewed as preying on the vulnerability of older persons, and are termed as both the problem and solution to these changes.

These policies to regulate intergenerational support indicate a distinct set of priorities relating to global aging in a neoliberal world, and that individuals, families, and communities will increasingly be held responsible for the care of the aged. However, the translation into policy and the political appropriation of these complex changes ignores research demonstrating that migration within families is not a single event or point of no return, nor always prompted only by the desires of the young, that old age support networks have persisted, and that interdependence is a better way to characterize these social changes than are metaphors of dependence and destitution.

Looking at and Looking Back at Global Aging

Debates on aging have become more widespread and local political voices on the topic have intensified in the global South partly because, over the past decade, the moorings of debates about how aging is understood and interpreted at the global level have changed in important ways. In April 2002, at the second World Assembly on Aging (WAA) in Madrid, held two decades after the first one in Vienna, world aging was rebaptized as global aging. Experts and participants from various nations observed that the world "had changed beyond recognition" since 1982.[8] The Madrid International Plan of Action on Ageing (MIPAA), termed a "global guiding document," was passed at the 2002 WAA; it prioritized the health and well-being of the old, including the provision of enabling environments for older persons.[9] The political declaration of the conference recognized the diversity of aging populations and espoused a "developmental" approach to aging that emphasized participation, inclusion, integration, and access to services for older persons to realize their full potential in a "society for all ages." The Assembly in Madrid also ended on an ambitious note, with a plan that was nonbinding on member states but nevertheless made 239 separate recommendations, offered a brave new world for the elderly and stated that aging was "one of the dominant themes of the century."[10]

The UN has now declared that aging is "pervasive"; it is seamless and present everywhere, influencing population structures and societies to a greater or lesser extent all over the world.[11] With aging framed as a common challenge confronting the whole globe, there is an effort to move away from the notion of a classical European paradigm and trajectory of modernization in the origins and path of population aging. The developing world is now at the heart of discussions on aging, marking a new turn in a field so long defined by industrialized and modern societies. Experts are hopeful that the broad vision for aging articulated in Madrid has found a broader canvas and strategic platform in the Sustainable Development Goals (SDGs) proposed by national governments and adopted in September 2015 by the United Nations as a global development agenda aimed to be achieved by 2030.[12]

The SDGs and their articulation and framing were based on input from wide-ranging "coalitions" of countries across the world advocating for the elderly. HelpAge International and its partner NGOs campaigned in over thirty countries to ensure that the interests of older persons were represented in national drafts.[13] Subsequently, a Stakeholders Group on Aging has been active in forming global and national partnerships—including with Age International, the AARP, the International Federation on Aging, Gray Panthers (an organization founded in 1970 by Maggie Kuhn to defend older persons' rights in the United States), and the NGO Committees on Aging, to name a few—to address national policymakers and work with specialized UN agencies such as the UNDP in promoting awareness of the breadth and diversity of the aging population.[14] Their activities have led to aging's being envisioned as part of the goals of "leave no one behind," and action on various SDGs related to poverty eradication, health and population dynamics, gender equality, economic growth, and empowerment are viewed as critical to promoting the wellbeing of older persons. The aims are to provide older persons with universal social protection, health care and income security, access to productive employment, and vocational training to improve employability; and to integrate older persons into frameworks relating to the treatment of chronic, noncommunicable diseases and management of the challenges posed by dementia.[15]

How did this happen? As I have brought out in this book, experts who founded the first gerontological associations perceived aging as a "world" idea that affected "modern societies" that had experienced industrialization, were culturally mature, and demonstrated a democratic political evolution. The last perception served to raise doubts about the membership of Soviet Russia and its allies in this select and "civilized" club of experts on aging. These ideas reflected a discourse of difference, which was supported by biomedical theories associating aging and decline with chronic diseases of old age related to modern lifestyles and cultures primarily rooted in Western Europe and North America. While gerontological experts based in Europe and the United States sought to expand their scientific networks through chronic disease research in developing countries, such research served partly to elucidate the prevalence and risks of chronic diseases in the developing world, and help them compare and reinforce the differences in, for instance, cancer typologies, age of onset, and risks between the developed and the developing worlds. At times, it also helped to contrast these patterns and vulnerabilities in white populations with other "backward" groups in Western society, such as African Americans. The axes of difference were therefore drawn as much as ever between the West and the rest, but also identified social distinctions in the West, such as between white and African American medical subjects in the United States. American and European medical researchers working on aging often differed in their prioritized research on diseases of aging in these years.

As scientists in Asia and Africa began entering debates around cancer and aging, some of them argued these diseases and aging in non-Western settings were distinct in their risk patterns and often defined by poverty, diet, and customs. However, while they argued that issues of aging and disease in backward societies were different compared to the West, at the same time, they observed that "tropical" paradigms of diseases and bodies needed to be challenged and that differences in development rather than geographical latitude determined these variances.

Chronological age thresholds were not necessarily the only marker of aging, and in countries with lower life expectancies, the same chronic diseases and decline could occur a generation or more earlier due to social and environmental factors. These experts in Asia and Africa tried to show that there was no linear trajectory of modernization linked to the infallible progression of demographic and social change or to disease patterns associated with aging, and they sought to recognize the more complex issues of aging in the context of both social and epidemiological changes. It was clear even in the early days, when chronic disease acted as a proxy for aging in the emerging international agenda for scientific gerontologists, that while aging as an issue bridged developed and developing nations, it also demonstrated structural differences and historical inequalities between the two worlds.

In the 1960s, a more inclusive field began to emerge for gerontology and its subfields, as social transition and change in societies beyond the West drew interest. Older persons were often seen as unable to adjust to modern times unless assisted by experts and, possibly, the new methods and promise of social gerontology. Influential experts in the United States and Europe argued that aging in society, or the study of its 'problems' through social gerontology, was relevant across the world for managing groups such as the old who were maladjusted—that is, unable to cope with rapid social changes.[16] In the decades of decolonization, anthropologists, missionaries, and urban sociologists surveying social changes in Asia and Africa observed that fast-paced urbanization, the gleam of industrial growth, and new solidarities among young nations seemed to lie ahead.[17] In their view, aging was not simply a challenge brought on by a shift in demographic structure or by chronological aging at an individual level; it was also caused, prematurely, by the material changes in the lives of communities struck by urbanization. They often characterized the old as a dependent group, mostly resident in villages, that made demands on the meager livelihoods youth earned in the cities. For some of these experts, the elderly's tendency to control families and labor constraints based on caste and other considerations also impeded the emergence of new, secular ties and industrial relations vital to modernizing young nations. At this stage, development was an aspiration and a means to a sought-after modern way of life in these nations.

Throughout the 1970 and 1980s, the aspirations to modernize had transformed into a deepening disenchantment with development efforts, and the first "worldview" of aging (expressed in Vienna in 1982) was colored by the failures of development and an inequitable, neoliberal international economic order. Aging and its "problems" were seen as emblematic of the social marginalization that occurred among vulnerable groups as a result of weakening family solidarity arising from adopting modern ways of living in smaller units as well as the uncertainties and challenges that dogged national development programs. By now, poverty programs were at the heart of development and its institutions, and the World Bank's participation in international development was growing. The condition of old persons was frequently expressed through the vocabulary of poverty, especially by urban sociologists who deftly tied aging with destitution, chronically poor health, and migration in a range of studies on slums and urban settlements. There was a shift in issues that defined older populations and captured their marginalization. The "abandoned" aged persons associated with the rise of factories and migration had been situated in rural areas in the 1950s, and formed part of the narratives regarding rapid social change, but the aged and poor subjects who formed the focus of new social work and urban reform narratives from the 1980s on were based in cities and urban settlements. Aging, at this point, became linked to larger international issues such as habitat and urbanization, and it remained so by the time of the Madrid Assembly in 2002.

This aged person in the city emerged as a key concern at the Madrid meeting. One of the three priority areas in the MIPAA emphasized the interrelation of aging and habitat. Reflecting these priorities, the World Health Organization (WHO) now runs a fast-growing program called "Global Age-Friendly Cities," which aims to make cities more habitable for people of all ages and specifically to develop an environment for "active aging." This perspective and its reception at a local level have resulted in, among other things, the expansion of healthcare services in cities in recent decades (while the countryside continues to be underserved), and an increased emphasis on urban planning.

Several countries have voiced a need to recast this emphasis. In the years following the Madrid summit, some countries that found the MIPAA challenging to implement have pointed out that the "social gap" between rural areas and the cities as well as the utter poverty of the old in rural areas have been overlooked by a focus on urbanization and the provision of social services in cities; these, they say, require urgent intervention. Countries such as China and India, with a majority of their aging populations in rural areas and separated from children who have migrated, are now addressing this challenge through rural employment generation plans and poverty alleviation schemes.[18]

Shaping the Global through Local Interests

This brings us to a crucial point: how can we meaningfully assess global aging as an agenda and what has a global, transnational vision of aging promised and delivered? How useful is the "global" in global aging, and what are the limits of a global agenda and of transnational institutions in spurring policy changes? What are the influences that have acted at the local level? What are the interconnections, the strengths and weaknesses of these local links that help us understand what aging means, beyond its totalizing, all-encompassing claims?

Even though the scope and agenda outlined by the first WAA in Vienna was widely criticized both before and after it was held, it offered an opening and opportunity for local and regional interventions rather than larger transnational alliances. The aging fund established to implement the Vienna recommendations did not draw large donations, and UN agencies were mostly able to work with local actors to plan national programs and fund small-scale projects and regional conferences. As discussed in Chapter 6, the ambitions of integrating aging into development policies did not immediately gain momentum, and the focus was instead on preventing catastrophes and securing a space for the rights and livelihoods for older persons among other vulnerable groups. Civil war, famines, floods, and conflicts in Africa and Asia for instance created the conditions for NGOs such as HelpAge International (HAI) to define a new approach to fundraising and charity that often capitalized on an ex-colonial public's conscience and attracted support through government disaster relief funds. The aim was to align with a global interest in humanitarian relief and build their visibility in sites and spaces associated with humanitarian crises.

Aside from both economic and humanitarian crises in the years that followed the Assembly in Vienna, social work institutions and NGOs in Asia and Africa began to adapt and recast the plan presented at the WAA in its local afterlives, as we have seen in the case of the local social work leadership in Zimbabwe leading to the drafting of a national plan on aging.

Often, the Vienna Assembly was invoked to create an entry point and leverage for criticizing a national government that was evading the need to recognize aging as a distinct policy agenda and issue; this was the case in India, as activists working in urban slums criticized the marginalization of vulnerable older persons.

The transnational vision that emerged during and after the WAA partly echoed a wider social solidarity and mobilization in this decade, reflecting a critique of development and modernization programs as well. Older persons and their reduced status and vulnerability were linked to the deep flaws in the power structures and economic inequities of international relations. Since the WAA was held in the 1980s, at the time of a global economic crisis, it also created a window of opportunity for seeing aging and its "problems" as related to the economic dependency and bankruptcy created by a failing international economic order. Many social workers and experts, as well as their partners in organizations such as the International Council for Social Welfare, shared the worldwide view that the end of the development decades (or the lack of anticipated economic growth and development in many developing countries) and the beginnings of neoliberal thinking implied that the poverty and marginalization of older persons were intimately linked with inequitable economic relations and more powerful, industrialized societies' subordination of poorer nations' interests. In Europe and the United States, some social scientists, such as Peter Townsend, Meredith Minkler, and Carol Estes were also voicing strains of critical gerontological thought in these years that argued that the old's "dependency" was rooted in social and historical conditions as well as institutionalized structures of society such as the labor market, and that patriarchy was conditioning the gender-biased and stigmatizing perspectives of older persons.[19]

However, it was at the national level that cross-country networks far more participatory than earlier began to emerge, and it was in these sites that a "global" imagination of aging was confronting local transformations. In South Asia, in countries such as Nepal, participatory action networks involved more than seventy local NGOs, and these networks contributed to shaping the national plan presented at the Second World Aging Assembly in Madrid.[20] The first President of the International Federation on Aging (IFA) from Asia, Sharad Gokhale, hosted the first global conference of the IFA held outside of Europe, near Bombay (1992), and the meeting served as a stage to honor the adoption in 1991 of the UN Principles on Older

Persons.[21] The principles had been moved by Julia Tavares de Alvarez, the Dominican Republic's Alternate Permanent Ambassador to the United Nations and a lifelong advocate of aging as an issue of concern. Alvarez joined the meeting in India to speak about her work both in her own country and with the UN Social Development Commission. She also underscored that the acceptance of a rights-based approach to aging was viewed as pathbreaking, but at the same time, it was clear that the participating nations' commitments were less firm than they might have been for a UN convention that would be ratified by member states.[22]

Throughout the 1990s, the global vision of aging seemed to be deepening and assuming wider support in terms of principles and advocacy networks, but Sharad Gokhale would repeat that the global situation was still inhospitable and there was a need to incorporate lessons from other fields, such as "the effective approaches adopted by women, children, youth, and disabled persons"—in other words, other groups who shared proximate social agendas but had greater success in garnering global support and resources.[23] The campaigns and networks concerned with aging in the 1990s, including the humanitarian campaigns stemming from moral concerns taken up by HAI, highlighted the vulnerability of the aged in general and of disadvantaged elders in particular. This was a reframing of an older strain of thought voiced by anthropologists, sociologists, and others in the 1950s regarding the social consequences of modernization in "traditional" societies. With the opening up of Asian and African societies to structural reforms and neoliberal social policies in the 1980s and 1990s, ideas that encouraged "the active and assertive participation" of older persons and the need for the better "situated" among them to be allowed to work in late life and empower themselves to relate to developmental issues (such as the environment and HIV/AIDS) were increasingly influential and focused on research and advocacy meetings on aging in the global North and South.

Two decades after Vienna, a range of stakeholders recognized that the Second World Aging Assembly in Madrid could not simply assert a common global agenda but also needed to offer concrete social planning that engaged and mobilized constituencies of older persons and families. The MIPAA advocated the empowerment of older persons, supported their access to jobs, and emphasized activity-focused healthy aging. It urged a focus on the entirety of the human life-course, rather than a distinct and late life focus on "old age," and the need for societies to foster intergenerational solidarity. The events preceding the Madrid meeting involved an extended planning process toward the agenda for the Assembly, involving older persons and a range of diverse organizations, especially from the global South. This approach was premised on the belief that involving older persons, NGOs, and activists on a large and intimate scale would also ensure that these local groups could pin governments down to ensure follow-up action after the meeting.[24] The plan also had a specific set of recommendations for governments to identify national focal points and other means to mark their progress toward meeting the plan's goals; it also advised integrating these recommendations with existing development policies and poverty eradication strategies.

Beyond Conferences

In my meetings with experts and advocates over the past few years, I have found that perspectives regarding notions of global aging and their diffusion, as captured by the MIPAA, vary greatly. International NGOs such as HAI have been influential in spreading awareness among policymakers in countries that lacked distinct policies for aging until the Vienna Assembly (1982). In the case of Ghana, for instance, by working with social policy activists, HAI was able to shape a national aging policy, and local experts, who had been influenced by discussions in Vienna, discussions in Dakar, and advocacy in the United States were ready to translate these developments to a national level. In India, however, some senior officials in the Social Welfare Ministry in New Delhi seemed less aware of the MIPAA Declaration and stated that they dealt with a slew of other national initiatives that have far more budgetary support than aging.[25] In Pakistan, a meeting hosted by HAI and the Society for Human Rights and Prisoner's Aid (SHARP) emphasized that awareness of aging issues was still weak and that the old were "invisible" in public life. Aging-related policies were not as well-developed and funded as, say, the Poverty Reduction Strategy Papers.[26] By contrast, municipal officials who are part of the South African Local Government Association (SALGA) have demonstrated an awareness of the MIPAA and stated that the challenge for them lies in the "translation" of its diverse objectives from national policies into local programs.[27]

Two of the MIPAA's chief objectives were reinforcing the links between aging populations and development, and integrating aging-related policies and programs with the broader goals of development programs. However,

linking aging to the agenda of development, when the latter has traditionally focused on youth and productivity, has been a challenge at the local
level. Even at a transnational level of policy framing, global priorities
voiced and voted for at aging assemblies have not been followed, even in
institutional initiatives within the UN. Often, it has taken sustained pressure
and pushback from activists to shift UN officials away from a "natural" focus
that entwines youth, development, and productivity. For instance, both the
goals relating to noncommunicable disease risks and the global Sustainable Development Goals, when they were being drafted, focused on "premature mortality" such as deaths among the young and those below forty
years of age.[28] Experts on aging critiqued the SDGs because of their emphasis on the health of children and youth instead of more holistic goals
involving health for all ages.[29] And as we have seen, rural aging has been
neglected in the MIPAA itself.

Local policies have also been shaped by impulses other than global
agendas, and regional influences have been a significant force in prompting
changes in aging policies among neighboring countries. Lesotho's adoption of universal social pensions for older persons was shaped closely by its
neighbor South Africa's adoption of social pensions.[30] The Parental Maintenance laws introduced at the state and federal levels in India from 2005
through 2007 were inspired by laws initiated in countries such as Singapore.[31] Regional influences and homogeneities, however, have their own
limitations. In West Africa for instance, there have been distinct traditions
of social security laws, pension regulations, and even attitudes toward older
populations that have been governed by local differences in ethnic politics and labor force requirements.[32] Even a few decades ago, scholars noted
that in West African countries, colonial legacies were shaping very different policy priorities toward social security for the old, for example in
British-influenced Nigeria as compared to Francophone Côte d'Ivoire.[33]

Regional differences or gaps, even at the level of communication, were
in evidence in the Dakar gerontology conference with which this narrative began. At the Dakar meeting, one of the participants noted: "This
week, I observed on several occasions the elaborate attempts of 'Francophone' Africans and 'Anglophone' Africans to find their words during private discussions on aging at the breaks from formal sessions. The outside
observer might find the gestures, the straining for words odd or amusing
but this is one of the realities of Africa."[34] Such differences have persisted,
and these gaps have partly reflected language barriers but also reflect a

wider lack of familiarity with priorities and programs between and within regions and a dearth of exchanges or prior partnerships. In 2002, at the meetings led by the Organization of African Unity to draft a regional policy framework preceding the Madrid declaration, there were debates and strong exchanges between Anglophone and Francophone delegates that also reflected differences in approaches to aging and its regional priorities. Anglophone Africa had a long-standing social work–related emphasis on aging that graduated into a "development" approach, but these delegates were unfamiliar with histories of social provisions and social changes in Francophone West Africa and the Lusophone countries, much less with the advocacy work relating to aging that had developed in Mozambique.[35]

Often, countries and states that have adopted aging policies have a long-standing advantage in being "models" of development programs that are difficult to replicate in other settings. In South Asia, countries or states that have been ahead in terms of enacting aging policies are difficult to emulate, as they have been consistently good performers in meeting development goals; aging has been just one more prioritized area with programs introduced to tackle it. Nations such as Sri Lanka, which has one of the fastest aging populations in South Asia, enacted policies relating to farmers' and fishermen's pensions even in the 1980 and 1990s, since informal workers are among the most vulnerable as they grow older. Similarly, states such as Kerala in India that have both a large aging population and high levels of migration, and that can draw from a tradition of community mobilization, have innovated care-giving for older persons through local NGOs and youth organizations; these state-level initiatives have often been far ahead of national policies, including in terms of support offered to unmarried older women, who are most often overlooked, and in terms of introducing dementia-friendly environments in some cities.[36]

Bottom-Up Approaches from Civil Society Groups

Efforts to implement the MIPAA have led to a growing role for international NGOs such as HelpAge International, through their national partners. In the years following Madrid, the International Association of Gerontology (IAG; now called the International Association for Gerontology and Geriatrics, or IAGG), the IFA, and HAI have continued to be influential in shaping national strategies for research and policies to implement the vision they helped frame in Madrid.[37] The IAG, for instance, was involved in promoting an Active Ageing Framework at its 18th Global Congress held in Brazil, which was attended by more than 4,000 participants, and works closely with the UN Program on Aging. Others have worked with national NGOs in helping frame policy interventions, such as the IFA's partnerships with NGOs in Cameroon, India, South Africa, and Uganda.[38]

Many of the international NGOs involved in aging today have been working on the issue since the 1970s. While this indicates an important continuity with the past, there are also noticeable changes in their more diverse membership and in their goals in the South. Experts from Asia and Africa are now increasingly filling up the leadership positions in the NGOs and building strong regional networks. Their ability to shape UN meetings, especially in Madrid where they were part of the negotiations, has expanded considerably, particularly as they are actively engaged in advocacy at the national and regional levels.

Yet how far these NGOs have influenced recent national-level aging policies is difficult to assess in concrete terms, as their impact has been uneven. They have the support of the UN agenda in the issues they advocate at a national level, but crucially, policy-related resources are still largely determined by national priorities. Despite considerable NGO-based advocacy in the South and Southeast Asia regions, funds for implementing national aging policies in these countries are still limited, according to a recent report.[39] NGO leaders, researchers, and health practitioners at a WHO-led forum in Valencia in 2002 urged governments to support "integrated health services" that would offer aging populations health and social services through community-based care, thus allowing older persons to be part of communities and families, but governments and see this as an NGO-led approach and have invested little in such services.[40] In Valencia, representatives from various countries agreed that this integrated approach was key to keeping older persons involved in activities or and ensuring their wellbeing, participation, and security, but inter-sectoral approaches, even between health and social welfare departments, have been difficult to coordinate and monitor.[41]

Thus the making of aging as a global issue needs to be judged less by the hubris of global conferences and leadership, of an expansive new order and intensity of engagements, and far more by continuities: colonial traditions in social and welfare policies, national networks and the experiences of local frictions and resistance in the sphere of social policies. Some

NGOs have moved toward this painstakingly by working with local institutions and experts. The influence of these NGOs in some cases is well entrenched, such as the early and persistent good relations HAI cultivated with governments such as Ghana's, relations which were mediated by local experts such as Professor Nana Apt, who attended IAG meetings in the 1980s, was exposed to international debates on aging, and, on returning to Ghana, conducted local studies and campaigned for aging programs.[42] This implies that even when funds were limited at a local level, because of this mix of experts and social workers, there were efforts to integrate services and programs for older persons within existing poverty alleviation programs and other development initiatives.

Further, the focus on national and regional resources is also significant because global aging as an agenda has lacked the large-scale, cross-sectoral funding and global health partnerships associated with other issues, such as HIV/AIDS and malaria. Large private foundations, such as the Bill and Melinda Gates Foundation, have so far not offered large grant opportunities for aging in global health. Rather, the support for large aging programs has inevitably come from development funds obtained mostly from national agencies that have often been pooled with grants from UN agencies and a few international NGOs.

Faith-Based Care and Private Partnerships

Both in global health and global social policy, there are actors whose influence has been underestimated, even though, in many societies, they represent the continuity of colonial networks and legacies. These groups, with old as well as new local connections, have been crucial in translating policies into practice and in providing services both in cities and in underserved areas. Christian charity has been reconfigured to offer, through faith-based networks, programs for poverty alleviation, livelihood training for older persons, and long-term care in the community. Some partnerships, such as those founded by Jesuit orders in Asia and Africa, have had strong and long-standing roots in caring for vulnerable groups, especially in urban settings, as we have seen in the case of social work training in Zimbabwe and the Indian Social Institute in New Delhi.[43]

The UN too had encouraged the Vatican to participate in deliberations on aging in the late 1970s to 1980s, partly since aging, as a new population issue distinct from the more divisive matter of population control, seemed less confrontational and more inclusive of Church views. With population control discussions failing to create common ground with the Holy See, for instance, the United Nations Population Fund (UNFPA) tried to involve Jesuit organizations in meetings preceding the Vienna Assembly. Monsignor Fahey, a Jesuit representative of the Holy See, recalled that, a few years after confrontations over population control at the World Population Conference in Bucharest (1974) had escalated, some of the UN leadership in New York wanted to let the church know "that we want them to be involved in aging initiatives such as at Vienna, and . . . we are not just interested in passing around contraceptives."[44]

At a meeting in Delhi in 1981, planned by Monsignor Fahey and supported by UNFPA funds, South Asian representatives from an urban social work background and from a Jesuit-supported research institute in India advanced a strong critique of national development policies' and international aid programs' failures. They identified poverty as the defining characteristic of the majority of the elderly in South Asia.[45] This intersection, between social experts in urban areas and Christian missions supporting research and training on aging, has been evident in the activities of the social work school Father Joseph Hampson led in Zimbabwe. Continuities in these services are evident all over Africa, in particular in the work of church orders in Francophone Africa.[46] The absence of religious organizations, which leads to a lack of religious or community services, can in fact pose a significant challenge to supporting families in caring for frail or sick old persons; experts in China organizing community services to support the aged and supplement family caregivers recently noted as much.[47]

Global aging has several scales and networks, and it continues to be characterized in some parts of the developing world by "sacred" rather than "secular" moorings, especially in the realm of caregiving. Professional associations such as the IAG, which promotes scientific and research-focused collaborations, and international NGOs such as HAI, which was rooted in Christian notions of humanitarian relief in the early years of its founding, work closely with the UN, are viewed as inhabiting the realm of mobilization and work, and are increasingly prominent in shaping policy advocacy. But it is clear that in many settings, the roles of faith-based organizations and even their cross-national networks are still barely recognized or studied. In nations where the state is still unable to provide basic social security or support, such as the Democratic Republic of Congo, where state-building efforts have been failing, the refuge provided by the Roman Catholic Church against elder abuse and witchcraft allegations in cities like Kinshasa has been notable. This is an under-researched field.[48]

In many developing countries, at sites and spaces where aging policies are being discussed, new players are now emerging—in particular, a second generation of private social entrepreneurs and experts, some from the private sector rather than the traditional fields of social work and government development programs. A "silver" market for drugs, devices, and care services is rapidly emerging in Asia. A few years ago, on a hot June afternoon, I attended the annual conference of the IFA in Hi-Tech City in Hyderabad, India. It was hosted by a motley group of organizers ranging from NGOs, founders of private hospitals, and "knowledge" partners consisting of the Tata Institute of Social Sciences, the Institute of Economic Growth, and the Indian Association of Gerontology.[49] I noticed a persistent and curious pattern of events at the meeting that was unusual in social policy conferences held in India: most sessions, papers, and presentations by experts were poorly attended, but a large number of participants at the conference met during, between, and outside of panel and pedantic discussions. A dense presence of enterprising small "social business" entrepreneurs and professionals made this conference vibrant beyond its formal agenda, attracting interest from India and abroad. Offerings of Ayurvedic therapy, health farms, services relating to telemedicine technologies for homecare, and information about innovative retirement communities jostled in an emerging new marketplace for a graying developing world. This is also at other conferences, such as at aging conferences in China, where the opening up of government regulations for investment in care services and institutions for older persons is leading to the entry of an influential market of private players, especially real-estate development companies and public-private partnerships founded between local officials and international investors.

Some questions, however, remain unanswered, even as these partnerships make inroads: What are the implications of these market-driven solutions, and how far will they bridge funding gaps in a sector such as aging that has already been seeing the retrenchment of public and welfare resources by the state? Are they possibly short-term solutions and injections of investments, awaiting long-term inputs from families, communities or governments, or does their growing presence imply that the UN is unlikely to invest more deeply in global aging as an agenda, given that global aging has had long-standing associations with decline, dependency, and care burdens and that it came of age in the 1970s and 1980s, when the UN system was already in decline or on a downturn?

At the same conference, however, there were also new alignments that have already been reflected in this study. The BRICS (Russia, China, India, South Africa, and Brazil, representing an alternative balance of global economic forces and governance) was the focus of presentations comparing aging policies in these emerging economies.[50] In recent years, experts and NGOs are discussing shared lessons between emerging economies as a means of understanding aging through new axes of geopolitical alignments and, possibly, of new resources.[51] Partners of the Global Alliance of International Longevity Centers, a network co-founded by Robert Butler, the first director of the National Institute on Aging in the United States, for instance, have been organizing meetings (since 2012) that have brought together debates on the role of BRICS nations and their aging programs.[52]

Change and Continuity

The politics of aging is now truly distanced from its earlier assumptions and paradigms, but it has also acquired new contradictions. In the past, Western preoccupations concerning decolonization, the Cold War, the burdens of social security and old age support ratios, or fears that the "productive" age groups were shrinking shaped narratives of age and aging. In Europe and North America today, these claims are increasingly contested with evidence that retirement-age thresholds need to be flexible, that enabling environments can be created for older persons, and that notions of chronological age need to be reviewed and replaced by other measures, such as functional and cognitive aging.[53]

New claims and interests from developing nations are also refashioning transnational politics relating to global aging. In considering aging in developing countries, the following aspects need to be kept in mind: it inevitably trains a spotlight on youth, who continue to form a large proportion of the population and promise what some term a "demographic dividend"; infectious disease burdens and chronic diseases coexist with aging; and families are both migrating but also continuing to provide support to the aged, although increasingly, they need more resources to fulfill their responsibilities. Migration has not immediately led to the neglect of older persons, who are often viewed as having been left behind, but the chief challenge remains that the states in Asia and Africa are, by and large, reluctant to take responsibility for pension funding and other social provisions, except perhaps for the poorest sections of population.[54] Moreover, the marginalized among the old—the rural poor, older women, and those employed mostly in the informal sector—are still seldom the main focus of these new interests, and programs to support active aging continue to be focused on urban populations.[55]

The need for a more universal approach through a binding international convention of human rights has been a growing focus of debate since 2012. UN member states and NGOs such as the IFA and HAI founded the Open-Ended Working Group on Ageing to begin addressing this need, but the debates are ongoing, and social protection and justice for the vulnerable sections of the aging population still fall by and large to national governments. Global aging's coming of age has not necessarily been based on more accurate information, nor has it triggered global alarm over the fate of the planet, as other issues, such as climate change, have. The Organization of African Unity document prepared for the Madrid meeting (2002) stated that, in several African countries, sharp gaps in information about who was old and the heterogeneous nature of the aging population persisted.

Aging has therefore made inroads as an international agenda in times of vulnerability. As a transnational agenda, it has waxed and waned based on perceived worries and crises produced by development in the global South, including during the 1970s and 1980s during the world economic crisis and, later, during humanitarian crises and disasters. In the 1950s, when Kingsley Davis and others expressed worries about aging as a new challenge, they were concerned about post–Second World War challenges regarding labor and productivity, and they feared the contamination of European models of welfare support for a dependent population of elders in the United States.

No doubt the Madrid Assembly had a powerful influence in shifting the discourse from an emphasis on dependence to claims regarding the productivity of older persons and on arguments about core aging issues concerning all generations. But moving away from the historical legacies, or what were perceived as "traditional" stigmas about the old being needy and dependent, has been challenging. And various groups and societies have experienced the price of "visibility" in making aging a global agenda differently. International NGOs and experts have certainly gained in terms of increasingly being "gatekeepers," managing local NGOs, leading old persons' mobilization at the grassroots level, and communicating their concerns at various levels. In a movement that has lacked an assigned UN agency to pursue its interests and budgets between conferences, these advocates have been remarkably proactive.

In terms of an intellectual history of ideas, the power and advocacy of experts has drawn attention to, and partly succeeded in redefining, the suffering of older persons, particularly in the Third World, in the language of human rights and of productivity and development. As we saw in the last chapter, HAI and the IFA identified new "political" spaces and distressing events, including older persons' abandonment in refugee camps or abuse within families. This has meant that international NGOs built a moral discourse of suffering using an emotive vocabulary and social science tools such as local surveys, reports, and assessments that have dramatized the near-permanent crises-ridden situations and precarity in these societies. By doing so, they could project distinct needs and put forth a blueprint for development that differs from development in the West. This has allowed critical spaces to emerge for debate about how development and modernization might have alternative trajectories.

Teleological narratives have sometimes been rejected only to be recast in new ways. An emphasis on an "alternative" pathway for societies in the global South still emphasizes the notion of a progress-based, evolutionary narrative of productive aging with a final end.[56] It promises that there are demographic, or in this case gerontological dividends to be collected globally in societies that manage aging successfully, even though reversals in development have often been in evidence. This addresses the stigma of dependence and marginality associated with aging and anxieties about slowing economies, especially in the global South, but it also raises questions—with few answers—about the availability of care for the frail and vulnerable and about whether governments will shoulder their fair share of responsibility along with families.

Aging thus emerges today as a global agenda that highlights a compelling moral discourse of humanitarian empathy, need, and vulnerability. Its votaries often lead advocacy campaigns promising that research and programs demonstrate continuing productivity and gerontological dividends in aging societies. Despite these assertions, aging populations are associated closely with development and modernization, and they continue to be viewed either as a sorry, marginalized fallout of these processes or as impeding them through old-age dependency on care and support. We find that this ideas and tropes have been cast and recast in new vocabularies for the past many decades. Aging policies still lag behind in global resources and campaigns as they compete for support in a world of global health that prioritizes magic bullet–like "cures" and technocentric interventions. Its complexities make many reluctant to address it, for its scope extends far beyond the confines of chronological age, and it requires local, contextual histories and knowledge of family roles, social disparities, and welfare. Aging needs to be seen as coupled with these issues rather than distinct from them, as these issues will make it, increasingly, the defining focus of our societies.

Abbreviations

AARP	American Association for Retired Persons
AGHE	Association for Gerontology in Higher Education
ASWEA	Association for Social Work Education in Africa
CRA	Club for Research on Aging
DFID	Department for International Development
ECAFE	Economic Commission for Asia and the Far East
FSA	Federal Security Agency
HAI	HelpAge International
HRAF	Human Relations Area Files
IAG	International Association of Gerontology
ICSG	International Center for Social Gerontology
IFA	International Federation on Aging
IGC	International Gerontological Congress
MDG	Millennium Development Goals
MIPAA	Madrid International Plan of Action on Ageing, United Nations
NIA	National Institute of Aging
NIEO	New International Economic Order
NIH	National Institutes of Health
NSP	Nathan Shock Papers
PIC	Population Investigation Committee

RLI	Rhodes Livingstone Institute
SDG	Sustainable Development Goals, United Nations
SSRC	Social Science Research Council
UICC	Union for International Cancer Control (earlier, International Union Against Cancer)
UNHCR	United High Commission for Refugees
WAA	World Assembly on Aging, organized by the United Nations, held in Vienna (First World Assembly, 1982) and in Madrid (Second World Assembly, 2002)
WFI	White Fathers' [Pères Blancs] inquiry
WL	Wellcome Library

Notes

Introduction

1. *Report, African Conference of Gerontology*, Dakar, December 10–14, 1984, under the patronage of HE Mr. Abdou Diouf, president of the Republic of Senegal, organized by the Government of Senegal with the International Center for Social Gerontology, in collaboration with the UN, UNESCO, and UNFPA (n.p., 1984), 9–21.

2. Several UN representatives posted in Africa and from Geneva were present in Dakar, as were experts from the NGO HelpAge International, leading American and European members of gerontological associations, and rural development experts and social workers from Senegal and across Africa. It was supported by funds from UN agencies and from international gerontological associations. Others heard about the Dakar meeting by word of mouth and tried to plan their own versions to discuss the needs of aging populations (interview with Father Joseph Hampson, missionary, social worker, and participant at the Dakar Conference, April and June 2015. Hampson is a founding figure of the School of Social Service in Harare, Zimbabwe; in 1985, he was the director of fieldwork at the School of Social Service).

3. I am grateful to my friend and colleague Isabella Aboderin, head of the Aging and Development Unit at the African Population and Health Research Center, for offering a discussion of these new Africa plans. The 2063 vision meeting began to be articulated in a series of consultations held in Addis Ababa, Ethiopia, in May 2013.

4. Massimo Livi-Bacci, *A Concise History of World Population*, 5th ed. (London: Wiley Blackwell, 2012); John Bongaarts, "Human Population Growth and the

Demographic Transition," *Philosophical Transactions of the Royal Society B: Biological Sciences* 364, no. 1532 (October 27, 2009): 2985–90. The change in the age structures of populations around the world and its demographic determinants are discussed in the *World Population Aging, 2015* report published by the United Nations, Department of Economic and Social Affairs, Population Division, ST/ESA/SER.A/390 (New York, United Nations).

5. David Bloom, David Canning, and Pia Malaney, "Demographic Change and Economic Growth in Asia," in *Population Change in East Asia*, a supplement to *Population and Development Review* 26 (2000), 257–90; P. N. Mari Bhat, "Mortality and Fertility in India, 1881–1961: A Reassessment," in *India's Historical Demography: Studies in Famine, Disease and Society*, ed. Tim Dyson (London: Curzon Press, 1989), 73–118.

6. United Nations, Economic Commission for Africa, *The State of Older People in Africa, 2007: Regional Review and Appraisal of the Madrid International Plan of Action on Aging* (New York: United Nations Division for Social Policy and Development Aging, 2007), 12. See also UN Department of Social Affairs and Economic Division, *World Population Aging 2015*, ST/ESA/SER.A/390 (New York: United Nations, 2015).

7. UN Department of Social Affairs and Economic Division, *World Population Aging 2015*, 1–2.

8. I use the word *dominant* here to indicate its influence in international mobilization around aging, although, as this book demonstrates, these ideas were being increasingly recast by experts in the South. Social policy experts such as Lloyd-Sherlock, writing on the eve of the Second World Assembly on Aging (2002) have said Western experiences' influence on global aging are shaped by concerns about withdrawal, dependency, physical frailty, and pensioner status—quite distinct from the concerns of many rapidly aging nations in the global South, where there is still a young labor force and social policies have mostly focused on other age groups, such as children and mothers, or on the poorest strata below the poverty line, leaving a gap in social and health policies that needs to include older persons as a distinct constituency for the first time. Lloyd Sherlock, "Social Policy and Population Aging: Challenges from North and South," *International Journal of Epidemiology* 31, no. 4 (2002): 754–57. See also Nana A. Apt, *Coping with Old Age in a Changing Africa: Social Change and the Elderly Ghanaian* (Aldershot: Avebury, 1996); Lawrence Cohen, *No Aging in India: Senility and the Family* (Delhi: Oxford University Press, 1999).

9. United Nations, *World Assembly on Aging* (henceforth WAA), A/CONF 113/22, Annex (New York: United Nations, 1982), 7–8.

10. The improvement in mortality rates due to improved nutrition, improved public health measures, and, more important, because of a decline in birth

rates resulted in an increasing proportion of persons surviving into the advanced stages of life across the world. UN projections noted that in 1950, there were about 200 million persons who were sixty years of age and over throughout the world; by 1975, this figure had increased to 350 million, with the rate of growth of older persons in developing countries increasing rapidly. See "International Plan of Action on Aging: I Introduction," UN Documents: Gathering a Body of Global Agreements, www.un-documents.net/ipaa-1.htm.

11. For a discussion of the influence of Bertillion, Alfred Sauvy, and other French demographers and statisticians had on the perception of "population aging," see Claudine Sauvain-Dugerdil, Henri Léridon, and C. G. N. Mascie-Taylor, *Human Clocks: The Bio-Cultural Meanings of Age* (Bern: Peter Lang, 2006), 264–67. The authors argue that nineteenth-century notions of the "immutability" of old age persisted and were associated with an unchanging "age of old age" or a "threshold age" with negative connotations relating to pensions, defense, and economic development, and that these notions colored even reports such as the Committee of Enquiry into the Problems of the Elderly's Laroque report later in the twentieth century. A "statistical category" increasingly began to prevail over any tendency to blur age categories. For a nuanced analysis of these questions relating to the emergence of population aging as a statistical category, see Patrice Bourdelais, "The Aging of the Population: Relevant Question or Obsolete Notion?," in *Old Age: From Antiquity to Postmodernity*, ed. Paul Johnson and Pat Thane (London: Routledge, 1998), 110–12. For other notions of aging, see Bernice Neugarten, ed., *The Meanings of Age* (Chicago: University of Chicago Press, 1996); Peter Laslett, "Societal Development and Aging," in *Handbook of Aging and the Social Sciences*, ed. R. Binstock and Ethel Shanas (New York: Van Nostrand Reinhold, 1976), 87–116; John Vincent, "Aging Contested: Anti-Aging Science and the Cultural Construction of Old Age," *Sociology* 40, no. 4 (2006): 681–98.

12. *Report, African Conference of Gerontology*, 9–10

13. Walter Fernandes, "Aging in South Asia as Marginalization in a Neo-Colonial Economy: An Introduction," in *Aging in South Asia: Theoretical Issues and Policy Implications*, papers presented at the Asian Regional Conference on Active Aging, Manila, 1982, sponsored by the UNFPA and Opera Pia International, ed. Alfred de Souza and Walter Fernandes (New Delhi: Indian Social Institute, 1982), 1–13. The cosponsor Opera Pia International was an international Catholic charity founded to mobilize church leadership throughout the world, especially in developing countries, to participate in the World Assembly on Aging (1982). One of its founders, Erdman Ballagh Palmore, wrote the *Handbook of the Aged in the United States* (Westport, CT: Greenwood Press, 1984). See Andrew W. Achenbaum and Daniel M. Albert, *Profiles in Gerontology: A Biographical Dictionary* (Westport, CT: Greenwood Press, 1995), 117

for a discussion of the role played by Father Charles J. Fahey from the Diocese of Syracuse, who was the representative of the Holy See at the WAA and founded institutions that promoted education and training in the "Third Age."

14. Fernandes, "Aging in South Asia as Marginalization in a Neo-Colonial Economy," 11.

15. Ibid., 8.

16. I have retained the term and category "developing countries" here based on its common and politicized usage in the 1980s, referring to decolonized, industrializing societies and distinct from industrially advanced, "developed" nations in the West. The term emerged during the development decades in the 1960s, replacing terms such as "backward societies" and "traditional societies," and was synonymous with the "Third World" as coined by the French demographer Albert Sauvy. I also borrow from the work of Dipesh Chakrabarty, in his analysis of the marginalization of non-European histories and of the remaking of Western knowledge in non-Western settings. Dipesh Chakrabarty, *Provincializing Europe: Postcolonial Thought and Historical Difference* (Princeton: Princeton University Press, 2000). I have used ideas from Ashis Nandy, ed., *Science, Hegemony and Violence: A Requiem for Modernity* (New Delhi: Oxford University Press, 1988), and from writings by Warwick Anderson on postcolonial science. Warwick Anderson, "Postcolonial Techno-Science," *Social Studies in Science* 32, nos. 5–6 (2002): 643–58.

17. Central Intelligence Agency, *Long-Term Global Demographic Trends: Reshaping the Political Landscape* (Langley, VA, July 2001); Richard Jackson and Neil Howe, *The Graying of the Great Powers: Demography and Geopolitics in the 21st Century* (Washington, DC: Center for Strategic and International Studies, 2008); Peter G. Peterson, *Gray Dawn: How the Coming Age Wave Will Transform America and the* World (New York: Three Rivers Press, 2000). For a framing of global demographic shifts, see *World Population Aging: Highlights, 2015* (New York: UN, DESA, 2015), 1–6, www.un.org/esa/population/publications/worldageing; *Global Aging: Aging in Africa*, www.global-ageing.eu/agafrica.html.

18. Mark L. Hass, "A Geriatric Peace: The Future of US Power in a World of Aging Populations," *International Security* 32, no. 1 (2007): 112–47.

19. David E. Bloom, David Canning, and Gunther Fink, "Implications of Population Aging for Economic Growth," NBER Working Paper no. 16705, January 2011, http://www.nber.org/papers/w16705.

20. United Nations, *World Population Aging: 1950–2050*, ST/ESA/SER.A/207 (New York: Department of Economic and Social Affairs, Population Division, UN, 2001).

21. Ibid.

22. I draw here primarily from the work of Matt Connelly and Alison Bashford on the subject of population control movements and their neo-Malthusian ethos

and geopolitics. Matt Connelly, *Fatal Misconception: The Struggle to Control World Population* (Cambridge: Harvard University Press, 2008); Alison Bashford, "Nation, Empire, Globe: The Spaces of Population Debate in the Interwar Years," *Comparative Studies in Society and History* 49, no. 1 (2007): 170–201. Other notable works on international development, the politics of population growth, and anxieties about imperial power and population decline include John Sharpless, "Population Science, Private Foundations, and Development Aid: The Transformation of Demographic Knowledge in the United States, 1945–65," in *International Development and the Social Sciences: Essays on the History and Politics of Knowledge*, ed. Fred Cooper and Randall Packard (Berkeley: University of California Press, 1997), 176–202; Michael Teitelbaum and Jay Winter, *The Fear of Population Decline* (Orlando, FL: Academic Press, 1985). Sharpless, Teitelbaum, and Winter discuss how France and Italy, among other nations, voiced fears of "denatalite" (de-natality) in the face of falling birth rates and feared threats to imperial power and "national grandeur" early in the twentieth century.

23. Several of Foucault's works discuss these efforts to impose a homogeneity on old age and to delimit it. See *Discipline and Punish* (London: Tavistock, 1977), 184–85 and *The History of Sexuality* (Harmondsworth: Penguin, 1976). For a discussion of his influences on gerontology and the place of the professional and intellectual power of gerontologists and gerontology and other aging fields, see Stephen Katz, *Disciplining Old Age: The Formation of Gerontological Knowledge* (Charlottesville: University of Virginia, 1996).

24. Ian Hacking, *The Social Construction of What?* (Cambridge: Harvard University Press, 2000).

25. Social policy advocates such as Carol Estes have critiqued those who projected aging as an "enterprise" or its commodification and suggested alternate vocabularies for and perspectives on aging. C. L. Estes and E. Binney, "The Biomedicalization of Aging: Dangers and Dilemmas," *Gerontologist* 29 (1989): 587–96; C. L. Estes, *The Aging Enterprise* (San Francisco: Jossey Bass, 1979). For other critiques, see Pat Thane, "Social Histories of Old Age and Aging," *Journal of Social History* 37 (2003), 93–111; Patrice Bourdelais, *L'Age de la Vieillesse: Histoire Du Vieillissement de la Population* (Paris: Editions O. Jacob, 1997); Anne-Marie Guillemard, *Aging and the Welfare Crisis* (Newark: University of Delaware Press, 2000).

26. Some notable historical studies offer critiques of the medical and technological paradigms that shaped colonial health history and the international development led by colonial authority, scientific experts, missionaries, local leaders, and international foundations; see David Arnold, "Introduction: Disease, Medicine and Empire," in *Imperial Medicine and Indigenous Societies* (Manchester: Manchester University Press, 1988), 1–26; Arnold, *Colonizing the*

Body (Berkeley: University of California Press, 1993); Arnold "Nehruvian Science and Postcolonial India," *Isis* 104, no. 2 (June 2013): 360–70; Alison Bashford, "Global Biopolitics and the History of World Health," *History of the Human Sciences* 19 (2006): 67–88; Heather Bell, *Frontiers of Medicine in the Anglo-Egyptian Sudan, 1899–1940* (Oxford: Clarendon Press, 1999); Sanjoy Bhattacharya, *Expunging Variola: The Control and Eradication of Smallpox in India, 1947–1977* (New Delhi: Orient Longman, 2006); Nandini Bhattacharya, *Contagion and Enclaves: Tropical Medicine in Colonial India* (Liverpool: Liverpool University Press, 2012); Marcus Cueto, *Cold War Deadly Fevers: Malaria Eradication in Mexico (1955–75)* (Baltimore: Johns Hopkins University Press, 2007); Andrew Cunningham and Bridie Andrews, eds., *Western Medicine as Contested Knowledge* (Manchester: Manchester University Press, 1997); John Farley, *To Cast Out Disease: A History of the International Health Division of the Rockefeller Foundation (1913–1951)* (New York: Oxford University Press, 2004); Achintya Kumar Dutta, "*Kala-Azar* in Assam: British Medical Intervention and People's Response," in *Maladies, Preventives and Curatives*, ed. A. K. Bagchi and K. Soman (New Delhi: Tulika Books, 2005), 15–31; Soma Hewa, "The Hookworm Epidemic on the Plantations in Colonial Sri Lanka," *Medical History* 38 (1994): 73–90; Sarah Hodges, "The Global Menace," *Social History of Medicine* 25 (2012): 719–28; Richard C. Keller, "Geographies of Power, Legacies of Mistrust: Colonial Medicine in the Global Present," *Historical Geography* 34 (2006): 26–48; Lenore Manderson, *Sickness and the State: Health and Illness in Colonial Malaya, 1870–1940* (Cambridge: Cambridge University Press, 1996); Laurence Monnais and H. J. Cook, eds., *Global Movements, Local Concerns: Medicine and Health in Southeast Asia* (Singapore: NUS Press, 2012); Randall Packard, *White Plague, Black Labor: Tuberculosis and the Political Economy of Health and Disease in South Africa* (Los Angeles: University of California Press, 1989); Gyan Prakash, *Another Reason: Science and the Imagination of Modern India* (Princeton: Princeton University Press, 1999); Amy Staples, *The Birth of Development: How the World Bank, Food and Agriculture, and World Health Organization Changed the World, 1945–1965* (Ohio: Kent State University Press, 2006); Sujit Sivasundaram, "Sciences and the Global: On Methods, Questions, and Theory," *Isis* 101, no. 1 (2010): 146–58; Megan Vaughan, *Curing Their Ills: Colonial Power and African Illness* (Stanford, Stanford University Press, 1991). For a discussion of the colonies such as the West Indies and India as sites and spaces of medical innovation, see Mark Harrison, *Medicine in the Age of Commerce and Empire: Britain and Its Tropical Colonies, 1660–1830* (Oxford: Oxford University Press, 2010).

27. Packard attributes these silos partly to the convenience of academic divisions in labor and calls for greater probing of "entanglements." See Randall M. Packard, *A History of Global Health: Interventions in the Lives of Other People*

(Baltimore: Johns Hopkins University Press, 2016), 1–14, 133–37. For an interesting discussion of the shifts in focus and politics from international to global health, see Allan Brandt, "How AIDS Invented Global Health," *New England Journal of Medicine* 388, no. 23 (June 6, 2013): 2149–52.

28. A few significant histories have focused on key intersectionalities in colonial and international health, traced regional/local perspectives, and provided critiques of ideological paradigms and normative epidemiological and policy assumptions in international and global health, such as Sunil Amrith, *Decolonizing International Health: India and Southeast Asia, 1930–65* (Basingstoke: Palgrave, 2006); Warwick Anderson, "Where Is the Postcolonial History of Medicine?" *Bulletin of the History of Medicine* 72 (1998): 522–30; Julie Livingston, *Improvising Medicine: An African Oncology Ward* (Durham: Duke University Press, 2012); Randall Packard, *A History of Global Health* (Baltimore: Johns Hopkins University Press, 2016); Anne-Emanuelle Birn and Theodore Brown, eds. *Comrades in Health: US Health Internationalists, Abroad and at Home* (New Brunswick, NJ: Rutgers University Press, 2013); Laurence Monnais and David Wright, eds., *Doctors Beyond Borders: The Transnational Migration of Physicians in the 20th Century* (Toronto: University of Toronto Press, 2016); Helen Tilley, *Africa as a Living Laboratory: Empire, Development and the Problem of Scientific Knowledge, 1870–1950* (Chicago: University of Chicago Press, 2011); and David Arnold, "Diabetes in the Tropics: Race, Place and Class in India, 1880–1965," *Social History of Medicine* 22, no. 2 (2009): 245–61.

29. Mark Nichter, *Global Health: Why Cultural Perceptions, Social Representations, and Biopolitics Matter* (Tucson: University of Arizona Press, 2008); see also Laëtitia Atlani-Duault and Laurent Vidal, "Le moment de la santé globale," *Revue Tiers Monde* 215, no. 3 (2013): 7–16.

30. In the West, aging in international policy debates has largely engaged attention as an issue related to social marginalization, pension reform, chronic disease, flows of capital, and financing of care and, until recently, far less in terms of intergenerational relations and disparities. Some significant exceptions to this perspective in the field of aging research apply. These include the work of Martin Kohli, Simon Biggs, Elise Feller, Sheila Neysmith, and Chris Phillipson, to name a few of the notable scholars working at the intersections of sociology, psychology, critical social gerontology, and social work on questions of intergenerational relations, social and ethnic identities, and unpaid family care in settings such as Germany, Australia, France, Canada, and the United Kingdom.

31. Ernest Burgess, ed., *Aging in Western Societies* (Chicago: University of Chicago Press 1960). See also Ethel Shanas et al., *Old People in Three Industrial Societies* (New York: Atherton, 1968); and Wilma Donahue and Clark

Tibbitts, "European Approaches to Aging," *Public Health Reports* 70, no. 6 (June 1955): 581–84.

32. Burgess, *Aging in Western Societies.*

33. The spread of civilization in this case was imbued with Cold War connotations of the spread of both democracy and development; both were interlinked in this thinking. Clark Tibbitts and Wilma Donahue, *Aging in Today's Society* (Englewood Cliffs, NJ: Prentice-Hall, 1960), xvii.

34. Abdel R. Omran, "The Epidemiologic Transition: A Theory of the Epidemiology of Population Change," *Milbank Memorial Fund Quarterly* 49, no. 4 (1971): 509–38.

35. Julie Livingston, *Improvising Medicine: An African Oncology Ward in an Emerging Cancer Epidemic* (Durham: Duke University Press, 2012); George Weisz, *Chronic Disease in the Twentieth Century: A History* (Baltimore: Johns Hopkins University Press, 2014).

36. The epidemiological transition originated as a model in demography and has had wide uptake in public health. It implies changing patterns of population-age distributions, mortality, fertility, life expectancy, and causes of death. Central to the model it represents are changes in patterns of mortality (including increasing life expectancy and reordering the relative importance of different causes of death, including a shift to chronic, "lifestyle" diseases). The rise of cancer and heart disease in the United States and Europe in the early twentieth century, for instance, reflected their transition from receding pandemics to degenerative and manmade diseases. There have been several critiques of it including by John Caldwell. Others have argued that it was advanced at a time of "naïve optimism" about the elimination of diseases and did not take into account nutrition, poverty, income inequalities, and "the global nature and historical sequence of the mortality transition as it spread." John C. Caldwell, "Population Health in Transition," *Bulletin of the World Health Organization* 79 (2001): 159–60; Robert E. McKeown, "The Epidemiologic Transition: Changing Patterns of Mortality and Population Dynamics," *America Journal of Lifestyle Medicine* 3, 1 Supplement (2009): 19S–26S; Abdel R. Omran, "The Epidemiologic Transition: A Theory of the Epidemiology of Population Change," *The Milbank Quarterly* 83, no. 4 (2005): 731–57; Omran, "The Epidemiologic Transition Theory Revisited Thirty Years Later," *World Health Statistics Quarterly* 51 (1998): 99–119. For contemporary references to these debates, see Richard Horton, "The Neglected Epidemic of Chronic Disease," *The Lancet* 366 (2005): 1514 and "Non-Communicable Diseases: 2015 to 2025," *The Lancet* 381 (February 2013): 509–10.

37. Julio Frenk, Joseé L. Bobadilla, Jaime Sepúlveda, and Malaquias López Cervantes, "Health Transition in Middle-Income Countries: New Challenges for Health Care," *Health Policy and Planning* 4, no. 1 (1989): 29–39; Lenore

Manderson and Carolyn Smith-Morris, *Chronic Conditions, Fluid States: Chronicity and the Anthropology of Illness* (New Brunswick, NJ: Rutgers University Press, 2010). See James Ferguson's work for explorations of alternative trajectories to these ideas in the context of Sub-Saharan countries that have been undergoing a "counter-transition" leading to a reversal of falling mortality trends. James Ferguson, *Expectations of Modernity: Myths and Meanings of Urban Life on the Zambian Copperbelt* (Berkeley: University of California Press, 1999).

38. Chakrabarty, *Provincializing Europe*.

39. Ibid.

40. John Sharpless, "Population Science, Private Foundations, and Development Aid: The Transformation of Demographic Knowledge in the United States, 1945–65," in *International Development and the Social Sciences: Essays on the History and Politics of Knowledge*, ed. Fred Cooper and Randall Packard (Berkeley: University of California Press, 1997), 21, 176–202; Matt Connelly, *Fatal Misconception: The Struggle to Control World Population* (Cambridge: Harvard University Press, 2008); Alison Bashford, "Nation, Empire, Globe: The Spaces of Population Debate in the Interwar Years," *Comparative Studies in Society and History* 49, no. 1 (2007): 170–201.

41. The following works focus on Peace Corps volunteers and social workers: Sunil Amrith, *Decolonizing International Health: India and Southeast Asia, 1930–65* (New York: Palgrave Macmillan, 2006); Sanjoy Bhattacharya, *Expunging Variola: The Control and Eradication of Smallpox in India, 1947–1977* (New Delhi: Orient Longman, 2006); Matt Connelly, *Fatal Misconception: The Struggle to Control World Population* (Cambridge: Harvard University Press, 2008); Frederick Cooper and Randall M. Packard, eds., *International Development and the Social Sciences: Essays on the History and Politics of Knowledge* (Berkeley: University of California Press, 1997); Nick Cullather, *The Hungry World: America's Cold War Battle against Poverty in Asia* (Cambridge: Harvard University Press, 2010); Inderjeet Parmar, *Foundations of the American Century: The Ford, Carnegie, and Rockefeller Foundations in the Rise of American Power* (New York: Columbia University Press, 2014); Daniel Immerwahr, *Thinking Small: The United States and the Lure of Community Development* (Cambridge: Harvard University Press, 2015); James Midgley, *Professional Imperialism: Social Work in the Third World*, Studies in Social Policy and Welfare, vol. 16 (London: Heinemann, 1981). I am grateful to Elana Sulakshana for having brought Nicole Sackley's work to my notice: Nicole Sackley, "Foundation in the Field: The Ford Foundation New Delhi Office and the Construction of Development Knowledge, 1951–1970," in *American Foundations and the Coproduction of World Ordering the Twentieth Century* (Göttingen, Germany: Vandenhoeck & Ruprecht, 2012). There are

many historically framed studies of the politics of expertise in international and global health; see for instance Johanna Tayloe Crane, *Scrambling for Africa: AIDS, Expertise, and the Rise of American Global Health Science* (Ithaca, NY: Cornell University Press, 2013).

42. For a discussion that shifts attention away from Cold War rivalries to French colonial experts and the WHO, see Jessica Pearson-Patel, "French Colonialism and the Battle against the WHO Regional Office for Africa," *Hygiea Internationals: An Interdisciplinary Journal for the History of Public Health* 13, no. 1 (2016): 65–80.

43. UN General Assembly, Declaration of Old Age Rights: Draft Resolution / Argentina: 30/09/1948A/C.3/213, September 30, 1948, UN Library, New York. See http://research.un.org/en/undhr/ga/thirdcommittee.

44. A lack of comparative research and disaggregated information based on age continued to nag international experts even at the Second World Assembly on Aging held in Madrid (2002). *United Nations, The Aging: Trends and Policies* (New York: United Nations, 1975); UN General Assembly, *Follow-up to the Second World Assembly on Aging Report of the Secretary-General*, 58th Session, Item 109, 17 July 2003, Document A/58/160 (New York: United Nations, 2003), 7–8.

45. An initial study of the aged was conducted in 1948 in recognition of the rights of old persons. Resolution 213-III, 1948 by the Economic and Social Council. See *Official Records of the Economic and Social Council*, Eleventh Session, Supplement no. 3, Chapter II, Section C (c) (UN Depository, New York) at Columbia University, Law Library for UN General Assembly Resolutions. For an outline of these studies, see *United Nations, The Aging: Trends and Policies*, 2–6, 5.

46. Florence Palmer, "The World Assembly on the Elderly and the World Health Organization," in *The UN World Assembly on the Elderly The Aging as a Resource: The Aging as a Concern and The Situation of the Elderly in Austria*, ed. Charlotte Nusberg, Proceedings of the Two Meetings Organized by the International Federation on Aging, May 27–29, 1980, Vienna, Austria (Washington, DC: International Federation on Aging, 1981), 8.

47. "Old" in these surveys was defined as sixty years and above in age, though it clearly conveyed little in terms of their functional condition, especially in the case of the rural or urban poor who died in old age in what some termed a "euphemism for death due to starvation." For a discussion of old age and the effects of poverty in the 1970s in South India, see Goran Djurfeldt and Staffan Lindberg, *Pills against Poverty: A Study of the Introduction of Western Medicine in a Tamil Village* (New Delhi: Macmillan, 1980), 94. See also a wider discussion in Alfred De Souza and Walter Fernandes, eds., *Aging in South Asia: Theoretical Issues and Policy Implications* (New Delhi: Indian Social Institute, 1982), 11–15.

48. John Illife, in his carefully nuanced work on poverty in urban Africa, describes a lack of "social identification" associated with those old people who had drifted to the city without families or other ties. Illife, *The African Poor*, 166.

49. Ibid.

50. Tout, *Aging in Developing Countries*, 47, 52.

51. For an interesting discussion on some of these challenges and approaches, see Maxine Berg, ed., *Writing the History of the Global: Challenges for the Twenty-First Century*, British Academy Original Paperback Series (Oxford: Oxford University Press, 2012).

52. I am grateful to Anne-Emanuelle Birn for discussions on these aspects, especially on social policy and equity debates relating to older persons in Latin America, in particular Argentina.

53. For an account of Latin American countries' ties with the International Association of Gerontology, such as the first regional meeting held in Mexico (1956), see Liliana Gastron and Gerardo Gastron, "Medio siglo de gerontología en Latinoamérica," *Revista Espanola de Geriatria y Gerontologia* 33, no. 5 (1998): 309–13; and *Revista Argentina de Gerontología y Geriatría Año* 28 (April 2011): 8–22. Peter Lloyd-Sherlock's work discusses population aging in Argentina and other sites in Asia and Africa. See *Population Aging and International Development: From Generalisation to Evidence* (Bristol, UK: Policy Press, 2010). In the case of Brazil, see Otávio T. Nóbrega, Vicente P. Faleiros, and José L. Telles, "Gerontology in the Developing Brazil: Achievements and Challenges in Public Policies," *Geriatrics & Gerontology International*, 2 (June 2009): 135–39; Silva Ana Lucia, "Population Aging in Brazil: Current and Future Social Challenges and Consequences," *Revista Brasileira de Geriatria e Gerontologia* 19, no. 3 (September 2016): 507–19.

1

Old Age in Young Nations

1. Robert R. Kuczynski, *Colonial Population* (1937; New York: Negro Universities Press, 1969), vii. In particular, in telling the age of a man you have never seen.

2. Emphasis added. Granville P. Edge, *Vital Records in the Tropics* (London: George Routledge and Sons, 1932), 45, 43. I am grateful to Helen Tilley for pointing me to Granville Edge's work. I want to thank Lawrence Cohen and Gregory Mann for their critical input on this chapter concerning the role of anthropologists, their early studies of social change, customary law, and the role of elders in African history.

3. Mario I. Aguilar, *The Politics of Age and Gerontocracy in Africa: Ethnographies of the Past and Memories of the Present* (Trenton, NJ: Africa World Press, 1998) and a later edited work on rethinking age in Africa published in Mario I. Aguilar,

Rethinking Age in Africa: Colonial, Post-Colonial and Contemporary Interpreta-tions of Cultural Representations (Trenton, NJ: Africa World Press, 2007); and Fred Cooper, *Citizenship between Empire and Nation: Remaking France and French Africa, 1945–1960* (Princeton: Princeton University Press, 2014). Many works discuss the fundamental importance of the politics of age and gerontoc-racies in Africa that shaped these categories; these works also tie the politics of age and gerontocracies in Africa with questions of disciplining and mobilizing labor. In these decades of decolonization, anxieties grew among colonial administrators in Africa about the erosion of gerontocratic discipline and values as well as the "blockages" of generations that were creating new and unstable identities.

4. David Victor Glass, *Population Policies and Movements in Europe* (1940; London: Frank Cass and Company, 1967), 1–85; Simon Szreter, *Fertility, Class and Gender in Britain, 1860–1940* (Cambridge: Cambridge University Press, 1996), 9–21.

5. C. P. Blacker, "The Future of Our Population," *Eugenic Review* 28, no. 3 (1936): 211.

6. Ibid.

7. Pat Thane's work discusses the anxieties about loss of power in the colonies that Keynes voiced. Pat Thane, *Old Age in English History: Past Experiences, Present Issues* (Oxford: Oxford University Press, 2000); Pat Thane, "The Debate on the Declining Birth-Rate in Britain: The 'Menace' of an Ageing Population, 1920s–1950s," *Continuity and Change* 5, no. 2 (1990): 283–305. See also Lesley Hall, "Malthusian Mutations: The Changing Politics and Moral Meanings of Birth Control in Britain," in *Malthus, Medicine and Morality*, ed. Brian Dolan (Amsterdam: Rodopi, 2000), 141–63.

8. Carr Saunders, "Europe's Falling Birth Rate," *Daily Telegraph*, September 15, 1937.

9. Recent historical research has explored the roles of demographic experts and population science in influencing a late colonial agenda of population policies and development, in particular the focus on mapping population growth and growth rates of African colonies. Karl Ittmann, "Demography as Policy Science in the British Empire, 1918–1969," *Journal of Policy History* 15 (2003): 426.

10. See Thane, *Old Age in English History*.

11. Fred Cooper, *Decolonization and African Society: The Labor Question in French and British Africa* (New York: Cambridge University Press, 1996), 58–60. The disturbances in the West Indies in particular catalyzed the passing of the Colonial Development and Welfare Act, 1940.

12. Karl Ittmann, *A Problem of Great Importance: Population, Race and Power in the British Empire, 1918–1973* (Berkeley: University of California Press, 2013); Karl Ittmann, Dennis D. Cordell, and Gregory H. Maddox, eds., *The Demo-*

graphics of Empire: The Colonial Order and the Creation of Knowledge (Columbus: Ohio University Press, 2010).

13. For a view from the colony, see Partha Chatterjee's discussion of colonial Bengal in his edited book *Texts of Power: Emerging Disciplines in Colonial Bengal* (Minneapolis: University of Minnesota Press, 1995), 1–29.

14. Pierre Gourou, "French Indo-China: Demographic Imbalance and Colonial Policy," *Population Index* 11 (1945), 68–81; Gourou, *Les Paysans du Delta Tonkinois*, Etude de Géographie Humaine (Paris: EFEO, 1936). For a discussion of Pierre Gourou's contribution to colonial geography, for instance, see John Kleinen, "Tropicality and Topicality: Pierre Gourou and the Genealogy of French Scholarship on Rural Vietnam," *Singapore Journal of Tropical Geography* 26, no. 3 (2005), 339–58.

15. *Congrès international de la population*, Paris, 1937 (Paris: Hermann, 1938). The meeting produced eight dense volumes of papers on demographic theories, historical demography, and demographic trends.

16. PIC, *The Future of Our Population*, PP/ROG/C.13/2 Series 2, Wellcome Library, London (henceforth WL).

17. Kuczynski mentions this in the preface of *Colonial Populations*.

18. Carnegie Grant Application, Copy 20.10.37, PP, WL.

19. Alison Bashford, "Nation, Empire and Globe: The Spaces of Population Debate in the Inter War Years," *Comparative Studies in Society and History* 49, no. 1 (2007): 170–201.

20. For an insightful discussion of the emergence of demography as a field in the postwar empire and for an analysis of the work and networks of the PIC, see Karl Ittmann, *A Problem of Great Importance*, 26–27, 30–45. I am grateful to Professor Ittmann and Helen Tilley for generously sharing their leads and notes relating to the PIC and its key members as well as their insights about Malcolm Hailey and the Africa Survey with me. Helen Tilley's work has been an invaluable resource in understanding this complex research agenda and its politics. Helen Tilley, *Africa as a Living Laboratory: Empire, Development and the Problem of Scientific Knowledge, 1870–1950* (Chicago: University of Chicago Press, 2011).

21. Reginald Coupland, "The Hailey Survey," *Africa* 12 (January 1939), 10.

22. I use the term sub-Saharan Africa here and in other parts of this book (in this case, as employed by those reviewing and supportive of Kuczynski's work) as indicative of the lingering politics of colonial categories and donor-led generalizations in international health. Scholars have argued that it is a confusing term trying to identify a vast region and that it represents, in part, a replacement of essentializing notions and geographies such as "tropical" Africa, with the implication that Africa is "one country."

23. R. R. Kuczynski, *The Cameroons and Togoland: A Demographic Study* (London: Oxford University Press, 1939); *Demographic Survey of the British Colonial*

Empire (London: Oxford University Press, 1948). See also A. D. Roberts, "Earlier Historiography of Colonial Africa," *History in Africa* 5 (1978): 156–60.

24. Quoted in Roberts, "Earlier Historiography of Colonial Africa," 159.

25. Bruce Berman and John Lonsdale discuss these changes in development policy after the Second World War in the context of Kenya. Bruce Berman and John Lonsdale, *Unhappy Valley: Conflict in Kenya and Africa*, vol. 2: *Violence and Ethnicity* (Columbus: Ohio University Press, 1992), 242–43.

26. Granville St. J. Orde-Browne's *The African Labourer* (New York: International Institute of African Languages and Cultures, 1933); Edgar B. Worthington, *Science in Africa: A Review of Scientific Research Relating to Tropical and Southern Africa* (Oxford: Oxford University Press, 1938); and other works such as William Macmillan's *Africa Emergent: A Survey of Social, Political, and Economic Trends in British Africa* (London: Faber and Faber, 1938). Cited in Roberts, "Earlier Historiography of Colonial Africa," 158–60.

27. Lord Hailey, *An African Survey: A Study of Problems Arising in Africa South of the Sahara* (Oxford: Oxford University Press, 1938), xxiv, 115, 113. Hailey's career as governor of the North-Western Provinces in India before he retired, and his refashioning as an Africa expert in his later years, allowed him to adopt a comparative perspective of the challenges in collecting demographic data on native populations in the colonies in Africa and British dominions such as India. He noted that unlike in Africa, where it was difficult to tell whether the population had increased or decreased over the past hundred years because of a lack of attention to population records, Indian census operations had been more comprehensive and dated back to 1872, partly because of the existence of an army of literate enumerators. This praise was not entirely accurate, because both British and, later, Indian census officials often had little faith in the native Indian enumerator and Indian respondents, as discussed later, in the case of age returns. See Timothy Alborn, "Age and Empire in the British Census," *Journal of Interdisciplinary History* 30, no. 1 (1999): 61–89.

28. This included the "non-self-governing areas" or colonial and mandated areas and not self-governing colonies such as British India. Cited by Kuczynski, *Colonial Population*, from pages xv–xvi of the *Statistical Year-Book of the League of Nations, 1935–6*, 19–24.

29. *Annual Public Health Report for India 1942*, 3, V/24/3742IOL, India Office Records and Private Papers Library, London.

30. Lord Hailey, *An African Survey*, 116–17.

31. Ibid.

32. Granville Edge, *Vital Records in the Tropics*, 23.

33. In India, for instance, census operations in the early twentieth century represented an effort to collect mostly social and physical data. For an interesting discussion on "imperial" demography, its making, and its travel

from domestic to colonial settings, see Karl Ittmann, "Demography as Policy Science in the British Empire," 432–33.

34. The old who were indigent and poor had always been in the margins of colonial administrative measures for poverty administration, though the politics of development brought in new aspects of welfare and rights to these debates. See Andreas Eckert, "Regulating the Social: Social Security in Late Colonial Tanzania," *Journal of African History* (2004), 467–89; for discussions on gerontocratic orders, see Omotade Adegbingin, "The Problem of Gerontocracy in Africa; The Yorùbá Perspective as Illustrated in the *Ifá* Corpus," *Human Affairs* 21 (2011): 454–69.

35. E. A. Gait, "Age," *Census of India, 1911* (Calcutta, 1913), chap. 5, 147–49; G. F. Hardy, *Memorandum on the Age Tables and Rates of Mortality of the Indian Census, 1901* (Calcutta: Government of India, 1905); 31-9-1 R 80 V Indian Census 1901, Age Table, 1–9, India Office Library Collections, British Library, London.

36. I refer here briefly to the extensive debates on "memory studies" among historians, sociologists, and psychologists. See Karen E. Till, "Memory Studies," *History Workshop Journal* 62 (2006), and the insightful work of Jay Winter, *Remembering War: The Great War between Historical Memory and History in the Twentieth Century* (New Haven: Yale University Press, 2006). There are critical views of the "memory industry" in Kerwin Lee Klein, "On the Emergence of 'Memory' in Historical Discourse," *Representations* 69 (2000); Elizabeth Tonkin, *Narrating Our Pasts: The Social Construction of Oral History*, Cambridge Studies in Oral and Literate Culture, vol. 22 (Cambridge: Cambridge University Press, 1992).

37. Gait, "Age," 147–49.

38. Ibid.

39. Ibid.

40. Age-related data was useful to colonial officials because it was relevant to marriage, education, and other practices that legally required regulation to ensure that age at marriage and other such laws were observed.

41. See Eleanor Newbigin, *The Hindu Family and the Emergence of Modern India: Law, Citizenship and Community* (New York: Cambridge University Press, 2013). For a broad overview of the Indian census and an interesting discussion on age in the Indian census, see editor Gerald Barrier's classic *The Census in British India: New Perspectives* (New Delhi: Manohar, 1981). See also Timothy Alborn, "Age and Empire in the British Census," *Journal of Interdisciplinary History* 30, no. 1 (1999): 61–89. Bernard Cohn and Arjun Appadurai discuss the meaning of the census, objectification of identities, and their shaping by administrators and by Indians.

42. This refers to the Census of 1911, and to those individuals aged sixty or over. Gait, "Age."

43. Kuczynski, *Demographic Survey of the British Colonial Empire*, vol. 1: *West Africa*, 173, 547, 630–32.

44. Drysdale Anderson, "An Empirical Age Scale," *Biometrika* 25, no. 1/2 (May 1933): 61–70.

45. For a fascinating discussion on the diverse meanings of age, see Claudine Sauvain-Dugerdil, Henri Leridon, and Nicholas Mascie-Taylor, eds. *Human Clocks: The Bio-Cultural Meanings of Age* (Bern: Peter Lang, 2006), 1–11, 33–36.

46. See Allan Brandt, "Racism and Research: The Case of the Tuskegee Syphilis Study," *The Hastings Center Report* 8, no. 6 (December 1978): 21–29; and *No Magic Bullet: A Social History of Venereal Disease in the United States Since 1880* (Oxford: Oxford University Press, 1985). There is a vast literature on representations of deficiencies in African American bodies and minds that were compared to "normal" Caucasian populations (based on attributing physical deviance, disability, and racial inferiority to the former) in epidemiological studies of diseases and health, in psychiatry, and in other fields. See for instance the works of Lundy Braun, Steve Epstein, Keth Wailoo.

47. Timothy Alborn, "Age and Empire in the British Census," *Journal of Interdisciplinary History* 30, no. 1 (1999): 61–89.

48. Mark Harrison, *Climates and Constitutions: Health, Race, Environment and British Imperialism in India, 1600–1850* (New York: Oxford University Press, 1999).

49. Dependents, Pensions for Parents of Deceased ECOs: Fixing of "Old Age" in India. L/MIL/7/4425 1946, Records of the India Office, The British Library, London.

50. *Home Department (Public), Government of India*, "Questions to be Asked in the Census of 1941," 45/9/40–Public, National Archives of India, New Delhi.

51. The demographic historian Sumit Guha argues that economic categories later replaced "ascriptive" ones in census operations; he also identifies financial and political factors that shaped these shifts. Sumit Guha, "The Politics of Identity and Enumeration in India c. 1600–1990," *Comparative Studies in Society and History* 45 (January 2003): 161; see also 148–67. R. Mansell Prothero, "Population Census of Northern Nigeria, 1952: Problems and Results," *Population Studies* 10, no. 2 (November 1956): 166–83. See also E. J. Arnett, "The Census of Nigeria in 1931," *Journal of the Royal African Society* 32, no. 129 (October 1933): 398–404.

52. Sripati Chandrasekhar, *Census and Statistics in India*, 8–15, Sripati Chandrasekhar Papers, Ward M. Canaday Center, Carlson Library, University of Toledo. I am grateful to Zachary Makowski, who assisted me with scans and lengthy searches at the Canaday Center.

53. Ibid. Sripati Chandrasekhar was a well-known Indian demographer, economist, sociologist, and scholar who published extensively on demography and population control, especially relating to India.

54. S. Chandrasekhar, *Census*, 15; quotes from *Indian Census Report for 1932*, Government of India (New Delhi, 1932), 82.

55. S. Chandrasekhar, *Census*, 29–30.

56. For a discussion on the debate about the bridge from memory and history and reliance on collective memories, see Pierre Nora, *Between Memory and History: Les Lieux de Mémoire Histories: French Constructions of the Past: Postwar French Thought*, vol. 1 (New York: New Press, 1995).

57. Cormac O'Grada, "The Greatest Blessing of All': The Old Age Pension in Ireland," *Past & Present* 175 (May 2002): 124–61. I am also grateful to Pat Thane for meeting me and discussing debates relating to aging and social and political change in Britain, and for offering advice on further searches.

58. Simon Szreter, Hani Sholkamy, and A. Dharmalingam, eds., *Categories and Contexts: Anthropological and Historical Studies in Critical Demography* (Oxford: Oxford University Press, 2004).

59. Sujata Patel, "The Nostalgia for the Village: M. N. Srinivas and the Making of Indian Social Anthropology," *South Asia: Journal of South Asian Studies* 21, no. 1 (1998): 49–61.

60. "The age-set system tends to stratify the population according to seniority, and the individual's position within the system constitutes an important index of social status and, to some extent, regulates his behaviour towards all other members of the society (whether seniors, equals, or juniors). The relations between age mates, and also in certain contexts between members of different age sets (within the age-set hierarchy), are not those of specific contractual commitments which are entered on voluntarily and which cease with the fulfilment of the commitment. They are of a much more diffuse type, involving general and permanent obligations of co-operation, solidarity, mutual help, &c.—closely resembling, in this respect, the family and kinship union." S. N. Eisenstadt, "African Age Groups: A Comparative Study," *Journal of the International African Institute* 24, no. 2 (April 1954): 101 and 100–13.

61. Paul Spencer, *Time, Space and the Unknown: Masai Configurations of Power and Providence* (London: Routledge, 2009).

62. A. C. Hollis, "The Masai," *Journal of the Royal African Society* 42, no. 168 (July 1943): 121.

63. Fred Cooper, *Citizenship between Empire and Nation. Remaking France and French Africa, 1945–1960* (Princeton: Princeton University Press, 2014): 148.

64. Berman and Lonsdale, *Unhappy Valley*, vol. 1: *State and Class*, 160–61. Lonsdale discusses the power of the local administrators in lending authority to precolonial chiefs or, based on local contingencies, to new, "progressive" groups. See also Jan-Bart Gewald, "Researching and Writing in the Twilight of an Imagined Conquest: Anthropology in Northern Rhodesia, 1930–1960," Working Paper, African Studies Center, Leiden (75/2007), 1–42.

65. James Ferguson terms this the "mythology of modernization" in Africa in *Expectations of Modernity: Myths and Meanings of Urban Life on the Zambian Copperbelt* (Berkeley: University of California Press, 1999), 14; see also chaps. 1 and 2.

66. G. W. B. Huntingford, "The Social Institutions of the Dorobo," *Anthropos* (January–April 1951): 1–48.

67. William O'Donnell, "Religion and Morality Among the Ibo in Southern Nigeria," *Primitive Man* 4, no. 4 (1931): 54–60.

68. Joe Hampson, *Old Age: A Study of Aging in Zimbabwe* (Harare: Mambo Press, 1982), 39–55. Hampson is a Jesuit missionary and founder of one of the earliest social work teaching and programs on aging in Zimbabwe with support from Help the Aged, UK.

69. B. Malinowski, "Introductory Essay: The Anthropology of Changing African Cultures," *Methods of Study of Cultural Contact in Africa*, International African Institute, Memorandum XV (1934; London: Oxford University Press, 1965), x–xi.

70. Isaac Schapera, ed., *Western Civilization and the Natives of South Africa: Studies in Culture Contact*, quoted in his article "The Old Bantu Culture," 3–36, 20–21.

71. "Changes were seeping in among some sections, but many traditional native institutions persisted both in memory and practice." Isaac Schapera, "Contact between European and Native in South Africa," in *Methods of Study of Cultural Contact in Africa*, 28–30, 32–34.

72. Isaac Schapera, *Migrant Labour and Tribal Life* (Oxford: Oxford University Press, 1947), 116–28.

73. Ibid., 169, 179–81.

74. Godfrey and Monica Wilson, *The Analysis of Social Change: Based on Observations in Central Africa* (1945; Cambridge: Cambridge University Press, 1965), 17–18, 40–44, 85–87. The Wilsons observed, "In primitive societies the golden age is in the past," 87–88.

75. Ibid., 23, 99, 141, 167.

76. Jomo Kenyatta, "Kikuyu Religion, Ancestor Worship, and Sacrificial Practices," *Africa* 10 (January 1937): 308, 322–25. See also Mwenda Ntaraangwi, David Mills, and Mustafa Babiker, eds., *African Anthropologies: History, Critique and Practice* (London: Zed Books, 2006), 14–41.

77. Berman and Lonsdale, *Unhappy Valley*, 1:217–18.

78. Schapera, *Migrant Labour and Tribal Life*, 14–16.

79. Andreas Eckert, "Regulating the Social: Social Security, Social Welfare and the State in Late Colonial Tanzania," *Journal of African History* 45, no. 3 (2004): 467–89.

80. H. A. Fosbrooke, "Can Labour Be Stabilized without Permanent Urbanization and Concomitant Social Security Measures?," in *Present Interrelations in*

Central African Rural and Urban Life, ed. R. J. Apthorpe, Proceedings of the Eleventh Conference of the Rhodes Livingston Institute held in Lusaka, Northern Rhodesia, January 14–17, 1958 (Cape Town: RDI, February 1958), 88–91.

81. Ibid. Fosbrooke, the director of the Rhodes Livingston Institute, argued at this meeting that the complexities in African social problems implied that a multiplicity of disciplines were required: "gone are the days of the 'lone wolf' anthropologist who chose a tribe according to his interest and inclination, succeeded in raising funds from some University or Foundation, came in and studied his tribe single-handed, and finally retired to University life or no chance of returning to field anthropology" (91).

82. Schapera, *Migrant Labour and Tribal Life,* 200.

83. Quote from W. H. Hutt, "The Economic Position of the Bantu in South Africa," in Schapera, *Western Civilization and the Natives of South Africa,* 201–2, 195–237. Hutt vigorously criticized the assumption by the South African government and press that the natives were uncivilized simply because they fell below an economic standard of civilization even if they were "way ahead of many White people from the standpoint of culture, intelligence, physique." In the same volume, Isaac Schapera's teacher at Witwatersrand, R. F. Alfred Hoernle, writing in the 1930s in protest against segregation policies regarding the mixture of races, argued that civilization and culture were not a function of "race," nor was the latter defined by skin color. Hoernle, "Race Mixture and Native Policy in South Africa," 272–76, 263–81.

84. B. S. Guha, "Progress of Anthropological Research in India," *Anthropos* 41/44, no. 4/6 (July–December 1946/1949): 607–613.

85. Arjun Appadurai, "Putting Hierarchy in Its Place," 40–43; Ferguson, *Expectations of Modernity,* 24–25. Some of the well-known works in this period included M. N. Srinivas, *Religion and Society among the Coorgs of South India* (Oxford: Oxford University Press, 1952); Iravati Karve, *Kinship Organization in India* (Poona: Deccan College, 1953).

86. D. N. Majumdar, *The Fortunes of Primitive Tribes* (Lucknow: Universal, 1944), 223–27, 25–26, 213. Majumdar completed his PhD from Cambridge and also attended Malinowski's lectures in London; he was influenced by both physical and social anthropological methods. In 1952 he attended the International Symposium on Anthropology in New York and was a UN delegate to the World Population Conference in Rome (1954). Shyamal Kumar Ray, *Bibliographies of Eminent Indian Anthropologists* (Calcutta: Anthropological Survey of India, 1974), 141.

87. D. N. Majumdar, *Social Contours of an Industrial City: Social Survey of Kanpur, 1954–56* (Westport, CT: Greenwood Press, 1960), 211, appendices 2 and 3, 224–42. Majumdar observed that "return migration" of the young back

to the village was not easy but even then, "workers long associated with factory life and its environment respond readily to the call of the village and migrate periodically to the villages even during their working life and permanently when they retire or when their services are terminated." But he noted that better educated postwar immigrants found the insecurities of village life, group dynamics, and lack of amenities did not offer a secure asylum, and as a result "the villagers have given but not received back talent" (ix–x).

88. M. N. Srinivas, *The Remembered Village* (New Delhi: Oxford University Press, 1976), 110.

89. Ibid., 109.

90. For an analysis of Karve's life and her links with the development of the anthropological field in India, see Nandini Sundar, "In the Cause of Anthropology: The Life and Work of Irawati Karve," in Patricia Uberoi, Nandini Sundar, and Satish Deshpande, *Anthropology in the East: The Founders of Indian Sociology and Anthropology* (New Delhi: Permanent Black, 2007).

91. Ray, *Bibliographies of Eminent Indian Anthropologists*, 162–74.

92. Iravati Karve, "The Care of the Aged in the Indian Joint Family," *Social Welfare* (September 1955): 12–13.

93. Ibid., 12–13, 32.

94. Sjoerd R. Jaarsma, "A Challenged Perspective: Missionary Ethnography in West New Guinea," in *Anthropologists and the Missionary Endeavour: Experiences and Reflections*, ed. Ad Borsboom and Jean Koomers (Saarbrucken: Nijmeegs Instituut Voor Comparatieve Cultuur-en Ontwikelingsstudies, 2000), 33:25–39.

95. The literature on the White Fathers (or the Society for Missionaries of Africa), founded in 1868 by Charles M. Lavigerie, archbishop of Algiers, is extensive and consists of histories of the missions and their expansion from Algeria to the Great Lakes, biographies of missionaries, and studies of the controversial role played by the White Fathers in colonial enterprise, in particular in Rwanda. See William Burridge, *Destiny Africa: Cardinal Lavigerie and the Making of the White Fathers* (London: G. Chapman, 1966); Glenn D. Kittler, *The White Fathers* (Edinburgh: Allen, 1957). For the interwar years, see Francis Nolan, *The White Fathers in Colonial Africa, 1919–1939* (Nairobi: Pauline Publications, 2012); Aylward Shorter, *Cross and Flag: The "White Fathers" during the Colonial Scramble (1892–1914)* (Maryknoll, NY: Orbis Books, 2006); Ian Linden, *Church and Revolution in Rwanda* (Manchester: Manchester University Press, 1977).

96. *Table d'enquête sur les mœurs et les coutumes indigènes (An Enquiry into the Indigenous Traditions and Customs of Peoples of West and Central Africa)*. I am especially grateful to Professor Ilan Meyer for helping me access additional research support to consult these records at UCLA. The inquiry is entirely in French, as are the responses, and the names of the respondents are rarely

given. This collection was consulted from the carbon copies kept at the Charles E. Young Research Library at UCLA, donated from the main headquarters of the Pères Blancs, Padri Bianchi/Via Aurelia 269, 00165/Roma, Italy (original carbon copy set of manuscripts bound in volumes). Chapter 8 ("Old Age and Death, Questions 303–348") of each questionnaire contains typed questions on old age and death; the responses were mostly collected in 1951–52. The translations of the interviews (in quotations) into English are mine. See www.oac.cdlib.org/findaid/ark:/13030/tf5b69n9kp/entire_text/.

97. WFI, *Sommaire de La Table D'enquête*—Deuxième *Fascicule*, Yoruba, Collection 246, Box 3, Folder 4, 303–5; WFI, *Sommaire de La Table D'enquête—Troisième Fascicule*, chap. 8, Vieillesse et Mort, Tribu de Malinké, Préfecture Apostolique de Kayes, 387.

98. Ibid.

99. WFI, *Sommaire de La Table D'enquête—Deuxième Fascicule, Bambara, Archevêché de Bamako, Mission de Belenko*, chap. 8, question 313, 280–81.

100. Monica Hunter Wilson, "An African Christian Morality," *Africa* (January 1937): 265–91.

101. Megan Vaughan, *Curing Their Ills: Colonial Power and African Illness* (Stanford: Stanford University Press, 1991), 70–75.

102. WFI, *Sommaire de La Table D'enquête—Deuxième Fascicule, Bambara, Archevêché de Bamako, Mission de Belenko*, chap. 8, Vieillesse et Mort, question 309, 277; WFI, *Sommaire de La Table D'enquête—*Troisième *Fascicule*, chap. 8, Vieillesse et Mort, Diocese of Kitega-Ngozi, Barundi tribe, question 309, 307.

103. The Xhosa elderly, Moffat and Livingston wrote, died outside of the family and were abandoned in the bush much like wild beasts. Andreas Sagner, "'The Abandoned Mother': Ageing, Old Age and Missionaries in Early and Mid-Nineteenth Century South-East Africa," *Journal of African History* 42 (2001): 173–74, 77, 192–93. These judgments about old age popularized the figure of the "abandoned mother" and of old age as a "lifecycle phase of degradation and misery," but were also somewhat ambiguous: they saw the old in Africa as posing a challenge to civilized progress but also as "objects of innocent suffering."

104. I am grateful to Professor Radhika Singha at Delhi University for bringing this to my attention and for guiding me to the relevant book and archival references. The "ghat" consisted of the steps leading down to the river. Peggs appealed to the Governor General to suppress these practices. Abhijit Dutta, *Nineteenth Century Bengal and the Christian Missionaries* (Calcutta: Minerva Associates, 1992), 78–80; "Hindu Idolatory a Root of Bitterness," *Church Missionary Intelligencer* 9 (1858): 40.

105. In the 1960s and 1970s, this was part of a moral language of social work which assumed that now that community life was strained and fractured in developing countries, case workers had to enable destitute and "maladjusted" old persons to

readjust in an environment of endemic poverty. Unlike in the West, Christian social workers were advised that the family always needed to be a part of the solution. See W. Clifford, *A Primer of Social Case Work in Africa* (Nairobi: Oxford University Press, 1966), 60–61. For a discussion of the politics of dependence and aging in India, see Kavita Sivaramakrishnan, "Aging and Dependence in an Independent Indian Nation," *Journal of Social History* (2013).

106. John Illife, *The African Poor: A History* (Cambridge: Cambridge University Press, 1988), 146–47.

107. Leo W. Simmons, *The Role of the Aged in Primitive Society* (New Haven, CT: Yale University Press, 1945). See also Leo W. Simmons, "Aging in Preindustrial Societies," in *Handbook of Social Gerontology: Societal Aspects of Aging*, ed. Clark Tibbits (Chicago: University of Chicago Press, 1960), 87.

108. Simmons, "Aging in Preindustrial Societies"; Dale Dannefer and Chris Phillipson, *The SAGE Handbook of Social Gerontology* (New York: Sage, 2010), 50–51. Simmons's work was widely reviewed, although most of the reviews by fellow anthropologists and sociologists, and especially experts in African studies, found his methodology ambitious but unreliable, and termed the conclusions highly questionable. See A. H. Gayton's review of *The Role of the Aged in Primitive Society* in *American Anthropologist* 48, no. 4 (New Series) (October–December 1946): 649–50; and Solon T. Kimball in *American Journal of Sociology* 52, no. 3 (November 1946): 287.

109. Simmons's work later traveled "back" to Asian experts as a view from the West about preindustrial cultures and the aged. Private Papers Collections of Philip Hauser, Robert J. Havighurst, Ernest Burgess, and Robert Redfield, Special Collections Research Center at the University of Chicago; Clark Tibbits Papers, History Research Center at the University of Michigan Library, Ann Arbor. See also Tibbits, *Handbook of Social Gerontology*.

110. Simmons, "Aging in Preindustrial Societies," 87.

111. See Kingsley Davis and J. W. Combs Jr., eds., *The Social and Biological Challenge of Our Aging Population* (New York: Columbia University Press, 1950), 149; emphasis added. Davis cited the study by Olga Lang, *Chinese Family and Society* (New Haven: Yale University Press, 1946). Other contemporary studies of families and generational ties in the "East" that were cited included Marion J. Levy, *The Family Revolution in Modern China* (Cambridge: Harvard University Press, 1949), 149.

112. Simmons, *The Role of the Aged in Primitive Society*, 51.

113. See Simmons, "Aging in Pre-Industrial Societies"; and "Aging in Primitive Societies: A Comparative Survey of Family Life and Relationships," *Law and Contemporary Problems* 27 (Winter 1962): 36–51.

114. Quoted in Simmons, "Aging in Primitive Societies," 43.

115. T. Lynn Smith, "The Changing Number and Distribution of the Aged Negro Population of the United States," *Phylon Quarterly* 8, no. 4 (1957): 340.

116. Leo Simmons is quoting the work of William H. Prescott, *History of the Conquest of Peru: With a Preliminary View of the Civilization of the Incas* (New York: Harper and Brothers, 1847); see also "Aging in Primitive Societies: A Comparative Survey of Family Life and Relationships," 42–3.

117. Smith, "Changing Number and Distribution," 339–54. Smith wrote often on this subject and quoted several influential reports to support his case. See "The Migration of the Aged," New York State Joint Legislative Committee on Problems of the Aging, Growing with the Years, Legislative Document No. 32 (Albany, 1954), 69–80; "The Migration of the Aged," in *Problems of America's Aging Population*, ed. T. Lynn Smith (New York: McGraw-Hill, 1948), 15–28, among others.

118. Proceedings of the World Population Conference, 1954, 91. See http://babel .hathitrust.org/cgi/pt?id=mdp. 39015015212932;view=1up;seq=103, and also the session on aging and its economic and social implications chaired by the French demographer Alfred Sauvy.

2

Growing Old in the Time of Chronic Disease

Note: This chapter has benefitted from feedback received from scholars at several academic meetings and seminars. In particular, it has been revised based on input from Cathy Burns, Julie Livingston, and Megan Vaughan relating to a panel on "Biomedicine, Body Parts, and Aging in Africa, India, and the United States" at the American Historical Association, January 3, 2015, and a meeting held at the University of Witwatersrand, in June 2014. I am also thankful to Laurence Monnais for our discussions of the social framing of cancers in Vietnam and Cambodia and on colonial and postcolonial networks of scientific expertise.

1. "Outline of a History of the International Association of Gerontological Societies: The Dawn of the History of the IAG," draft of chap. 1, 1–2A. Nathan Shock Papers, Bentley Historical Library, University of Michigan (henceforth NSP).

2. "Early in 1954 the trustees of the CIBA Foundation decided to embark on special measures in support internationally, of basic research relevant to the problems of ageing, so that the conference already arranged became the first in what it is hoped will be a series of conferences on subjects in this field." G. E. W. Wolstenholme and Margaret P. Cameron, eds., *CIBA Foundation Colloquium on Aging* (henceforth *CIBA*) (London: Little, 1955), 1:title page.

3. T. Gillman, "Nutrition, Liver Disease and Some Aspects of Ageing in Africans," *CIBA*, 104–6.

4. Alexis Carrel Papers, Folder 317, 31, Rockefeller Archive Center, Sleepy Hollow, New York.

5. Kathleen Hall, "Obituary Notice of Deceased Members: Vladimir Korenchevsky," *Journal of Pathology and Bacteriology* 80 (1960): 451–61.

6. Memo regarding Foundation for Research on Old Age, April 25, 1950, from Dr. V. Korenchevsky to E. V. Cowdry. IMG 0913, E. V. Cowdry Papers, Becker Medical Library (henceforth EVCP). The societies he mentions ranged over Europe and the United States as well as one each in Argentina, Canada, and Australia.

7. Ibid.

8. Nathan Shock, "The International Association of Gerontology: Its Origins and Development," Opening Session, draft 2, 6/26/85, IAG History, Folder 1, 1–2, NSP.

9. Edward J. Stiglitz, "Chronic Illness and Senescence," *Journal of the American Medical Association* (henceforth *JAMA*) 150, no. 5: 87 (Commission on Chronic Illness, Special Article).

10. George Weisz, *Chronic Disease in the Twentieth Century: A History* (Baltimore: Johns Hopkins University Press, 2014).

11. V. Korenchevsky, "The War and the Problem of Ageing," *Annals of Human Genetics* 11, no. 1 (January 1941): 314–32. There is a dense literature on gerontology's early theories, including debates around the aging of tissues and the making of the scientific boundaries of gerontological research in these years. See Hyung Wook Park, "Edmund Vincent Cowdry and the Making of Gerontology as a Multidisciplinary Scientific Field in the United States," *Journal of the History of Biology* 41, no. 3 (September 2008): 529–72. For Cowdry's contribution, see Hannah Landecker, "Edmund Vincent Cowdry," in *The New Dictionary of Scientific Biography*, ed. Noretta Koertge, vol. 2 (Farmington Hills, MI: Gale, 2007); Albert Lansing, "Edmund Vincent Cowdry, 1888–1975," *Gerontologist* 15, no. 477 (1975): 477.

12. V. Korenchevsky, "The Problems of Ageing, and the Ways and Means for Achieving the Rapid Progress of Gerontological Research," in *The Social and Biological Challenge of an Aging Population*, ed. Kingsley Davis and J. W. Combs, Proceedings of the Eastern States Health Conference, March 31–April 1, 1949 (New York: Columbia University Press, 1950), 11–12.

13. Hyung Wook Park, "'Senility and Death of Tissues Are Not a Necessary Phenomenon': Alexis Carrel and the Origins of Gerontology," *Korean Journal of Medical History* 20 (June 2011): 181–208.

14. For a discussion of the emergence of biogerontology and its debates, in particular the challenges in terms of "boundary work" in establishing it as a new scientific field and its less credible past due to antiaging research, see T. F. Gieryn, "Boundary-Work and the Demarcation of Science from Non-Science: Strains and Interests in Professional Ideologies of Scientists," *American*

Sociological Review 48 (1983): 781–95; J. Kempner, C. S. Perlis and J. F. Merz, "Forbidden Knowledge," *Science* 307 (2005): 854; Jennifer R. Fishman, Robert H. Binstock, and Marcie A. Lambrix, "Anti-Aging Science: The Emergence, Maintenance, and Enhancement of a Discipline," *Journal of Aging Studies* 22, no. 4 (December 1, 2008): 295–303.

15. Speech by Professor Enrico Greppi, president of the Fourth Congress of the International Association of Gerontology, Merano (Bolzano), Italy, July 14–19, 1957, vol. 1.

16. Korenchevsky, "The Problems of Ageing," 12.

17. Korenchevsky, "The War and the Problem of Ageing."

18. E. V. Cowdry, "Gerontological Conferences in the Summer of 1950 in Europe," *Journal of Gerontology* 6, no. 1 (1951): 60, 61. After the Second World War there were an estimated 75,000 veterans receiving payments. See Louis I. Dublin (in collaboration with Mortimer Spiegelman), *The Facts of Life: From Birth to Death* (New York: Macmillan, 1951), 415, 431–32.

19. Cowdry, "Gerontological Conferences," 59; Korenchevsky, "The Problems of Ageing," 20–21. See also "Man and His Years: An Account of the First National Conference on Aging," sponsored by the Federal Security Agency, Health Publications, North Carolina, 1951, 1–13.

20. Fourth Congress of the International Association of Gerontology, 1:15–28.

21. Cowdry, "Gerontological Conferences," 61.

22. Letter from V. Korenchevsky, Oxford University, to E. V. Cowdry, St. Louis, October 20, 1947, EVCP. Each of these international meetings would find support from local universities and often from the U.S. government for funding the travel of individual delegates; the travel of the U.S. delegation was mostly supported by the Macy Foundation and the FSA. Final Report, Second Gerontological Congress, 60, EVCP.

23. See Keith R. Benson, Jane Maienschein, and Ronald Rainger, eds., *The Expansion of American Biology* (New Brunswick, NJ: Rutgers University Press, 1991), 5–8; Gregg Mitman's discussion of the role played by social assumptions in ecological studies and biochemical research in the 1930s, in the context of social roles and the Depression, in Gregg Mitman, "Evolution as Gospel: William Patten, the Language of Democracy and the Great War," *Isis* 81 (1990): 446–63; and Richard E. Brown, *Rockefeller Medicine Men: Medicine and Capitalism in America* (Berkeley: University of California Press, 1979).

24. D. H. Stapleton, *Creating a Tradition of Biomedical Research: Contributions to the History of Rockefeller University* (New Brunswick, NJ: Rutgers University Press, 2004), 10–11. See also Jane Maienschein's work on the expansion of cytology as a collaborative field in the 1920s with Cowdry as one of its leaders. Jane Maienschein, "Cytology in 1924: Expansion and Collaboration," in Benson, Maienschein, and Rainger, eds., *The Expansion of American Biology*,

23–51; Daniel J. Kevles, *The Physicists: The History of a Scientific Community in Modern America* (Cambridge: Harvard University Press, 1995).

25. Cowdry, "Gerontological Conferences," 60–61. For a discussion of postwar UN agencies such as UNESCO and visions of a "universal epistemology of scientific collaboration," see Perrin Selcer, "The View from Everywhere: Disciplining Diversity in post–World War Two International Social Science," *Journal of the History of the Behavioral Sciences* 45, no. 4 (Fall 2009): 309–29.

26. Nathan Shock, "History of Gerontology," draft, corrected by hand, Box 5, NSP. The report, produced by the IGC, was titled *Old Age in the Modern World: Report"* (Edinburgh: E. & S. Livingstone, 1955).

27. Pichat's later work discussed changing stages in the evolution of mortality in developing countries; J. E. Bourgeois-Pichat, *The Concept of a Stable Population: Application to the Study of Populations of Countries with Incomplete Demographic Statistics* (New York: United Nations, 1968). For a short discussion of Pichat's changing views on the evolution of mortality in three stages in developing countries, see Graziella Caselli, Jacques Vallin, and Guillaume Wunsch, *Demography, Analysis and Synthesis: A Treatise in Population Studies* (Burlington, VT: Academic Press, 2006): 71–72.

28. This is my translation of his speech in French. Fourth Congress of the International Association of Gerontology, 1:36. See also "The Works of Jean Bourgeois-Pichat: Some Guidelines," in *Population: An English Selection* 3 (1991): 1–13.

29. Claudine Sauvain-Dugerdil, Henri Léridon, and C. G. N. Mascie-Taylor, *Human Clocks: The Bio-Cultural Meanings of Age* (Bern: Peter Lang, 2006).

30. Keith Wailoo, *How Cancer Crossed the Color Line* (Oxford: Oxford University Press, 2011); Barron H. Lerner, *The Breast Cancer Wars: Hope, Fear, and the Pursuit of a Cure in Twentieth-Century America* (New York: Oxford University Press, 2001).

31. Clark Tibbitts, "Gerontological Research and the Universities," in *Academic Gerontology: Dilemmas of the 1980s* (Ann Arbor, MI: Institute of Gerontology, 1980), 51–52. See also Henry S. Shryock Jr., "The Changing Age Profile of the Population," in *The Aged and Society*, ed. Milton Derber (Champaign, IL: Industrial Relations Research Association, 1950), 7.

32. Profile of E. V. Cowdry, in W. Andrew Achenbaum and Daniel M. Albert, *Profiles in Gerontology: A Biographical Dictionary* (Westport, CT: Greenwood Press, 1995), 90–91.

33. Letter from O. J. Pollak, Secretary Treasurer, American Society for the Study of Arteriosclerosis, to Dr. Henry Simms, CRA, December 26, 1950, EVCP.

34. Office memo from Harold F. Dorn to Norman Topping, PH Service, U.S. Government, September 27, 1951, NSP.

35. Report of the Second International Gerontological Congress, meeting program, in folder on International Gerontological Meetings, Box 5, NSP.

36. E. V. Cowdry, ed., *Problems of Ageing: Biological and Medical Aspects*, foreword to the second edition (printed with support from the Josiah Macy Jr. Foundation, 1942; first edition 1939), xvi.

37. "Note prepared by Chairman William MacNider for the Executive Committee of the Club for Research on Aging," Folder 12: Club for Research on Senility, 1939–1947, Box 41, EVCP; emphasis added.

38. Leon S. Medalia and Paul Dudley White, "Diseases of the Aged: Analysis of Pathological Observations in 1.251 Autopsy Protocols in Old Persons," *JAMA* 149, no. 16 (August 16, 1952): 1433–35. See also Leon Medalia, "Fellows and Members of the Gerontological Society," *The Gerontologist*, August 15, 1956, 451.

39. Korenchevsky, "The War and the Problem of Aging," 314–32.

40. Oscar R. Ewing, *Man and His Years: An Account of the First National Conference on Aging*, sponsored by the Federal Security Agency (Raleigh, NC: Health Publications, 1951), 1–2.

41. Nathan Shock, ed., *Conference on Problems of Aging: Transactions of the Twelfth Conference*, February 6–7, 1950, New York (New York: Josiah Macy Jr. Foundation, 1951).

42. Ann Pollock, *Medicating Race: Heart Disease and Durable Preoccupations with Difference* (Durham: Duke University Press, 2012).

43. Wailoo, *How Cancer Crossed the Color Line*; Lerner, *The Breast Cancer Wars*. I am grateful to James Colgrove for discussing the literature in this area with me.

44. Wailoo, *How Cancer Crossed the Color Line*.

45. Stephen Katz, *Disciplining Old Age: The Formation of Gerontological Knowledge, Disciplinarity and Beyond* (Charlottesville: University of Virginia Press, 2009), 82–83.

46. Wolstenholme and Cameron, eds., *CIBA*, title page.

47. Nathan Shock produced a self-conscious history of international gerontology that differs from the "spirit of internationalism" marking Korenchevsky's accounts of the birth of the IAG. While conceding that this was "a period of ferment," with growing numbers of societies and new scientific disciplines as well as government funding to help matters, he notes that Korenchevsky saw the United States as a source of primary funding for the IAG, and this made many at the 11th Macy Conference less than enthusiastic in the beginning. Nathan Shock, "IAG and the History of Gerontology," draft, corrected by hand, Box 5, 2A, 3A, NSP.

48. Oral History Recordings, Harold Leroy Stewart transcripts from interview, consulted at the Columbia University Libraries.

49. Johannes Clemmensen, ed., *Symposium on Geographic Pathology and Demography of Cancer* (Oxford: Oxford University Press, 1950), supported

by WHO and UNESCO, Wellcome Library Collections, London. Articles and commentaries by V. R. Khanolkar and Joseph Gillman who attended the symposium are on pages 58–59 (Khanolkar) and pages 108–9 (Gillman).

50. Discussions on geographic pathology were led by Leroy Stewart of the National Cancer Institute and Jacques May of the American Geographic Society. See elaborations on this framework in ibid., 7–8; Harold Leroy Stewart, "Geographic Pathology," paper presented at the International Symposium of the Control of Cell Division and the Induction of Cancer, Lima, Peru, and Cali, Colombia, July 1–6, 1963, 303–8; Jacques May, "The Ecology of Human Disease," *Annals of the New York Academy of Sciences* 84, no. 17 (1960): 789–94.

51. Wailoo, *How Cancer Crossed the Color Line*; Keith Wailoo, *Drawing Blood: Technology and Disease Identity in Twentieth-Century America* (Baltimore: Johns Hopkins University Press, 1997), 145.

52. Dipesh Chakrabarty, *Provincializing Europe* (Princeton: Princeton University Press, 2008).

53. Letter from Joseph Gillman (JG) to E. V. Cowdry, April 28, 1952, EVCP. Cowdry enjoyed close relations with the American Cancer Society and was a founding member of a research commission to initiate international cancer studies. E. V. Cowdry, "The Fourth International Cancer Research Congress," *JAMA* 135, no. 16 (1947): 1067–72. The E. V. Cowdry Papers capture his consultancies on cancer with the government of India, his work in South Africa, and his networks in China and East Asia.

54. Over the next decade Gillman built collaborations with cancer researchers all over Africa to investigate liver cancers and explore the role of infectious diseases and environmental factors in cancer etiology.

55. In Africa, researchers argued that the problem of cancer could be explained, for example, as "part of the wider problem of the biology of the African" that was affected by diet, malnutrition and other environmental challenges. In that sense, Africa not only provided a need for cancer-related research "but an opportunity for fundamental work which will contribute to medical science as a whole." Report of the Committee on Geographic Pathology of Cancer of the Research Commission of the International Union Against Cancer, Rome, Italy, July 1956, by Harold Leroy Stewart (HLS), Chairman, Box 56, Folder 1, 29, Harold Leroy Stewart Papers.

56. Charles Berman, "Malignant Disease in the Bantu of Johannesburg and the Witwatersrand Gold Mines," *South African Journal of Medical Science* 1 (1935): 12–30; Charles Berman, *Primary Carcinoma of the Liver: A Study in Incidence, Clinical Manifestations, Pathology and Aetiology* (London: H. K. Lewis, 1951).

57. J. Higginson, "Primary Carcinoma of the Liver in South Africa," *British Journal of Cancer* 10, no. 4 (1956): 609–22; and J. Higginson and Oettle, "Cancer Incidence in the Bantu and 'Cape Colored' Races of South Africa: Report of a

Cancer Survey in the Transvaal (1953–55)," *Journal of the National Cancer Institute* 24, no. 3 (1960): 561–89.

58. T. Gillman, "Nutrition, Liver Disease and Some Aspects of Ageing in Africans," *CIBA*, 104–6; emphasis added. Gillman quotes Charles Berman's study, conducted in 1951, in the footnotes. This incidence was also because the African liver was injured severely and with greater frequency and "on repeated occasions, virtually from birth," and this was clear from studies undertaken among Africans in Durban. The clinical features were completely different from those among Europeans and could be attributed to the accumulation of excessive iron in all tissues due to a "nutritionally based derangement," 114.

59. For a general background, see Leonard Thompson, *A History of South Africa*, 4th ed. (New Haven: Yale University Press, 2014); Diana Wylie, *Starving on a Full Stomach: Hunger and the Triumph of Cultural Racism in Modern South Africa* (Charlottesville: Virginia University Press, 2001). For a nuanced discussion of the politics of science in South Africa, see Saul Dubow, ed., *Science and Society in Southern Africa* (Manchester: Manchester University Press, 2000). I am grateful to Renee Van Der Wiel for her meticulous searches at the libraries and collections at the University of Witwatersrand and to the audience and scholars at a conference held at WISER, in April 2014 at the Body and Ageing Symposium for their feedback on my research on Gillman and cancer research in South Africa.

60. See Charles Berman's work on liver cancers, supported by the mining industry; Gillman drew from this early research (1920–40s). For a background on Charles Berman, see, E. J. Verwey, ed., *New Dictionary of South African Biography* (Pretoria: Pretoria HSRC Publishers, 1995), 1:17; and A. P. Cartwright, *Doctors of the Mines: A History of the Mine Medical Officers' Association of South Africa* (Cape Town: Purnell, 1971), 13–15. Randall Packard, "The Invention of the 'Tropical Worker': Medical Research and the Quest for Central African Labor on the South African Gold Mines, 1903–36," *Journal of African History* 34, no. 2 (1993): 271–92.

61. Packard, "The Invention of the 'Tropical Worker,'" *Journal of African History* 34, no. 2 (1993): 271–92.

62. Mervyn Susser, "A Personal History: Social Medicine in a South African Setting, 1952–5, Part 2: Social Medicine as a Calling: Ups, Downs, and Politics in Alexandra Township," *Journal of Epidemiology and Community Health* 60 (2006): 662–68, 664.

63. Higginson and Oettle, "Cancer Incidence in the Bantu," 589–605.

64. Higginson, "Primary Carcinoma of the Liver in Africa," 620–21.

65. Higginson and Oettle, "Cancer Incidence in the Bantu," Figure 2, 600–605, 603.

66. A contemporary observed, "Although the faculty in general were not particularly activist in regard to the disparities and inequities existing between the

South African whites and nonwhites, there were notable exceptions, such as Raymond Dart, Joseph Gillman, and his brother Teddy (Theodore)." Under Dart's leadership, faculty at Wits spoke up to allow the presence of nonwhite students, who had been accepted since 1940, when Dart was Dean, and to allow access to nonwhites beyond the segregated nonwhite hospitals. Quote from Morris J. Karnovsky, "A Pathologist's Odyssey: Mechanisms of Disease," *Annual Review of Pathology* 1 (2006): 1–22. See also P. V. Tobias, "In Memoriam: Joseph Gillman," *South African Medical Journal* (December 18, 1982): 1007–8.

67. I am thankful to David Rosner for discussing the literature on occupational tumors and exposure to asbestos in the 1950s and 1960s in the United States and aspects of this debate—or its gaps—in South Africa.

68. As had other inspiring colleagues such as Sydney Kark, who left for Israel after the social medicine "experiments" supported by the Gluckman Commission had been marginalized, shortly before the nationalist government came to power in 1948. Damien Droney, "Ironies of Laboratory Work during Ghana's Second Age of Optimism," *Cultural Anthropology* 29, no. 2 (2014): 363–84, http://dx.doi.org/10.14506/ca29.2.10.

69. Felicitation (Souvenir) Volume *Vasant Ramji Khanolkar*, published in July 1963, Bombay, on his sixty-eighth birthday. Copied from Tata Library, Bombay; contains no other publishing details. Leading medical and political figures in India and abroad, such as India's first health minister Maharani Amrit Kaur, E. V. Cowdry, and others, contributed to this work.

70. "In India where so many people die of cancer, we do not even have a scientific name for it." Khanolkar's opening address, December 1952. The report was also cited in *Townsville Daily Bulletin* January 5, 1953 ("Cancer Talks in Bombay: 260,000 Deaths in India Yearly"); *Times of India*, Nehru Memorial Museum and Library, Newspaper Archive, New Delhi.

71. R. N. Chaudhuri, "Tropical Medicine—Past, Present, Future," Presidential Address, Indian Science Congress, held in Hyderabad, *BMJ* 2 (1954): 429.

72. Frederick Hoffman, "Cancer in India, Persia and Ceylon," *Sankhya: Journal of the Indian Statistical Institute* 2, no. 3 (1936): 292. Khanolkar refuted the claims made by the American epidemiologist Frederick Hoffman who cited evidence to show that the "restricted" foods in the Indian diet tended to impede the onset of cancers even in a population that chewed betel nut, for instance, and would have been susceptible to oral cancers.

73. V. R. Khanolkar, presidential address, "Habits and Customs as Causative Agents of Cancer," Proceedings of the National Institute of Science, India, Part A, Physical Science 2 (1967), 312–13. This talk was published earlier as "Habits and Customs as Causal Factors of Cancer," *Patholgie und Bakteriologie* 18, no. 4 (1955): 423–28.

74. Ibid.

75. Ibid.

76. Ibid.

77. C. G. Pandit, "As I Know Him," in *Vasant Ramji Khanolkar*. See also www
.tatacentralarchives.com/history/biographies/21%20Meherbai%20Tata.html, on
Lady Meherbai, consulted on July 9, 2014; V. R. Khanolkar, "India's Contribution to Cancer Research: Years of Steady Progress," *Times of India*, Bombay
Edition, December 31, 1952, 8.

78. See K. Wailoo's discussion of breast cancer as the paradox of modern white
women's lives and notions of "civilized Whiteness" in the early twentieth
century. Wailoo, *How Cancer Crossed the Color Line*, 14–16, 145.

79. "History of the Anti-Cancer Movement in this Province" (pamphlet) regarding
the cancer movement led by middle-class women since 1935 and deepening
with the death of "many a useful prominent citizen" and others after 1946.
Series 126, Box 120, Folders 12–14, EVCP; Cowdry's visit to Madras and
reception by the head of the All India Women's Conference, Muthulakshmi
Reddy, which was mobilizing against cancer, was reported in the February 25,
1952 edition of the *Hindu* newspaper in "Treatment of Cancer."

80. V. R. Khanolkar, "The Susceptibility of Indians to Cancer," *Indian Journal of
Medical Research* 33, no. 2 (1945): 299–314.

81. Ibid., 308, 310.

82. Prasenjit Duara, "The Discourse of Civilization and Decolonization," *Journal
of World History* 15, no. 1 (March 2004): 1–5.

83. Sta. Cruz from Brazil, in a meeting on September 16, 1954. Box 56, Folder 1,
H. L. Stewart Papers, National Library of Medicine, Bethesda.

84. Homi K. Bhabha, "Preface," in *Vasant Ramji Khanolkar*, 1–4. Bhabha was then
chairman of India's first Atomic Energy Commission.

85. This is based on an ongoing review of Khanolkar's later correspondence with
E. V. Cowdry and interviews with experts at the Tata Memorial Cancer
Hospital, Mumbai.

86. WHO, WHO SEARO Report, Minutes of the Fourth Meeting, Section 2
(WHO, Delhi, 1964), 111, WHO SEARO Library, New Delhi.

87. See the discussion in Stephen J. Kunitz, *The Health of Populations: General
Theories and Particular Realities* (Oxford: Oxford University Press, 2006).

3

The Emergence of the International Gerontologist

1. Tibbitts, "Old Age," *International Social Science Journal* 15, no. 16 (1963): 39–54.

2. Kingsley Davis and J. W. Combs Jr., "The Sociology of an Aging Population,"
in *The Social and Biological Challenge of Our Aging Population* (New York:
Columbia University Press, 1950), 146–47.

3. Oscar J. Kaplan to E. V. Cowdry, April 21, 1951, Folder on Second IGC, Nathan Shock Papers, Bentley Historical Library, University of Michigan (henceforth NSP).

4. Letter from Ethel Shanas, Associate Professor, Department of Human Development, University of Chicago, to Nathan Shock, Chief Gerontology Branch, National Heart Institute, Baltimore, September 29, 1964, Folder II, Sixth International Gerontological Congress, Vienna, NSP.

5. See Chapter 5 and, in particular, the section discussing preparations for the World Assembly on Aging, Vienna (1982) and the role U.S. politicians and experts played.

6. Andrew Achenbaum, *Crossing Frontiers: Gerontology Emerges as a Science* (Cambridge: Cambridge University Press, 1995), 105–12. See also James Birren, "A Brief History of the Psychology of Aging," *The Gerontologist* 1, no. 2 (June 1961): 69–77.

7. Elaine Cumming and William E. Henry, *Growing Old* (New York: Basic Books, 1961). Achenbaum discusses these views and differences and offers a nuanced summary. Andrew Achenbaum, *Crossing Frontiers*, 106–8.

8. Cumming and Henry, *Growing Old.*

9. Clark Tibbitts, "The Older Generation in an Aging Population," draft written in 1955, when he was chairman of the Committee on Aging, United States Department of Health, Education, and Welfare.

10. Office of Defense Mobilization, "Productivity at Any Age," Health Resources Advisory Committee. (No author, circa early 1950s), Clark Tibbitts Papers, Bentley Historical Library Collections, University of Michigan. Tibbitts and Wilma Donahue were active contributors to these debates; these views were echoed by Tibbitts in his other works, such as "Social Contributions by the Aging," *Annals of the American Academy of Political Science* 279 (January 1952).

11. Ruth Shavan, in Albert Lansing, ed., *Cowdry's Aging*, 103–4. Shavan was a close associate of Burgess and Havighurst.

12. Wilma Donahue and Clark Tibbitts, "European Approaches to Aging," *Public Health Reports* 70, no. 6 (June 1955): 581–84.

13. At that point, Wilma Donahue was the chairman of the Division of Gerontology at the University of Michigan and organized the annual national conferences on aging supported by federal, state, and other agencies. Tibbitts was representing the United States Department of Health, Education, and Welfare at the congress and had been vice president of the second IGC.

14. Ernest Burgess, *Aging in Western Societies* (Chicago: University of Chicago Press, 1960). See also Ethel Shanas, Peter Townsend, Dorothy Wedderburn, Henning Friis, Poul Milhøj, and Jan Stehouwer, *Old People in Three Industrial Societies* (New York: Atherton, 1968).

15. Burgess's eminent colleague, Robert Park, had drawn on the work of others, such as W. I. Thomas and Forian Znaniecki's *The Polish Peasant in Europe and America* (Boston: Gorham, 1918–1920), 5 vols., and Louis Wirth's *The Ghetto* (Chicago: University of Chicago Press, 1928), who had compared shifts in social processes in Europe and the United States. Albert Hunter, "Why Chicago? The Rise of the Chicago School of Social Science," *American Behavioral Scientist* 24 (1980): 214, 218–19.

16. Ibid.

17. Townsend made it clear that they were challenging the assumptions (or misinterpretations), in the work of Talcott Parsons (1949), that the function and destiny of families in industrialized societies and the lack or absence of families aided technological and occupational changes. Peter Townsend, "The Place of Older People in Different Societies," *Lancet*, January 18, 1964, 159–61.

18. See Davis and Combs, "The Sociology of an Aging Population."

19. Philip M. Hauser and Raul Vargas, "Population Structure and Trends," in Ernest Burgess, *Aging in Western Societies*, 29–31, 51–52.

20. Kingsley Davis and J. W. Combs Jr., "The Sociology of an Aging Population," in *The Social and Biological Challenge of Our Aging Population* (New York: Columbia University Press, 1950), 166–68.

21. Ibid.

22. Ibid., 52.

23. Burgess, *Aging in Western Societies*.

24. Ibid.

25. Ibid.

26. Ibid., 384.

27. Ibid., 375.

28. Kingsley Davis, "Trends in the Ageing Population," in *Problems of Ageing: Biological and Medical Aspects*, ed. E. V. Cowdry (1939; Baltimore: Williams and Wilkins, 1952), 976–77.

29. Louis I. Dublin, "Longevity in Retrospect and Prospect," in Cowdry, ed., *Problems of Ageing*, 214–15.

30. Davis, "Trends in the Ageing Population," 976–77.

31. Howard Jensen, "Sociological Aspects of Aging," *Public Health Reports* (1896–1970) 73, no. 7 (July 1958): 569–76. See G. H. Halsey, "Implications of Aging as Predicted by Population Changes," *Geriatics* 14, no. 1 (January 1959): 1–7; Leonard D. Cain Jr., "The Sociology of Ageing: A Trend Report and Bibliography," *Current Sociology* 8 (1959): 57.

32. Tibbitts, "Old Age." All quotes from Tibbitts in this segment are from this editorial.

33. About the social gerontological enterprise in the United States, Tibbitts noted the significant impetus given by the activities of the sixteen-member

Inter-University Council of Social Gerontology, working under the chairman-
ship of the University of Michigan, which had been supported by the National
Institute of Health; handbooks and curricula on aging had been prepared on a
large scale, and a large number of American universities were now offering
aging-related curricula and research programs. Tibbets, "Old Age," 39–54.

34. See the table of contents, Fourth Congress of the International Association of
Gerontology, Merano, Italy, July 14–21, 1957, 4:3–4; "Areas of Gerontological
Interest as Reflected by Papers Presented at Three International Congresses of
Gerontology" discusses the spike in social themes relating to aging presented
at IAG meetings in 1954–60; table 3, in Tibbitts, "Old Age," 141.

35. Nathan W. Shock, *Classified Bibliography of Gerontology and Geriatrics:
Supplement Two, 1956–1961* (Stanford: Stanford University Press, 1963), 10.

36. Abstracts of papers presented at the Sixth International Congress of Gerontology, Copenhagen, Denmark, August 11–16, 1963 (Amsterdam: Excerpta
Medica Foundation, 1963).

37. There is an extensive correspondence regarding these funds and UNESCO
participation and advice on the IGC in Copenhagen. Letter from Sven Hyden,
Stockholm, January 22, 1963, to DG, UNESCO, regarding contribution
from the UNESCO to a gerontological seminar, 3-053.9A 06 (485) "63"
AMS–Sweden, UNESCO Archives, Paris. There were about 100 participants
at the UNESCO meeting and more than 800 at the IGC.

38. Ibid.

39. J. A. Huet, "Opening Address," in *First International Course in Social Geron-
tology* (Paris: International Center of Social Gerontology, March 16–20, 1970), 10.
Experts from France, Germany, Great Britain, Italy, the Netherlands,
Portugal, and the United States assembled to frame and deliver this course.

40. Ibid., 10–13.

41. Ibid., 13.

42. Todd Shepard, *The Invention of Decolonization: The Algerian War and the
Remaking of France* (Ithaca: Cornell University Press, 2006), 59–60.

43. Sauvy was also the long-time director of the French National Institute of
Demographic Studies. Alfred Sauvy, "The Passage from Activity to Inactivity
as it was in the Past as it was Today," in *First International Course in Social
Gerontology*, 50–51, 56. Others, such as Wilma Donahue, director of the
Institute of Gerontology at the University of Michigan, reiterated the same
focus around retirement and financing; see "Financing and Practical Applications of Training" (86–87).

44. Sauvy was referring primarily to a population of French males.

45. Sauvy, "Passage from Activity to Inactivity," 56.

46. U.S. Senate Committee on Aging, *The Graying of Nations: Implications*
(Washington, DC: Government Printing Office, 1978), 169.

47. Biological research on aging had some networks with Russian researchers and issues of retirement were seen as being addressed by the socialist commitment to the well-being of all citizens.

48. Jim Ogg and Catherine Gorgeon, "Social Gerontology in France," *Ageing and Society* 23, no. 6 (2003): 797–814.

49. The Report was titled *Rapport* de la *commission d'étude* des problèmes de la vieillesse, dit Report Laroque (Paris: Documentation Française, 1962). The report stressed the need to avoid the segregation of older persons, but it also reinforced the chronological thresholds to determine aging, urged the integration of the elderly who were portrayed as resisting integration, and associated aging with conservatism, attachment to habits, and impaired mobility.

50. Patrice Bourdelais, *L'Age De La Vieillesse* (Paris: Odile Jacob, 1993).

51. Jean Auguste Huet, "The Third Age: A Political Problem: Demographic Evolution in the World," *American Behavioral Scientist* 14, no. 1 (September–October 1970): 91.

52. "Application from International NGO for admission of relations with WHO," WHO Executive Board, EB 73/NGO/6, September 21, 1983, 5.

53. Ibid.

54. He continued to play a significant role in later years in the IAG. Dmitriy F. Chebotarev, "International Association of Gerontology," *Gerontologist* (June 1975): 276–77.

55. D. F. Chebotarev and Yu K. Duplenko, "The 9th International Congress of Gerontology: A Summary of the Scientific Program," *Gerontologist* (Summer 1973): 251–56; see also D. F. Chebotarev, ed., *Proceedings of the Ninth International Congress of Gerontology*, July 2–7, 1972, Kiev, vol. 1: *Plenary and Section Sessions* (Kiev, 1972).

56. Among prominent U.S. gerontologists attending the meeting in Kiev were James Birren, Nathan Shock, Walter Beattie, Ruth Binstock, and Jacques Huet of the ICSG, Paris; well-known European gerontologists, in particular renowned experimental gerontologists such as F. Verzar from the Institute of Gerontology in Basel, Switzerland, attended as well. Chebotarev and Duplenko, "The 9th International Congress of Gerontology"; Chebatorev, *Proceedings of the Ninth International Congress of Gerontology.*

57. "Gerontology and Modern Medicine," in Chebotarev, ed., *Proceedings of the Ninth International Congress of Gerontology*, 22–23. Alexander A. Bogomolets, president of the Academy of Sciences of Ukraine and director of the Institute of Physiology in Kiev, was an influential scientist in his generation in Russia. A later generation of biologists such as Zhores Aleksandrovich Medvedev claim that they were influenced by his book *The Prolongation of Life* (trans. Peter V. Karpovich and Sonia Bleeker [New York: Essential Books, Duell, Sloan &

Pearce, 1946]). Interview with Dr. Zhores Medvedev, February 21, 2006, at his home in Mill Hill, London, www.genmedhist.info/interviews/Medvedev, consulted in July 2015.

58. Ethel Shanas, "Self-Reports of Physical Capacity of Old People: A Six-Country Comparison," in Chebotarev, ed., *Proceedings of the Ninth International Congress of Gerontology*, 196–98. Shanas studied Denmark, Britain, the United States, Israel, Poland, and Yugoslavia based on data collected in the 1960s.

59. Shock revealed that 120 travel grants were raised, for instance, for U.S. delegates traveling to the IGC in Kiev. IAG History, "9th International Congress of Gerontology," Folder III, 23, NSP.

60. Zhores Medvedev had been a trenchant critic of the controversial genetic theories of Trofim Lysenko, director of the Institute of Genetics, which found support from the establishment under Stalin and also under Nikita Krushchev. I am grateful to Nikolai Krementsov for his framing of some of these debates in a personal conversation and over emails; these debates are explored more closely in his book *Stalinist Science* (Princeton: Princeton University Press, 1997). "International Association of Gerontology," Box 33, Correspondence with D. F. Chebotarev, NSP.

61. *Report of the World Assembly on Aging*, A/CONF.113/31 (New York: United Nations, 1982), 30.

62. Didier Fassin, *Humanitarian Reason: A Moral History of the Present* (Berkeley: University of California Press, 2012).

63. Representative of the Federal Republic of Germany, quoted in *Report of the World Assembly on Aging*, 33.

64. Peteris Zvidrins and Rudzata, "Reasons and Consequences of Population Aging in the USSR," in Chebotarev, ed., *Proceedings of the Ninth International Congress of Gerontology*, vol. 1, *Plenary and Section Sessions: Reports and Introductory Lectures Condensations of Papers*, 277. About two hundred papers concerned with social gerontology and gerohygiene were read at the plenary session, symposia, and section sessions at this meeting. See also Chebotarev and Duplenlko, "The 9th International Congress of Gerontology," 251–76. Contemporary analysts in the West were already analyzing these shifts, in particular the decline of the Great Russian population (in contrast to the increasing numbers of the population of Muslim origin or high non-Slavic fertility), policies to increase the work-life of individuals after pension age, and family and fertility policies. See Murray Feshbach, "Demography and Soviet Society: Social and Cultural Aspects," colloquium paper presented at the Kennan Institute, Wilson Center, February 19, 1981, www.wilsoncenter .org/sites/default/fi in les/op123_demography_soviet_society _feshback_1981.pdf.

65. Regarding conference discussions about pensions, "pension bankruptcy," and its associated "trauma," see Chebotarev and Duplenko, "The 9th International Congress of Gerontology," 256.

4
New Frontiers

1. Personal Papers, "Aging Around the World," Box 5, Donald O. Cowgill Papers, University of Missouri Library Collections, St. Louis. Letters in this box refer to the founding of the Kansas Association for Aging in Higher Education and related initiatives at the state level that brought Cowgill in touch with Beattie.

2. George L. Maddox, "The Future of Gerontology in Higher Education: Continuing to Open the American Mind About Aging," speech delivered at the 1988 AGHE accepting the Clark Tibbitts Award for 1987, *The Gerontologist* 28, no. 6 (1988): 748–52.

3. Cowgill would later refine this framework. Donald O. Cowgill, "Aging and Modernization: A Revision of the Theory," in *Communities and Environmental Policy*, ed. Jaber F. Gubrium (Springfield, IL: Charles Thomas, 1993), 124–46. See also Erdman Palmore and Kenneth Manton, "Modernization and Status of the Aged: International Correlations," *Journal of Gerontology* 29 (1974): 205–10.

4. Review of Donald O. Cowgill and Lowell D. Holmes, "Aging and Modernization" (1972) by Marilyn Johnson and Joseph Curran Jr., in *Contemporary Sociology* 2, no. 5 (September 1973): 530–32. Later critiques include Nancy Foner, "Age and Social Change," in *Age and Anthropological Theory*, ed. David I. Kertzer and Jennie Keith (Ithaca: Cornell University Press, 1984), 195–216.

5. Donald O. Cowgill and Rosemary A. Orgren, "The International Development of Academic Gerontology," paper prepared for AGHE Dallas, revised, hand-corrected draft dated 5/14/78, Box 5, "Aging Around the World"; Box 11, "Aging—Major Projects" has files on "Comparative Gerontology," Donald O. Cowgill Papers.

6. This included in particular Irene Taeuber's well-known *The Population of Japan* (Princeton: Princeton University Press, 1958) and demographic studies produced by the Office of Population Research at Princeton University.

   Margaret Lock discusses this in her work on aging and menopause in Japan and North America, when she refers to the work of Dona Haraway on situated knowledge and notes that several sets of knowledge do not always intersect consistently, and that disciplines (based on their histories) can often ignore others. Margaret Lock, *Encounters with Aging: Mythologies of Menopause in Japan and North America* (Berkeley: University of California Press, 1993), xxii. See also Donna Haraway, "Situated Knowledges: The Science Question in

Feminism and the Privilege of Partial Perspective," *Feminist Studies* 14, no. 3 (1988): 575–99.

7. Ibid.

8. Letter from Mere N. Kisekka, Senior Lecturer, Department of Sociology, Ahmadu Bello University to Donald Cowgill, Joint Centers for Aging Studies, University of Missouri, on March 2, 1974, in Box 5, Personal Papers, "Aging Around the World," Donald O. Cowgill Papers.

9. Box 5, Personal Papers, "Aging Around the World," Donald O. Cowgill Papers.

10. "Famous Scientist Addresses Opening Session on Congress" quoted Cowdry's speech and the speech by Roswell B. Perkins, Assistant Secretary, Department of Health, Education and Welfare and Chairman, Federal Council of Aging, titled "The Role of the United States Government in Aging," in El Diario De Los Congressos, Mexico, September 18, 1956, 6. In International Gerontological Meetings/Congresses, First Pan-American Congress of Gerontology, 1956, Nathan Shock Papers, Bentley Historical Library, University of Michigan (henceforth NSP).

11. Walter Beattie, background paper on "Aging: A Framework of Characteristics and Considerations for Cooperative Efforts Between Developing and Developed Regions of the World," in *The Graying of Nations: Implications: Hearing before the Special Committee on Aging*, United States Senate, Ninety-fifth Congress, First session, Washington, DC, November 10, 1977, United States Congress Senate Special Committee on Aging (Washington, DC: U.S. Government Printing Office, 1978), 163, 167.

12. Susan Greenhalgh and Edwin A. Winckler, *Governing China's Population: From Leninist to Neoliberal Biopolitics* (Stanford: Stanford University Press, 2005), 99–105, 157–58, 220, 318–22.

13. Jean Haley, "Chinese Still Respect Elders," *Kansas City Times*, February 3, 1979, 2D. In Donald W. Cowgill Papers.

14. Greenhalgh and Winckler, *Governing China's Population*, 220, 320–21.

15. Susan L. Grosser, *Chinese Visions of Family and State, 1915–1953* (Berkeley: University of California Press, 2003).

16. For a discussion of these debates and changing notions of filial piety and intergenerational relations, see "Introduction" and the chapter by Martin Whyte, "Filial Obligations in Chinese Families: Paradoxes of Modernization," both in *Filial Piety: Practice and Discourse in Contemporary East Asia*, ed. Charlotte Ikels (Stanford: Stanford University Press, 2004); Deborah Davis and S. Harrell, eds., *Chinese Families in the Post-Mao Era* (Berkeley: University of California Press, 1993); Myron Cohen, "Family Management and Family Division in Contemporary Rural China," *China Quarterly* 130 (June 1992): 307–33. For a contrast with the demographic transition in Europe and changes in family roles and relations, see Peter Laslett and Richard Wall, eds., *House-*

hold and Family in Past Time (Cambridge: Cambridge University Press, 1972); Michael Mitterauer and Reinhard Sieder, *The European Family: Patriarchy to Partnership from the Middle Ages to the Present,* trans. Karla Oosterveen and Manfred Horzinger (Oxford: Basil Blackwell, 1982); Jerome Silbergeld and Dora C. Y. Ching, eds., *The Family Model in Chinese Art and Culture* (Princeton: Princeton University Press, 2013), see especially the chapter by Rubie S. Watson, "Families in China: Ties That Bind?" for an overview of changing family ties under different political regimes in China. Generalizations about the ubiquity of filial piety since a hoary past—irrespective of class, social changes and time period, often used by authors to contrast with the growing needs and gaps in health care for the old—continue to be made. See for example, "For Thousands of Years, Filial Piety was China's Medicare, Social Security and Long-Term Care, all Woven into a Single Family Value," in A. E. Sher, *Aging in Post-Mao China: The Politics of Veneration* (Boulder, CO: Westview Press, 1984).

17. Kingsley Davis and J. W. Combs, "The Sociology of an Aging Population," in *The Social and Biological Challenge of Our Aging Population,* Proceedings of the Eastern States Health Conference, March 31–April 1, 1949 (New York: Columbia University Press, 1950), 148. Davis was not an expert on China of course, and he in turn quoted further from contemporary works such as Olga Lang's *Chinese Family and Society* (New Haven: Yale University Press, 1946); Land had collected both sociological data and used historical sources to trace the transformation of "old China into New China." A reviewer had criticized her work for its poverty of historical perspective in understanding traditional patterns and their complexity and for surmising on this basis regarding contemporary change. See Tung Tsu-Chu's review in *American Anthropologist* 49, no. 3 (1947): 476–77.

18. Watson "Families in China: Ties That Bind?"

19. Haley, "Chinese Still Respect Elders."

20. Correspondence between Donald Cowgill and Judith Treas, a sociologist at the Adrus Gerontology Center, Los Angeles, October 21, 1973, Donald W. Cowgill Papers. These arguments attracted interest, and others built on these investigations and presented them at the annual meetings of the Gerontological Society, Washington, DC, held in November 1979. See Ralph L. Cherry and Scott Magnuson-Martinson, "Modernization and the Status of the Aged in China: Decline or Equalization?," *Sociological Quarterly* 22, no. 2 (March 1981): 253–61.

21. Wu Cangping, *Cong ren kou xue dao lao nian xue: Wu Cangping zi xuan ji* [From demography to gerontology: Selected essays of Wu Cangping] (Beijing: Shou du shi fan da xue chu ban she, 2010), 412–19; Wu Cangping and Du Peng, *Ren kou lao ling hua guo cheng zhong de Zhongguo lao nian ren*

[The elderly in the process of population aging in China] (Shanghai: Hua dong shi fan da xue chu ban she, 1996), 92. This section is based on interviews conducted with Professor Wu Cangping and Professor Du Peng and on a review of their publications. I am thankful to Dongxin Zou at Columbia University and Shilpa Sharma at the University of Taipei for their careful searches, translations, and scholarly insights, to Arunabh Ghosh at Harvard University for our discussions on demographic exchanges between China and India, and to Susan Greenhalgh for input regarding further contacts of experts currently working in aging in China.

22. These discussions, the beginnings of gerontological expertise in China, are also tied to China's participation in the World Aging Assembly in Vienna (1982) (see Chapter 5), but Wu Cangping and others also argue that it was their studies, travel, and improved demographic analyses that made them frame an early gerontological agenda from "within," and UN directives and collaborations intensified this existing discourse.

23. Communication from Professor Du Peng, director of the Institute of Gerontology at the Renmin University of China, November 2015. I am also grateful for a collaborative award from the Dorothy Borg Fund of the Weatherhead East Asian Institute, Columbia University, that supported these exchanges and a pilot project comparing gerontological research in the Chinese-Indian context (2015–16).

24. Sun Juanjuan, "Academic Thoughts of Professor Wu Cangping," *Social Science of Beijing* 3 (2007): 3–8. Juanjuan writes that Wu was among the first demographers to advocate the control of population growth in 1979. In the same year, "he predicted that aging was the inevitable trend and it was not far ahead."

25. Cangping, *Cong ren kou xue dao lao nian xue*, 14–15.

26. Lan Hongwen, "On How Professor Wu Cangping Does Research, *Xuewei yu yanjiusheng jiaoyu* [Journal of academic degrees and graduate education] 3 (1995): 38–41. Lan notes, "He [Wu] says, the Marxist mode of thinking, in particular, helps him to observe and analyze problems." Lan comments that Wu's writings are always "dialectical, analyzing the problems in their concrete contexts."

27. Kang Liu, *Socialism with Chinese Characteristics* (Hawaii; University of Hawaii Press, 2004), 46–47. I am grateful to Eugenia Lean, Director of the Weatherhead East Asian Institute at Columbia University, for discussing the genesis of these ideas with me, and to the Institute for a grant to research the politics of Chinese gerontology with a collaborator, Professor Du Peng at Renmin University (2015–16).

28. Cangping and Peng, *Ren kou lao ling hua guo*, 86–88.

29. He wrote three essays on "aging while not yet affluent" (Wei fu xian lao). Wu coined this term after the 1982 census. He considered it an important charac-

teristic of China's aging problem. Wu Cangping, *Cong ren kou xue dao lao nian xue*, 469–495, 483.

30. Wu Cangping and Mu Guangzong, *China's Population Situation and Policies*, (Beijing: Foreign Languages Press, 2004), 51.

31. For a background on the changes in social and family support policies for older persons and their long-term care between the 1980s and the present in China, see Shengu Gu and Jersey Liang, "China: Population Aging and Old Age Support," in *Aging in East and West: Families, States, and the Elderly*, ed. Vern L. Bengtson, Kyong-Dong Kim, George C. Myers, and Ki-Soo Eun (New York: Springer, 2000), 59–93; X. Shang, "Moving toward a Multilevel and Multi-Pillar System: Changes in Institutional Care in Two Chinese Cities, *Journal of Social Policy* 30, no. 2 (2001): 259–81; R. J. Chou, "Filial Piety by Contract? The Emergence, Implementation, and Implications of the "Family Support Agreement in China," *Gerontologist* 51, no. 1 (2011): 3–16; Elizabeth J. Croll, "Social Welfare Reform: Trends and Tensions," *China Quarterly* 159 (1999): 684–99.

32. Wu Cangping, *Cong ren kou xue dao lao nian xue*, 14.

33. Susan Greenhalgh, *Just One Child: Science and Policy in Deng's China* (Berkeley: University of California Press), 19–20, 128–29, 296–97.

34. See comment by Qian in "A Letter to Wu Cangping on the Problem of Gerontology," *Journal of Renmin University of China* 3 (1988): 67. Qian was referring in particular to Wu's article "On the Formation of Gerontology, its Objects of Study, and Scientific Nature" published in the same journal (2 [1987]: 1–11).

35. Ibid.

36. Interview with Wu Cangping. See also Wu Cangping, "Theoretical Analysis of Active Response to Population Aging," *Laoling kexue yanjiu* [Scientific Research on Aging] 1 (2013): 4–13.

37. In 1980, life expectancy in India was estimated to be about fifty-five years; by 2015 in Sri Lanka, it was sixty-eight years, even though age-specific mortality after the reproductive years for women and for those above seventy years was comparable to that of the West. Regarding age-specific mortality in rural areas, the authors of *Aging in South Asia* quoted Goran Djurfeldt and Staffan Lindberg, *Pills against Poverty: A Study of the Introduction of Western Medicine in a Tamil Village* (Delhi: Macmillan, 1982); Walter Fernandes, "Aging in South Asia as Marginalization in a Neo-Colonial Economy: An Introduction," in Alfred de Souza and Walter Fernandes, *Ageing in South Asia: Theoretical Issues and Policy Implications*, Papers presented at the Asian Regional Conference on Active Aging, Manila, 1982, sponsored by the United Nations Population Fund and Opera Pia International (New Delhi: Indian Social Institute, 1982), 5–6.

38. Fernandes, "Aging in South Asia as Marginalization in a Neo-Colonial Economy: An Introduction," 5.

39. Ibid.

40. Kirpal Singh Soodan, *Aging in India* (Calcutta: Minerva Associates, 1975).

41. Lawrence Cohen, *No Aging in India: Alzheimer's, the Bad Family and Other Modern Things* (Berkeley: University of California Press, 1998), 89, 92–93.

42. Soodan, *Aging in India*, 112–13.

43. De Souza and Fernandes, *Ageing in South Asia*, 23. A background in social work also influenced their ideas, as there was a strong critique of inequality and of development paradigms among social workers in Latin America, Asia, and Africa. See James Midgley, "Social Welfare Implications of Development Paradigms," *Social Service Review* 58, no. 2 (June 1984): 181–98.

44. Letter to Donald Cowgill from Professor Peerasit Kamnuansilpa, National Institute of Development Administration, Research Center, Thailand, dated February 6, 1978: "the present concern of the country is with youths rather than the aged . . . but as population aging increases through longevity there should be serious consideration of gerontological studies," but only if there are jobs available as well. A letter to Donald Cowgill on February 24, 1978 from Dr. Yahya El-Haddad, University of Kuwait, refers to Professor Naji, who had returned from being trained in the United States. "Paper on World System Perspective on Aging," Box 20, Donald Cowgill Collections.

45. Paul Chowdhry, "The Aged and the Infirm," in *Encyclopaedia of Social Work in India* (New Delhi: Government of India, 1963), 24–29; C. B. Mamoria, *Labour Problems and Social Welfare in India* (Allahabad: Kitab Mahal, 1966). A discussion of anxieties about aging, social work, and the erosion of family solidarities in India can be found in Kavita Sivaramakrishnan, "Aging and Dependency in a Young Indian Nation: Migrant Families, Workers and Social Experts (1940–60)," *Journal of Social History* (March 2014): 1–26.

46. For a discussion of the influence of colonial priorities on social work and newer paradigms, including the role of modernization theory and critiques of poverty, see Margaret Hardiman and James Midgley, *The Social Dimensions of Development: Social Policy and Planning in the Third World* (Chichester: Wiley, 1982).

47. Ibid. For a discussion of U.S. influence on social work in India, see K. S. Mandal, "American Influence on Social Work Education in India," *Indian Journal of Social Work* 32, no. 4 (1989): 303–9, 305.

48. Issachar Ilan and Mirian Hoffert, "Training Social Workers for East Africa: A Personal Account," *Kidma* 1, no. 2 (1973): 24–28.

49. UNICEF was often supportive of the development of meaningful teaching materials for African contexts. See Shawky, "Social Work Education in Africa," *International Social Work* 15, no. 3 (1972): 3–16.

50. ASWEA Papers, 1971–83, AG 3303, Curricula of Schools of Social Work and Community Development Training Centres in Africa, Document 7, 1974; for other examples, see Nsamizi Training Institute's Diploma Course in Social Development, Uganda (established in 1954), 88; and the Oppenheimer Department of Social Service (established in 1965) in Zambia and its Social Work Course (for four years) that included urban destitution, public assistance programs, and social problems of modern Zambia. For specific references, see pages 35 (Ghana), 44 (Tanarive), 16–17 (Central African Republic), 18 (Cairo), 60–61 (Mauritius School of Administration, University of Mauritius). For a background to this social work archive, see Linda Kreitzer, *Social Work in Africa: Exploring Culturally Relevant Social Work Education and Practice in Ghana* (Calgary: University of Calgary Press, 2012).

51. De Souza and Fernandes, *Ageing in South Asia.*

52. Interview with Joseph Hampson (Jesuit missionary; as of 1985 Hampson was the director of fieldwork at the School of Social Service in Harare), September 2015, about the networks and models for the Social Work School in Zimbabwe. He observed that the ASWEA network meetings were inspiring and many like him, and others from sub-Saharan Africa and other countries, saw the courses in Ethiopia and Egypt as "models" to emulate. Hampson, with a network of social and welfare work partners, was also a key figure in developing a national plan of action for aging in Zimbabwe.

53. ASWEA Partners, *Challenges of Training: Guidelines for the Development of a Training Curriculum in Family Welfare*, AG 3303, 4, no. 1, 1971–83.

54. United Nations, *Report of Habitat: United Nations Conference on Human Settlements*, Vancouver, May 31–June 11, 1976, A/Conf.70/15 (New York: United Nations, 1976).

55. J. M. Kumarappa discusses the early focus of social workers in India in "Social Problems of India," National Conference of Social Work, Official Proceedings of the Annual Meeting, Atlantic City, New Jersey, April 17–23, 1948, Selected Papers of the Annual Meeting, 1874–1948 (New York, 1949), 74, 74–78. University of Michigan Libraries, Digital Collection, ACH 8650.

56. United Nations, *Improvement of Slums and Uncontrolled Settlements* (New York: United Nations, 1972).

57. United Nations, *The Aging in Slums and Uncontrolled Settlements* (New York: United Nations, 1977).

58. Ibid.

59. United Nations, Improvement of Slums and Uncontrolled Settlements, 10, 38.

60. The All Africa Conference of Churches reinforced the need to train social workers to deal with vulnerable refugee populations. Lars-Gunnar Eriksson, Göran Melander, and Peter Nobel, eds., *An Analysing Account of the Conference on the African Refugee Problem* (Uppsala: Scandinavian Institute of

African Studies [now the Nordic Africa Institute, NAI], 1981), 192; Peter Nobel, ed., *Refugees and Development in Africa* (Uppsala, Scandinavian Institute of. African Studies, 1987), 110.

61. Chris Chogugudza, "Social Work Education, Training and Employment in Africa: The Case of Zimbabwe," Ufahamu: Journal of African Studies 35, no. 1 (2009): 1–2; the author also cites further discussion in O. N. Moyo, Tramped No More: Voices from Bulawayo's Townships about Families, Life, Survival, and Social Change in Zimbabwe (Lanham, MD: University Press of America, 2007); E. Kaseke, "Social Work Practice in Zimbabwe," Journal of Social Development in Africa 6 (1991): 33–45.

62. W. Clifford, *A Primer of Social Case Work in Africa* (Nairobi: Oxford University Press, 1966), 48.

63. The author noted that the state had complete discretion in changing eligibility rules for pensions, and criteria such as good conduct as well as a range of burdensome requirements could be imposed for collecting for "old" persons. R. Singh, "Welfare of the Aged," *Indian Journal of Social Work* 30 (1970): 327–33.

64. Clifford, *A Primer of Social Case Work in Africa*, 10–11.

65. Ibid., 40.

66. Ibid., 40–41, 42.

67. There is an extensive literature on ideas relating to female bodies and aging; the work of Carol Bledsoe, Sarah Lamb, and Margaret Lock are of particular relevance here. See Sarah Lamb, *White Saris and Sweet Mangoes: Aging, Gender, and Body in North India* (Berkeley: University of California Press, 2000); Margaret Lock, *Encounters with Aging: Mythologies of Menopause in Japan and North America* (Berkeley: University of California Press, 1993).

68. Andreas Sagner, " 'The Abandoned Mother': Ageing, Old Age and Missionaries in Early and Mid-Nineteenth Century South-East Africa," *Journal of African History* 42, no. 2 (2001), 173–98; Andrea Menefee Singh, "Rural-Urban Migration of Women among the Urban Poor in India," *Social Action* 28 (October–December 1978): 326–56.

69. Most of the social casework focus in newer nations was therefore on youth, since they were unemployed and unskilled, and the social group worker was seen as assisting the caseworker and working with groups. Malcolm J. Brown, *An Introduction to Social Group Work in Africa*, Special Publication (n.p.: University of Zambia, Oppenheimer Department of Social Service, 1969), 64–65, 67.

70. Brown, *An Introduction to Social Group Work in Africa*, 67–68.

71. R. Singh, "Welfare of the Aged," 327–33.

72. Ibid.

5

The Birth of Global Aging and Its Local Afterlives

1. Report of the World Assembly on Aging, Vienna, July 26–August 6, 1982, A/CONF.113/13 (1982).

2. For more on this, see Chapter 4.

3. *Report of the World Population Conference, 1974* (held in Bucharest, Romania, August 19–30, 1974), E/CONF/60/19 (New York: UN, 1975). The year 1974 was declared World Population Year.

4. This was inserted in a section titled World Health Organization, "For a Just World," in *Report of the United Nations World Population Conference, 1974* (New York: United Nations, 1975), 32.

5. Report of the World Assembly on Aging, Vienna, July 26–August 6, 1982, A/CONF.113/13 (1982): 8–10.

6. Ibid.

7. "Some Quantitative Aspects of the Aging of Western Populations," *Population Bulletin* 1 (December 1951): 42–43, United Nations, New York. The writer noted that Latin America, Japan, and the Soviet Union were beginning to see a small fall in fertility and mortality, but they were distinct from the West, which had witnessed a long-term decline in both mortality and fertility.

8. Though the discussions in Bucharest in 1974 were to undermine and critique these notions.

9. Simon Szreter, "The Idea of Demographic Transition and the Study of Fertility Change: A Critical Intellectual History," *Population and Development Review* 19, no. 4 (December 1993): 659–701.

10. Matt Connelly, *Fatal Misconception: The Struggle to Control World Population* (Cambridge, MA: Harvard University Press, 2008).

11. Alison Bashford, *Global Population: History, Geopolitics and Life on Earth* (New York: Columbia University Press, 2014), 308–17.

12. Irene B. Taeuber, "Future Population Trends and Prospects," *Proceedings of the World Population Conference, Belgrade*, vol. 1, Summary Report, August 30–September 10, 1965 (New York: United Nations, 1966), 193. She noted that Japan and Argentina were in stages of advanced demographic transition, and the former was in a stage of high fertility, and this only reinforced the "hazards" of regional generalizations (195). Irene B. Taeuber Papers, 1912–1981, C2158, The State Historical Society of Missouri. See "Research and Data: Japan," F 2331–2446, F2267; "Audio Cassette Series," A. C. 2, Speech on "Growth Paths of Asian Population" at the World Population Society meeting on February 9, 1974 in Washington, DC, State Historical Society of Missouri, University of Missouri. I am grateful to the Historical Society and its archivist for allowing me to consult these papers.

13. Ibid., 193.
14. Ibid., 195–96; R. Bachi, "Statement by the Rapporteur," Meeting A4 on Future Population Trends and Prospects, 201–5.
15. Taeuber, "Future Population Trends," 196.
16. The ECAFE in these years was a meeting place for regional countries that were trying to achieve economic independence; regional demographic projections were closely tied to these development aspirations. See Nicholas J. White, "The Development and Activities of the Economic Commission for Asia and the Far East (ECAFE), 1947–1965," in *The Transformation of the International Order of Asia: Decolonization, the Cold War, and the Colombo Plan*, ed. Shigeru Akita, Gerold Krozewski, and Shoichi Watanabe (London: Routledge Studies in the Modern History of Asia, 2005), 93–94.
17. *Population Aspects of Social Development*, Report of the Regional Seminar and Selected Papers, Asian Population Studies Series (Bangkok, Thailand, January 11–20, 1972), 2, 12, 83–87.
18. Ibid.
19. United Nations Bureau of Social Affairs, "Implications of Population Trends for Planning Urban Development and Housing Programmes in ECAFE Countries," APC/WP/4, in *Population Aspects of Social Development*, 97, 97–114.
20. Ibid., 103–4.
21. Nearly 72 percent of Japan's population was living in cities with 20,000 or more inhabitants in 1960, but the UN report said this was overestimated. In most Asian countries, the urban population was growing at twice the rate of the total population. Over 17 percent of the population in the ECAFE region was living in urban areas. *Population Aspects of Social Development*, 16, 99–101.
22. Ibid., 13, 16.
23. Information on fertility and mortality were available for East Africa, but other countries (such as Portuguese Africa) had partial information or lacked fertility and mortality information (Nigeria and Liberia) and were "demographic *terra incognita*" (Ethiopia). Etienne Van De Walle, "The Availability of Demographic Data by Regions in Tropical Africa," in *The Population of Tropical Africa*, ed. John C. Caldwell and Chukuka Okongo (Hong Kong: Longman, 1968), 28–33. This book is a record of the First Population Conference sponsored by the Population Council at the University of Ibadan, Nigeria, January 3–7, 1966.
24. J. C. Caldwell, "Introduction," in Caldwell and Okongo, eds., *The Population of Tropical Africa*, 9.
25. There was an assumption that these linear trends in demographic (life expectancy, death rate, and fertility) and disease patterns would continue, but by the 1990s, uncertainties and reversals due to the catastrophic effects of the

HIV/AIDS epidemic were manifesting. John Caldwell's own research focus would shift considerably within the next two decades; John Caldwell, "Rethinking the African AIDS Epidemic," *Population and Development Review*, 26 (March 2000), 117–35.

26. Ibid., 14–15.

27. Report of the Secretary General, Economic and Social Progress in the Second Development Decade (New York: United Nations Department of Economic and Social Affairs, 1977), 22–23.

28. P. Sadasivan Nair, "Population Bomb: Its Demographic and Economic Implications," *Social Welfare* 20, no. 3 (June 1973), 19, 21.

29. Ibid.

30. V. K. R. V. Rao, "Planning the Demographic Transition," in "Proceedings of the National Conference on Population," ed. R. K. Sanyal and A. K. Nana. Supplement 1, *Journal of Population Research* (January–June 1975): 52. The conference members worried about the slow progress of the family planning movement and stated that the government's goals were ambitious. Ashish Bose, in "Findings of the Conference," stated that the illiterate masses in rural areas of India would not opt for family planning unless there was the provision of old age security combined with the emancipation of women. In an oft-quoted statement, India's then health minister, Karan Singh, observed that the demographic transition could not come about "unless there is comprehensive economic growth and social transformation" and noted that "population policy . . . was too important to be left to demographers. Karan Singh, "Adequate Funds Needed for Package Inputs," Valedictory Address, ibid., 55.

31. Karen Litfin, *Ozone Discourses: Science and Politics in Global Environmental Cooperation* (New York: Columbia University Press, 1997); Peter M. Haas, "Epistemic Communities and International Policy Coordination," *International Organization* 46, no. 1, Knowledge, Power and International Policy Coordination (Winter 1992): 1–35.

32. Arturo Escobar, *Encountering Development: The Making and Unmaking of the Third World* (Princeton: Princeton University Press, 1994).

33. Hong Chang Ping, "Ageing Problem and Our [efforts to] Mitigate Ir," August 20, 1984, 4. I am thankful to my colleague Professor Du Peng and his research assistants at Renmin University for having helped trace material on the history of gerontology in China, and to Shilpa Sharma in assisting in translating interviews conducted in July 2014 in Beijing; Johnson, D. Gale "Effects of Institutions and Policies on Rural Population Growth with Application to China," *Population and Development Review* 20, no. 3 (1994): 503–31. See also Jiali Li, "China's One-Child Policy: How and How Well Has It Worked? A Case Study of Hebei Province, 1979–88," *Population and Development Review* 21, no. 3 (1995): 563–85.

34. Ibid.

35. Interview conducted at Professor Wu's home in Beijing, July 8, 2015.

36. "That's why I used to travel widely. During the 1980s and 1990s I traveled almost to a hundred countries, many times particularly to those countries such as India, where I also observed their population policies, visited the population center in Bombay where I had many friends and went to rural areas to understand education of rural Indian people in family planning." Interview conducted at Professor Wu's Home in Beijing, July 8, 2014.

37. The CSDHA (a division of the ECOSOC) was located until the 1990s in Vienna. It dealt broadly with social and economic issues, and later, its mandate broadened to include environmental and sustainable development issues as well. It was subsequently relocated to New York and renamed the Division for Social Policy and Development, and is currently associated with the Department of Economic and Social Affairs (DESA), which forms part of the UN secretariat. I am grateful to Robert Venne and Dr. Srinivas Tata at DESA, New York, for their input on the changing profile and work of this division and its engagement with aging-related policies and programs, and for sharing its published reports (2011–2015). All views expressed about these bodies and their projects are my own. See www.un.org/development/desa/en/.

38. The IFA was founded in 1973 after a meeting of the American Association of Retired Persons (AARP), when some representatives expressed an interest in international mobilization, and had its headquarters in Canada. At the time of this meeting, preceding the Vienna Assembly, it had few partnerships in Asia, Africa, and Latin America, with loose links with pension bodies, government departments of aging, and medical experts in aging in India, South Africa, Bangladesh, Brazil, Mexico, and Costa Rica. Its leadership—including its president (Robert Prigent), vice presidents (from the United States and Belgium), and others—was mostly from the United States. See Charlotte Nusberg, ed., *The UN World Assembly on the Elderly: The Aging as a Resource, The Aging as a Concern and The Situation of the Elderly in Austria*, Proceedings of the Two Meetings Organized by the International Federation on Aging, May 27–29, 1980, Vienna, Austria (Washington, DC: International Federation on Aging, 1981), colophon.

39. Evener Ergun, "The World Assembly on the Elderly: The UN's Point of View," and Tarek Shuman, "The World Assembly on the Elderly and Non-Governmental Organizations," in Nusberg, ed., *The UN World Assembly on the Elderly*, 3–5, 6–7. Evener Ergun represented the UN Social Development Administration (1982).

40. Ergun, "The World Assembly on the Elderly"; Shuman, "The World Assembly on the Elderly and Non-Governmental Organizations."

41. Ibid., 7.

42. For a discussion of the critiques expressed by intellectuals in the global South during the "third development decade" in the 1970s and the 1980s as a "lost decade," see Arturo Escobar, *Encountering Development: The Making and Unmaking of the Third World* (Princeton: Princeton University Press, 2011), 89–92. Escobar traces how the postwar discourse on development was created, how the Third World emerged as a distinct social reality, and how Western experts offered specific technical solutions to address its problems. For one of many UN statements, see United Nations, Department of Economic and Social Affairs, *The United Nations Development Decade: Proposals for Action* (New York: United Nations, 1962).

43. In the 1980s, some believed that the UN had become the principal forum for the South, unlike the IMF and the World Bank, where power and vote were financially weighted. Peter Stephenson, *Handbook of World Development: The Guide to the Brandt Report* (New York: Holmes and Meir, 1981), 62–63.

44. Eduard Pumpernig, "The UN World Assembly on the Elderly from the Point of View of the EURAG," in Charlotte Nusberg, ed., *The UN World Assembly on the Elderly*, 18; emphasis added.

45. Ibid.

46. Ibid.

47. Almost two decades later, the EURAG and other such associations have shown an increasing commitment to the rights of older women workers, essentially women in the informal sector where women predominate, and to supporting their increased labor participation. However, the integration especially with the UN Commission on the Status of Women has been recent, and it has been argued that mainstreaming gender into aging policies, despite the recommendations of the Madrid International Plan of Action on Ageing produced by the Second World Assembly held in Madrid in 2002, is still slow. See the speech by Aparna Malhotra of UN Women, speaking on a panel sponsored by the Commission for Social Development, the EURAG, the Baha'i International Community and other NGOs at the United Nations Commission on the Status of Women 56, New York, February 27–March 9, 2012, www.own-europe.org.

48. EURAG Newsletter, *The Aging: Their Integration and Social Security in the Productivity Society of Europe*, June/September 1976, nos. 6/7, 8th International Congress of EURAG, Belgrade, June 1–4, 1976 (EURAG, General Secretariat, Austria).

49. R. Schubert, "Tasks and Aims of Research on Aging," 8, 9, 1–15, and E. Pumpernig, "The Situation of the Elderly Employee,"111–17, 113, in ibid.; emphasis added.

50. See the article by the influential French social policy expert and member of French Council of State, Pierre Laroque, "Women's Rights and Widow's Pensions," *International Labour Review* 106 (July 1972): 1–10.

51. Leopold Rosenmayr, "Help and Self-Help: Some Problems of Aging Policy," in Nusberg, ed., *The UN World Assembly on the Elderly*, 40–45.
52. Ibid., 42–43.
53. Ibid.
54. Ibid., 43.
55. His research on the aged in Vienna explored the dynamics of three-generation families. See Leopold Rosemayr, "The Family: A Source of Hope for the Elderly," in *Family, Bureaucracy and the Elderly*, ed. Ethel Shanas and M. Sussman (Durham, NC: Duke University Press, 1977), 132–57.
56. For an exploration of the cofounding of the IASW in 1928 by Rene Sand, a Belgian social worker and physician, and its links with the International Committee on Social Work (1929), see James Midgeley, *Social Welfare in the Global Context* (New York: Sage, 1997) and Walter A. Friedlander, *International Social Welfare* (Englewood Cliffs, NJ: Prentice-Hall, 1975); on social work's colonial roots, see James Midgeley, *Professional Imperialism: Social Work in the Third World* (London: Heinemann Educational Books, 1981). Sand was also on an expert committee that contributed to designing the foundational framework of the WHO; he had close ties with leaders and activists in developing nations.
57. These views had been echoed elsewhere at ICSW meetings to stress its action-oriented agenda, which was focused worldwide. Its leadership believed that conferences were unwieldly and their value lay in their capacity to assemble persons who could in turn meet others of diverse backgrounds and social realities. Speech by Zena Harman, Chairman of Program Committee, of the XIX International Conference on Social Welfare, Jerusalem, Israel, August 18–24, 1978; see *Human Well-Being: Challenges for the 1980s Social and Economic and Political Action, Proceedings of the XIX International Conference on Social Welfare, 1978* (New York: Columbia University Press, 1979), viii. Ingrid Gelinek, "The World Assembly on the Elderly from the Point of View of the International Council on Social Welfare," in Nusberg, ed., *The UN World Assembly on the Elderly*, 12, 12–18.
58. It also worked closely with several UN bodies involved in matters of labor relations, health care, and social development. Gelinek, "The World Assembly on the Elderly," 13.
59. Ibid. See Sybil Francis, "Social Needs in a Changing Society," *Caribbean Quarterly* 8, no. 2 (June 1962): 130–31; see also Denise Eldermire-Shearer, "Aging: The Response Yesterday, Today and Tomorrow," *West Indian Medical Journal* 57, no. 6 (2008): 577–87; Denise Eldermire-Shearer, "Ageing: A New Challenge to Health Care in the New Millennium, *West Indian Medical Journal* 50 (2001), 95–99; *The Status of the Jamaican Elderly*, report (Kingston: Planning Institute of Jamaica Report, 1995); and "The Elderly and the Family:

The Jamaican Experience," *Bulletin of Eastern Caribbean Affairs* 19 (1994): 31–46. Jamaica had strong links with the international social work community, and in the 1970s and later there were efforts to indigenize the scope of social welfare in the Caribbean, as part of a larger movement of "reconceptualizing" social work and turning away from Western models. Others have subsequently built on this legacy of aging-related programs in the Caribbean, leading to the continued leadership of the Caribbean Community countries in introducing social legislation relating to global aging and human rights. This includes activists such as Denise Eldermire-Shearer at the Department of Community Health and Psychiatry, University of the West Indies, who also founded Mona Ageing and Wellness. For a social work perspective of these events in the Caribbean and other parts of the global South, see Lynne M. Healy, *International Social Work: Professional Action in an Interdependent World*, 2nd ed. (Oxford: Oxford University Press, 2008), 135–233, chaps. 6–8, and also the references to the contribution of Sybil Francis (154–55).

60. Gelinek, "The World Assembly on the Elderly," 13–14.

61. Ibid., 14.

62. Ibid., 15.

63. "On situation of aging, prepare national plans, strengthen activities of regional bodies to increase awareness and to collect basic data for regional preparatory meetings." United Nations General Assembly Resolution 34/153, "Question of the Elderly and the Aged," in *Aging, Bulletin on Aging* 5, no.1 (1980): 5, 8.

64. Ibid.

65. Social Development Branch, "1982: World Assembly on Aging—Preparatory Activities," *Aging, Bulletin on Aging* 6, no. 1 (1980): 8.

66. Ibid., 2–3. Presumably, influenced by the notion of decline in family relations and the status of elders associated with modernization theory.

67. Ibid.

68. Reports on various meetings were summed up in ibid., for example, Regional Meeting in Manila (Asia and Pacific), October 19–23, 1981. A regional strategy was proposed, "to maintain the capacity of the extended family system in order to provide adequate care to the elderly. The family was recognized in developing countries and developed countries as having the greatest caring capacity." The elderly and their role in integrated rural development, utilizing social security funds to develop developmental projects that could benefit the aged were proposed, 9–10. It is not clear if any "lay" older persons were invited to these meetings, and most likely they were confined to "local experts" such as sociologists, social workers, NGO leaders, scientists, and policymakers whose names and designations are listed in the appendices to these reports.

69. United Nations Economic and Social Council, Economic Commission for Latin America, Report of the Latin American Regional Preparatory Meeting

for the World Assembly on Aging, San Jose, Costa Rica, March 8–12, 1982, E/CEPAL/G.1201, E/CEPAL/Conf.74/L.4 (March 31, 1982, UN Documents), 3–4.

70. Ibid., 3–5.

71. Debates at the meeting stressed that "especially in developing countries, the basic welfare requirements of the elderly were often distinguishable from the basic needs of the population as a whole . . . that the Plan of Action on Aging should presuppose the existence of the necessary international conditions to ensure the realization of the right to development and a fair and equitable international economic order" ("Summary of the Debates," ibid., 5).

72. Florence Palmer, "The World Assembly on the Elderly and the World Health Organization," in Nusberg, ed., The UN World Assembly on the Elderly, 8.

73. WHO, Declaration of Alma Ata, International conference on primary health care, Alma Ata, USSR, September 6–12, 1978, Geneva, www.who.int/hpr/NPH /docs/declaration_almaata.pdf. The advocates of selective primary health care summed up their views in J. A. Walsh and K. S. Warren, "Selective Primary Health Care: An Interim Strategy for Disease Control in Developing Countries," New England Journal of Medicine 301, no. 18 (1979): 967–74. There was widespread criticism of this departure from the Alma Ata vision; see Ben Wisner, "GOBI versus PHC? Some Dangers of Selective Primary Health Care," Social Science and Medicine 26, no. 9 (1988): 963–69.

74. Ibid.

75. A motion to consider "the question of the elderly" was raised in 1969 at the United Nations General Assembly in Resolution 2599 (XXIV), and to assist further discussions various studies began to be planned, resulting in a report titled The Aging: Trends and Policies, Department of Economic and Social Affairs (New York: United Nations, 1975), 2–3.

76. UN General Assembly, 28th Session, "Question of the Elderly and the Aged," Report of the Third Committee, A/8591 (December 14, 1971), UN Microfilms, held at the Diamond Law Library, Columbia University; emphasis added.

77. Alexandre Sidorenko and Alan Walker, "The Madrid International Plan of Action on Ageing: From Conception to Implementation," Ageing and Society 24 (March 2, 2004): 147–65. Carol Estes discusses it in her work as well.

78. Michael G. Schechter, The UN Global Conferences (London: Routledge, 2005), 90, 92.

79. Jeffrey Harrod and Nico Schrijver, eds., The UN Under Attack (Aldershot: Gower, 1988), 8–13, 21. In his contribution to this volume, titled "Developments in Decision Making in the United Nations," Johan Kaufman noted that even though the UN had begun hosting global conferences under its auspices, and the first of these was the Stockholm Conference on the Environment (1972),

these conferences' plans of action were "almost ritually adopted" but had "only been partly implemented, if at all." The UN secretariat too was less and less trusted, as some groups, such as the UN Conference on Trade and Development, were seen as supporting the interests of developing countries as confrontations over the NIEO deepened in these years (ibid., 24).

80. Letter from Ethel Shanas, sociologist at the University of Chicago, to Harold Brody, president of the American Gerontological Society, discussing the plans for a WAA, December 19, 1974, 1, Box 16, Folder 270, 121, Ethel Shanas Collection, University of Illinois in Chicago. I am thankful to the librarians for scanning the relevant correspondence and reports Shanas produced in the 1960–1980s. See references also in the Frank Church Papers, MSS 56 (special collections). I am grateful to the Boise State University Library in Idaho for allowing me to consult these papers. For a background on debates on federal policy and aging in these years, see Robert H. Binstock and Martin A. Levin, "The Political Dilemmas of Intervention Policies," in Robert H. Binstock and Ethel Shanas, eds., *Handbook of Aging and the Social Sciences* (New York: Van Nostrand Reinhold, 1976); Caroll L. Estes, *The Aging Enterprise: A Critical Examination of Social Policies and Services for the Aged* (San Francisco: Jossey-Bass, 1976); Robert J. Samuelson, "Busting the US Budget: The Costs of an Aging America," *National Journal* 10 (February1978): 256–60.

81. Theodore Schuchat, "Retirement Revolution Becoming a Major Force," *Sarasota Journal* (December 15, 1972), 8, news.google.com/newspapers?id =2nUoAAAAIBAJ&sjid=I4oEAAAAIBAJ&pg=7346%2C3857545.

82. Mildred M. Seltzer, "New Directions for Social Services: Much Ado about Nothing," originally published in *Journal of Gerontological Social Work* 4, nos. 3–4 (Spring/Summer 1982), republished in the same journal, 59, no. 2 (2016): 140–48.

83. Ibid.

84. Warren Weaver Jr., "Poll Detects Myths about Problems of Aged," *New York Times*, November 19, 1981, www.nytimes.com/1981/11/19/us/poll-detects-myths -about-problems-of-aged.html.

85. Also in shaping the draft plan presented to world delegates at the Vienna Assembly.

86. This Expert Group Meeting on Aging, held May 6–17, 1974, shaped the report produced for the UN on aging, its trends, and its policies, which in turn served as guidelines and recommendations for national and international policies. There were a few representatives from beyond Europe and North America at the meeting, including of a member each from Lebanon, Nigeria, Japan, and Argentina. Ethel Shanas Papers, Box 16, Folder 260, File 121, document on "Expert Group Meeting on Aging, May 6–17, 1974, Provisional List of Participants." The collection (Ethel Shanas Papers, 011-22-24) is housed at the

University of Illinois in Chicago, and I am grateful to the librarians for allowing me to consult and scan certain papers. *The Aging: Trends and Policies*, 50–80. D. F. Chebotarev in turn hosted a few regional meetings, bringing in delegates from Eastern Europe to Kiev, to discuss these plans; personal communication from Tarek Shuman, May 6, 2015. Views regarding the influential role played by Shanas and others in the US are my own, based on my research, and do not reflect Dr. Shuman's recollections of the Assembly.

87. Letter from Ethel Shanas to Harold Brody, Department of Anatomical Sciences, SUNYAS School of Medicine, December 16, 1974, in the Ethel Shanas Papers, Box 16, Folder 260, File 121.

88. *The Aging: Trends and Policies*; "Progress in Developing an Understanding of Aging Processes," Annexure, 83.

89. See n. 38 above for more details about the IFA and its links with the AARP. "The problem of aging is a relatively new one. . . . Although the field of gerontology is a relatively new one and is still in the process of defining its character, broad divisions of subject-matter have already appeared and, within them, various specialties related to particular problems and aspects of aging." Note prepared by the WHO on the "Health Concerns of the Elderly and the Aged," Annexure, 69.

90. Ethel Shanas Papers, Box 16, Folder 260, File 121, notes.

91. Ethel Shanas Papers, notes. This was also integrated into the meetings' recommendations. Commission for Social Development, 24th Session, January 6–24, 1975, Report of the Secretary General on the Expert Group Meeting on Aging held at the United Nations, May 6–17, 1974, E/CN.5/509, 3. Copy of UN Document in the Ethel Shanas Papers.

92. The general debates at the WAA took place over thirteen plenary meetings between July 26 and August 3, 1982. Delegates commented on the introductory papers, which had been prepared over several years by advisory committees and meetings, and on the text of the draft version of the international plan of action on aging, drafted by the UN and aging experts. See A/CNF.113/11, UNWAA (1982), 7–11 at the UN Library, New York. See also the final report, Report of the World Assembly on Aging, Vienna, July 26 to August 6, 1982, A/CONF.113/31 (United Nations, New York, 1982), 28–44. U.S. leadership watched the conference closely, since the United States substantially funded the Assembly Trust Fund. Michael G. Schechter, *The UN Global Conferences*, 90. The United States also submitted a detailed country report on the situation of the aged to establish its clear interest in the agenda of the conference, and Ronald Reagan was one of a handful of leaders who sent a message to the Assembly.

93. He was speaking to a writer from the UN Newsletter, UN WAA, Journal Newsletter no. 2, spring 1982, issued by the Division for Economic and Social

Information (UN Library and Archives, New York), 3. The Vienna plan did not result in more than a handful of immediate commitments to aging programs based on international funding, instead relying mostly on local initiatives and collaborations.

94. The Plan of Action of the Vienna Declaration noted, "The developing countries are in this sense about to 'age' without all the sectors necessary to ensure balanced and integrated development being able to follow at the same pace and guarantee a decent living standard for the dramatically increasing numbers of elderly people foreseen for the next few generations. Focused on a preparation for retirement in a gradual and individual process of aging, and to encourage policies for a more 'active' aging and enhance their capacity to continue interacting with society. Changing dependency ratios—in terms of the number of old people depending for their material safety on younger, economically active and wage-earning people—are bound to influence the development of any country in the world. . . . Problems of a social nature are likely to emerge in countries and regions where the aging have traditionally benefited from the care and protection of their next of kin or the local community." *Vienna International Plan of Action on Aging* (New York: United Nations, 1983), 16–17, www.un.org/en/events/elderabuse/pdf/vipaa.pdf.

95. Ibid.

96. All spellings as in original text, Kenya, UN World Assembly on Aging General Assembly, Statements, vol. I (New York: United Nations, 1982), consulted at the UNSA Collection, UN Library and Depository, New York), 2–4. These are volumes with a compilation of country papers.

97. Ibid.

98. Malawi, UN World Assembly on Aging General Assembly, Statements, 1:2–3.

99. WAA, GA, 1982, Statement by Sri Lanka, UNA Conference, 113 Statements, UN Library, New York City.

100. WAA, GA, 1982, Statement by Nigeria, UNA Conference, 113 Statements, UN Library, New York City.

101. The former comment was made by the representative from South Korea, and a lengthy description of the integration of those over the age of 60 years into primary care services, such as those already available for maternal and child care in rural areas, was provided by a paper submitted by the Botswana government. UN World Assembly on Aging General Assembly, Statements, 1:3–5 (Korea); Botswana paper submitted to the World Assembly on Aging, Vienna, Austria, July 26–August 6, 1982, 1–4. The Botswana government also proposed an extension of the pension scheme (so far available to government pensioners) to all older persons in the country.

102. UN World Assembly on Aging General Assembly, Statements, 1:3–5 (Korea), 1–2 (Japan).

103. UN World Assembly on Aging General Assembly, Statements, Speech by Yu Guanghan, Chairman of the Chinese Delegation, at the World Assembly on Aging, Vienna, July 1982, 1:3. See also, Mr. Jaroslav Havelka, Czechoslovak Socialist Republic, address to the World Assembly on Aging, UN World Assembly on Aging General Assembly, Statements, 1:1–6.

104. UN World Assembly on Aging General Assembly, Statements, speech by Yu Guanghan, 1:3–4, 1–5.

105. Except for the work of a committee on aging that had recently been founded.

106. Kenneth Tout, *Aging in Developing Countries* (Oxford: Oxford University Press on behalf of HelpAge International, 1989), 243–44.

107. Kevin O'Sullivan, "A Global 'Nervous System': The Rise and Rise of European Humanitarian NGOs, 1945–1985," in *International Organizations and Development, 1945–90*, ed. Marc Frey, Sonke Kunkel, and Corinne R. Unger (Basingstoke: Palgrave Macmillan, 2014), 196–219. See also 197–98, 204–5.

108. There was a session before the main meeting where NGOs were invited to air their views, and were allowed to attend but not to record their opinions as the meeting was only open to UN agencies and member states.

109. Didier Fassin, *Humanitarian Reason: A Moral History of the Present* (Berkeley: University of California Press, 2011).

110. Walter Fernandes, "Aging in South Asia as Marginalization in a Neo-Colonial Economy: An Introduction," in Alfred de Souza and Walter Fernandes, *Ageing in South Asia: Theoretical Issues and Policy Implications* (New Delhi: Indian Social Institute, 1982): 1–2, 1–23.

111. See discussion in Chapter 1.

112. This was brought out in a discussion with Monica Ferreira on June 9, 2015 and came up indirectly in several e-mail exchanges between October 2014 and June 2015. Dr. Ferreira is the founder of the African Gerontology Center in Cape Town, and president of the International Longevity Center, Africa. She was present in Madrid and was in charge of drafting the African Union (AU) declaration to be sent to the United Nations based on the recommendations made in Madrid, and she recollected these differences and tense moments at that AU meeting. For the Madrid Plan on Aging, see www.un.org/en/events/pastevents/pdfs/Madrid_plan.pdf.

113. The ICSG's work is discussed in Chapter 3. Pierre Paillat, "The Organization of Research on Aging in Certain Countries," in "Old Age," special issue, *International Social Science Journal* 15, no. 3 (1963): 464–65. In this UNESCO-supported special issue, there was a review of research centers for aging across the world. Paillat's survey mentioned the Centre de Gérontologie Claude Bernard and Institut National d'Études Démographiques in Paris, but no mention was made of the Institute of Social Gerontology in Paris that supported teaching courses in social gerontology in the late 1970s and held

meetings on social gerontology in Dakar, Morocco, Bogota, and Taiwan in the 1980s.

114. Interview with Father Joseph Hampson in Zimbabwe, May 2015.

115. Letter from M. Nussbaumer to Mr. Adossama and Mr. Jain, "Réunion d'experts sur le vieillissement en Afrique Centre Internationale De Géron-tologie Sociale, Paris, Versailles, 4–6 Mai 1983," ILO, NGO 796, May 3, 1983. Consulted at the ILO (BIT) archives and library, Geneva.

116. This recommendation (R162 Older Workers Recommendation, 1980 [no. 162]) applied to all workers likely to encounter difficulties in employment and occupation because of advancement in age. It was aimed at providing them information on retirement benefits and planning for it, and it encouraged national policymakers to implement it in a "manner consistent with national practice and taking account of national economic and social conditions." It had been passed at the ILO but had not been ratified by countries. See www.ilo.org /dyn/normlex/en/fp=NORMLEXPUB:12100:0::NO::P12100_ILO_CODE:R162.

117. Participants noted, "The need for income security is hardly felt in a subsis-tence economy in a family, clan or community setting. In the context of an urban lifestyle, the need grows in relative importance. . . . In the industrial-ized countries, very elaborate systems of social security have been developed concerning the whole or large majority of the population. Social security systems in Africa were introduced in the public sector . . . but only a small minority benefit from [them]. It appears urgent to gradually extent the scope of the modern social security system by initiating . . . at least provisional coverage" (29, 31).

118. Bates, Mudimbe, O'Barr, eds., *Africa and the Disciplines* (Chicago: University of Chicago Press, 1993), xi; Kwame Anthony Appiah, *In My Father's House: African Philosophy of Culture* (New York: Oxford University Press, 1992), 45.

119. Rogers Brubaker and Frederick Cooper, "Beyond 'Identity,'" *Theory and Society* 29, no. 1 (2000): 5.

120. Kenneth Tout, *Aging in Developing Countries*, 58, 59; also email communica-tions from London and phone conversation in March 2013. Tout, who is now ninety-three years old (in 2017), was a tank commander during the First World War and participated in the Normandy / D Day landings. He worked for many decades at Help the Aged after serving in the Salvation Army. He is now writing a book on PTSD, and he wrote to a mutual friend: "I still instinctively duck away from fast low-flying aircraft after a bitter experience with Hitler's Luftwaffe in 1944. That indeed is life. I have limited stamina at 91 so will close this epistle now with warmest greetings and wishes for the many fascinating days to come—the 80 and 90 birthdays are not to be feared."

121. Interview in May 2015 with Father Joseph Hampson in Zimbabwe; he de-scribes his approach as being "from below, from the field."

122. *Zimbabwe Action Plan on Elderly* (ZAPE), edited proceedings of the Workshop (School of Social Work, Harare, 1987), 7.

123. As narrated in an interview with Father Joseph Hampson in May 2015.

124. Message from Dr. G. L. Monekosso, Regional Director of the WHO for Africa, to the national workshop on care of the elderly, Harare, December 15, 1986, in ZAPE, 3, 3–5.

125. The Mexico City Declaration in 1984 had made a reference to aging, and this was seen as endorsing the agenda of aging. Message from Dr. G. L. Monekosso, ZAPE, 3.

126. ZAPE, 7–8.

127. UNDP Report, 1999.

128. Speech by the Prime Minister, Comrade R. G. Mugabe, at the official opening on Planning for the Needs of the Elderly, ZAPE, 1–2.

129. Hampson describes the violence surrounding war communiqués and Kaunda's speech against the Muzorewa government as being in strong contrast to the silent coming apart of society fractured by violence and war in Zimbabwe. His book was based on a study supported by Help the Aged. The conditions around him, Hampson admits, made him throw off his cloak of "scientific neutrality," and he describes himself instead as an involved observer attempting to get behind the experiences of the elderly amidst this chaos. Joe Hampson, *Old Age: A Study of Aging in Zimbabwe* (Harare: Mambo Press, 1982), 5–6.

130. Ibid., 6.

131. "By this I mean that nobody has studied the process of aging in African society, no-one has said very much about how people adapt to the changes brought on by aging." He did not see the anthropological studies in South Africa as being studies of aging, as they were studying larger movements of social change. Ibid., 8.

132. Abosede George, in her work on girl hawkers in Lagos, argues that this was a means partly to control the labor of a segment of the unregulated working population. Abosede George, "Within Salvation: Girl Hawkers and the Colonial State in Development Era Lagos," *Journal of Social History* 44, no. 3 (Spring 2011), 837–59.

133. Hampson, *Old Age*, 74. Scholars have argued that that citizens' rights in Zimbabwe were extended to loyal party workers rather than to citizens. See Stephen Chan, "The Memory of Violence: Trauma in the Writings of Alexander Kanengoni and Yvonne Vera and the Idea of Unreconciled Citizenship in Zimbabwe," *Third World Quarterly* 26, no. 2 (2005): 369–82.

134. D. R. Kohli, "Challenge of Aging," in *Aging in India: Challenge for the Society*, ed. M. L. Sharma and T. M. Dak (New Delhi: Ajanta, 1987), 3–4.

135. UN World Assembly on Aging General Assembly, Statements, statement of Mr. M. C. Narasimhan, Leader of the Indian Delegation at the World Assembly on Aging, 1:5, 1–6.

6
International NGOs and the Aged in the Developing World

1. United Nations, *Report of the World Assembly on Aging, Vienna, July 26–August 6, 1982* (New York: United Nations, 1982), 25, 56, 51–52.
2. Ibid., 11.
3. Center for Social Development and Humanitarian Affairs, "Meeting on Fund Raising Strategies for Aging," *Bulletin on Aging* 2 (1989): 1–2.
4. Ibid.
5. Center for Social Development and Humanitarian Affairs, "United Nations Trust Fund for Aging," *Bulletin on Aging* 2 (1989): 7.
6. Ibid.
7. Center for Social Development and Humanitarian Affairs, "Belize: Opportunities for the Visually Impaired Elderly," *Bulletin of Aging* 2 (1989): 8; Center for Social Development and Humanitarian Affairs, "India: Hearing and Speech Therapy," *Bulletin of Aging* 2 (1989): 10; Center for Social Development and Humanitarian Affairs, "Dominican Republic: Seeds of Commitment," *Bulletin of Aging* 3 (1989), 7; Center for Social Development and Humanitarian Affairs, "Vegetable Gardening for Oromo Refugees," *Bulletin of Aging* 3 (1989): 11 (supported by the Oromo Relief Association in London, UK).
8. No doubt some meetings such as a symposium on aging and developments in the Middle East reported that in terms of principles, "Aging should be considered a state of ability and not disability," but their focus continued to be on medicine and geriatric care or on stressing that the elderly were living with their families "in keeping with traditional Islamic culture," and they did not elaborate on enabling and empowering older persons. Center for Social Development and Humanitarian Affairs, "Aging and Developments in the Middle East" (paper prepared by Dr. Al'Banna, Ministry of Social Affairs, Cairo, reporting on a symposium [June 18–23, 1989] held at the Fourteenth International Congress of Gerontology in Acapulco), *Bulletin on Aging* 2 (1989): 5.
9. For an account of the Gray Panthers, see Sanjek Roger, *Gray Panthers* (Philadelphia: University of Pennsylvania Press, 2011), 3–5, 140, 220, including chap. 4, which discusses their support of social gerontologists in California, and a later mention of a UN delegation of the Panthers that represented the Panthers at the Second WAA. I also draw from Andrew Achenbaum's valuable

account of the founding of the National Institute on Aging and its dynamic founder, Dr. Robert Butler, in *Crossing Frontiers: Gerontology Emerges as a Science* (Cambridge: Cambridge University Press, 1995), 214–16, where which he describes the emergence of gerontology as a "big science" and the growing funds for research (with a budget of $420 million in 1994).

10. In 1980, the UNHCR had reported that his budget (fixed at an unprecedented figure of 120 million pounds only three months earlier) needed to be doubled. Ben Whitaker, *A Bridge of People: A Personal View of Oxfam's First Forty Years* (London: William Heinemann, 1983), 98; Gil Loescher, "The UNHCR's 'New Look,' Financial Crisis, and Collapse of Morale Under Jean-Pierre Hocke and Thorvald Stoltenberg," in *The UNHCR and World Politics: A Perilous Path* (Oxford: Oxford University Press, 2001), chap. 7.

11. Barry N. Stein, "Durable Solutions for Developing Country Refugees," in "Refugees: Issues and Directions," special issue, *International Migration Review* 20, no. 2 (Summer 1986): 264–82.

12. Didier Fassin, *Humanitarian Reason: A Moral History of the Present* (Berkeley: University of California Press, 2012).

13. Ken Tout, "The Aging Dimension in Refugee Policy: A Perspective from Developing Nations," *Aging International* (June 1990): 6.

14. HelpAge International was founded in 1983 and was affiliated with Help the Aged in the UK. Initially it did not deliver programs, until the 1990s, when refugee relief in the Horn of Africa began to consume more effort. Apart from publications and reports, this chapter is based on conversations with several experts who have worked with HelpAge International or been involved with its partners or in its campaigns in the UK. These include Mark Gorman, Director of Strategic Development, HelpAge International (one of the earliest employees who joined HelpAge International, in 1988), interviewed in June 2015 and September 2015; Baroness Sally Greengross, International Longevity Centre (ILC), UK; Monica Ferreira, ILC, South Africa; Mathew Cherian, Chief Executive Officer, HelpAge, India; Isabella Aboderin, Head of Aging and Development Program, African Population and Health Research Center, Nairobi; Tavengwa Nhonga, Regional Representative for Africa, HelpAge International, Nairobi.

15. Tout, "The Aging Dimension in Refugee Policy," 6.

16. Ibid.

17. "Older people are often at least as vulnerable as other population groups, such as women and children. They also have unique contributions to make to the protection of their communities. Yet they are frequently invisible in all stages of the response"; *AgeWays*, Practical Issues in Development, 66 (December 2005): 2, 6–7 and "Older People Neglected in Darfur: Survey," *Sudan Tribune*, September 2005. Based on a survey by HelpAge Kenya,

www.sudantribune.com/spip.php?article9096 (September 2015). See also David Hutton, *Older People in Emergencies: Considerations for Action and Policy Development* (Geneva: World Health Organization, 2008).

18. Tout, "The Aging Dimension in Refugee Policy," 7–8.

19. In lesser numbers in El Salvador, the aged were left behind by militant younger members. Ibid., 6. The delivery of humanitarian aid and its politics has been discussed extensively; a few of the works used as background in this chapter are Barbara Harrell-Bond, *Imposing Aid: Emergency Assistance of Refugees* (Oxford: Oxford University Press, 1986) on Ugandan refugees in Sudan; Gil Loescher, *Beyond Charity: International Cooperation and the Global Refugee Crisis* (New York: Oxford University Press, 1993); John Rogge, ed., *Refugees: A Third World Dilemma* (Totowa, NJ: Rowman & Allanheld, 1987) to cite a few early and influential works.

20. Tout observed that special projects to meet the needs of elderly refugees had already been set up in Egypt, Chile, Brazil, Peru, Venezuela, and Colombia.

21. Such as Uganda, Chad, and Sudan in Africa, and many others in Central America and lingering refugee exodus in parts of Asia. Peter Nobel ed., *Refugees and Development in Africa*, Seminar Proceedings no. 19, The Nordic Africa Institute (Sweden: Bonuslaningens Boktrychkeri A B, 1987), 19–20.

22. Ibid., 19–20; UNHCR, *The State of the World's Refugees: In Search of Solutions* (Oxford: Oxford University Press, 1995), 48.

23. Margaret E. Keck and Kathryn Sikkink, *Activists beyond Borders: Advocacy Networks in International Politics* (Ithaca, NY: Cornell University Press, 1998).

24. Help the Aged had a remarkable history of fundraising and charitable work and was perceived widely not simply as an influential charity but as an iconic British institution like "Marks and Spencers or the British Museum" that served as "the most stimulating and creative centre in the world for the study and practice of everything that affects the welfare of old people"; Kenneth Hudson, *Help the Aged: Twenty-One Years of Experiment and Achievement* (London: Bodley Head, 1982): 7–8. Matthew Hilton, James McKay, Nicholas Crowson, and Jean-François Mouhot, *The Politics of Expertise: How NGOs Shaped Modern Britain* (Oxford: Oxford University Press, 2013), 69, 154.

25. See Chapters 2, 3, and 4.

26. UN General Assembly, December 3, 1982, A/RES/37/51. See www.un.org /documents/ga/res/37/a37r051.htm. There was an appeal "to Member States to make voluntary contributions to the Trust Fund" that aimed to, among other things, "encourage greater interest among developing countries in matters related to aging and to assist Member States, at their request, in formulating and implementing policies and programmes for the elderly [and] use the Trust Fund for technical co-operation and research related to the aging of populations and for promoting co-operation among developing countries in the

exchange of relevant information and technology," but both the Fund and agencies, such as the UNFPA, that were urged to raise funds for aging did not generate funds or evince interest in addressing this directive.

27. The ironies of this comment Whitaker quoted from the *Daily Telegraph* are telling in view of the Syrian refugee crisis in Europe (2015), where politicians are debating much the same issues. Ben Whitaker, A *Bridge of People: A Personal View of Oxfam's First Fifty Years* (London: William Heinemann, 1983), 137.

28. Hudson, *Help the Aged*, 64.

29. Ibid., 143–44. About Oxfam as well, Maggie Black, reflecting on its early decades in the 1950s, wrote that it was a barometer of how people in Britain and elsewhere viewed other societies over time, and especially a barometer of the least privileged and the challenges posed by what she terms the "Black Man's Burden." Maggie Black, A *Cause for Our Times: Oxfam the First 50 Years* (Oxford: Oxfam and Oxford University Press, 1992), 2, 236–64.

30. Interview with Mark Gorman, Director of Strategic Development, HelpAge International, June 2015, September 2015.

31. Kevin O'Sullivan, "A Global Nervous System: The Rise and Rise of European Humanitarian NGOs (1945–85)," in *International Organizations and Development, 1945–1990*, edited by Marc Frey, S. Kunkel and C. R. Unger (Basingstoke: Palgrave Macmillan, 2014), 196–97, 199–200.

32. Kevin O'Sullivan, "A Global Nervous System," 200–201.

33. Christian Aid records, The British Council Aid for Refugees, "Notes on the Elderly Refugee Campaign," November 1968, CA/I/9/5, School of Oriental and African Studies (SOAS) Archive, London. This series has several other references to relief work with elderly refugees aside from those who were part of the Hungarian Relief Fund.

34. In November 1983, five organizations—Help the Aged in UK and Canada, Pro-Vida Colombia, and Help the Aged in India and Kenya—came together to form HelpAge International. See www.helpage.org/who-we-are/our-history.

35. Nobel, *Refugees and Development in Africa*, 9, 19; Fassin, *Humanitarian Reason.*

36. Term for militia in Darfur, parts of Sudan and Chad consisting of Sudanese Arab tribes.

37. *Ethiopia and Eritrea: Lives on the Borderline*, directed by Raffaele Masto (Nova-T, 2000), http://search.alexanderstreet.com/view/work/2442651.

38. Didier Fassin, in his discussion about the Sangatte reception center in Calais, cites Mochel Agier's and Giorgio Agamben's work to analyze the notion of "the camp" and its internment. Fassin notes that Agamben argues that it actually opens up an apparently innocuous space and discusses how it becomes a biopolitical space and regime of exception "for the worlds undesirables"

(Agier); Fassin adds that Sangatte was both a reception center and detention camp for deportation depending on the refugees' assigned status. Fassin, *Humanitarian Reason*, 136–40.

39. Nancy Godfrey, "The Health Needs of Elderly Refugees: A Field Study in Eastern Sudan, 1985," *Report to Help the Aged*, September 1986 (London: London School of Hygiene and Tropical Medicine, Evaluation & Planning Centre for Health Care, Refugee Health Group, 1986). Godfrey was associated with the WHO Collaborating Center for the Health of Refugees and Other Displaced Communities at the London School of Hygiene and Tropical Medicine.

40. Aging around the World, "Winds of Social Change Reach Elderly in Zaire," *Ageing International* (1984).

41. Alex De Waal, *Famine That Kills: Darfur, Sudan* (Oxford: Oxford University Press, 1989), 177–82. De Waal estimated that child deaths in the age group 1–5 showed the largest rise in age-specific mortality from normal levels, in excess of all other age groups, with the age-specific death rate for children jumping from 15.7 to 79.5 per 1,000. Older people were more at risk than before, but the data was complex, and it differed between those who were in their fifties, who had a small increase from 14 to 21 per 1,000 in the death rate, and those above seventy years, for whom the death rate exceeded 70 per 1,000.

42. Fassin, *Humanitarian Reason*.

43. Dodo Thandiwe Motsisi, "Elderly Mozambican Women Refugees in the Tongogara Refugee Camp in Zimbabwe: A Case Study," *Refuge* 14, no. 8 (January 1995): 7–11.

44. "Behind God's back" refers to Alan Paton's implying international indifference to conditions and needs in the African continent. Cited in *World Refugee Report*, 1974, the Annual Survey Issue (published by U.S. Committee for Refugees), 3.

45. Andreas Sagner, "'The Abandoned Mother': Ageing, Old Age and Missionaries in Early and Mid-Nineteenth Century South-East Africa," *Journal of African History* 42, no. 2 (2001), 173–98.

46. This led experts at a meeting convened to discuss the protection of African refugees (1994) to observe that the Western media looked only at negative aspects of refugees and humanitarian aid. Protection of the African Refugees and Internally Displaced Person, seminar convened in Harare, February 16–18, 1994 (Harare, Southern African Research and Documentation Centre and African Commission on Human Rights, 1995), 18.

47. Tout, "The Aging Dimension in Refugee Policy," 8.

48. Ben Whitaker, *A Bridge of People*, 153. Statement by Poul Hartling, United Nations High Commissioner for Refugees, to the meeting of the Standing Conference on Refugees, December 8, 1980, www.unhcr.org/print/3ae68fcf38 .html.

49. Ibid.

50. The AARP agreed to fund the IFA and hosted its secretariat at its headquarters in Washington, DC (starting in 1973) for several years in order to give the new organization a strong start, and its secretariat was later moved to Montreal (1993). Bernard Nash (AARP) became the IFA's first president. Subsequent presidents were David Hobman of Age Concern England; Robert Prigent of Centre de liaison, d'etude, d'information, et de recherche sur 1es probiemes des personnes age's (CLEIRPPA) in France; and Sharad Gokhale of the Community Aid and Sponsorship Program in India. The IFA had supported the call for a WAA (1982), and the IFA's General Secretary at the time, William Kerrigan, became secretary general of the World Assembly—the first time in UN history that a representative of an NGO had become the director of a single-focus world conference. See www.ifa-fiv.org/wp-content/uploads/2012/11/057_IFA-Narrative-Final-edited.pdf.

51. They were involved in productive activities such as "growing vegetables, making sandals, basketry, mat-weaving."

52. Rhoda Immerman, "Help for the Elderly," *Refugee Participation Network* (November 1988): 1–3. Immerman was also director of the HelpAge Refugee Program in Zimbabwe; emphasis added.

53. Ibid., 2. "It was difficult for the social workers to establish their credibility with the elderly refugees as, initially, the latter suspected them of being researchers coming to exploit them. . . . However, the social workers persisted in offering their professional skill and concern and were able to intervene effectively on behalf of the elderly and disabled at the clinic."

54. R. Mupedziswa, "Elderly Camp Refugees and Social Development: Traditional Status A Salient Dimension Compromised?" (paper presented at a HelpAge workshop on "Change and Development through Workshops," September 11–12, 1989), 1–7.

55. Ibid., 5–7.

56. Dodo Thandiwe Motsisi, "Elderly Mozambican Women Refugees in the Tongogara Refugee Camp in Zimbabwe: A Case Study," *Refuge* 14, no. 8 (January 1995): 7–11.

57. K. B. Wilson, "Internally Displaced Refugees and Returnees from and in Mozambique," *Studies on Emergencies and Disaster Relief* (Stockholm: Nordiska Afrikainstitutet, 1994), 1–61.

58. This was true even among church bodies that were offering aid to refugees, as admitted at the All Africa Conference of Churches. See Lars-Gunnar Eriksson, Göran Melander, and Peter Nobel, eds., *An Analysing Account of the Conference on the African Refugee Problem* (Uppsala: Scandinavian Institute of African Studies [now the Nordic Africa Institute, NAI], 1981), 192.

59. For a discussion of these developmental claims, including of a birth control study in North India in the case of the population control programs, see Mahmud Mamdani, *Myth of Population Control: Family, Caste and Class in a North Indian Village* (New York: Monthly Review Press, 1972). R. Mupedziswa, "Elderly Camp Refugees and Social Development: Traditional Status A Salient Dimension Compromised?" (paper presented at a HelpAge workshop on "Change and Development through Workshops," September 11–12, 1989), 1–7.

60. The UNHCR's statement needs to be reviewed critically; it is hard to believe that all women in refugee camps were not vulnerable to sexual and gender-based violence and risks, even though some cases would have required more support than others. For a discuss of the UNHCR's "idealization" of some refugee women (and neglect of other women and girls) in their donor rhetoric, see Elena Fiddian-Qasmiyeh, "'Ideal' Refugee Women and Gender Equality Mainstreaming in the Sahrawi Refugee Camps: 'Good Practice' for Whom?" *Refugee Survey Quarterly* (2010) 29, no. 2: 64–84.

61. UNHCR, 200c, Statistics and Registration: A Progress Report, EC/50/SC/CRP. 10, February 7, 2000, quoted in Desiree Nilsson, "Internally Displaced Refugees and Returnees from and in the Sudan: A Review," *Studies on Emergency and Disaster Relief* (Copenhagen : Nordiska Afrikainstitutet, 2000), 17; S. Forbes-Martin, *Refugee Women* (London: Zed Books, 1992).

62. Nancy Godfrey and Alexandre Kalache, "Health Needs of Older Adults Displaced to Sudan by War and Famine: Questioning Current Targeting Practices in Health Relief," *Scientific Medicine* 28, no. 7 (1989): 707–13; and Nilsson, "Internally Displaced Refugees and Returnees," 16–17. Regarding scarcity of data regarding women in conflict situations, see Samia El Nagar, "The Impact of War on Women and Children in the Sudan," in *Conflicts in the Horn of Africa: Human and Ecological Consequences of Warfare*, ed. Terje Tvedt (Uppsala: EPOS, 1993), 99–113.

63. Statement by chief executive officer of HelpAge International, in *United Nations: Difficult Situation of Africa and Countries in Conflict in Support of Older People Highlighted at Ageing Assembly in Madrid* (UN Report, NAICS, Coventry, Normans Media Limited, 2002).

64. The funds for disaster relief available to HelpAge International are large, almost $10 million a year. Interview with Isabella Aboderin, Head of Aging and Development Program, African Population and Health Research Center, Nairobi, June 2015. All views expressed in this case relating to HelpAge's interest in disaster relief activities are my own.

65. *Hidden Victims: New Research on Older, Disabled and Injured Syrian Refugees*, www.helpage.org/newsroom/latest-news/hidden-victims-new-research-on-older-disabled-and-injured-syrian-refugees/.

66. This was the Conference on Legal, Economic and Social Aspects of African Refugee Problems, Adis Ababa, October 9–18, 1967. Excerpts published in Eriksson, Melander, and Nobel, eds., *An Analysing Account of the Conference on the African Refugee Problem*, 87.

67. "That special consideration should be given to marginalized groups in refugee settlements and camps, such as the very young, *the elderly*, pregnant women, the disabled and the sick." See Article 92, Peter Nobel, ed., *Report of the Meeting of the OAU-Secretariat and Voluntary Agencies on African Refugees*, Arusha, March 1983 (Uppsala: Scandinavian Institute of African Studies, 1983), 28.

68. Experts at HelpAge International and the UN Open Ended Working Group on Aging have written extensively on this subject of the "gaps" and how even the Madrid International Plan on Ageing (2001), the "successor" to the World Assembly on Aging, is not a human rights treaty and governments have no obligation to enforce it. The nine core international human rights treaties are the International Covenant on Civil and Political Rights, the International Covenant on Economic, Social and Cultural Rights, the International Convention on the Elimination of All Forms of Racial Discrimination, the Convention on the Elimination of Discrimination against Women, the Convention against Torture and Other Cruel, Inhuman or Degrading Treatment or Punishment, the Convention on the Rights of the Child, the International Convention on the Protection of the Rights of all Migrant Workers and Members of their Families, the International Convention for the Protection of All Persons from Enforced Disappearance, and the Convention on the Rights of Persons with Disabilities. See HelpAge International, "International Human Rights Law and Older People: Gaps, Fragments and Loopholes," 2012, www.helpageusa.org/what-we-do/rights/rights-policy/un-openended-working-group-on-aging/human-rights-policy-papers.

69. Doron and Apter, "The Debate Around the Need for a New Convention on the Rights of Older Persons," *Gerontologist* 50 (2010): 586–93; Bridget Sleap, "Why It's Time for a Convention on the Rights of Older People," HelpAge International, 2009, www.helpage.org/download/4c3cfa0869630/.

70. Ken Tout, "Reflections on Perspectives on Aging," *Bold* 17, no. 3 (2007): 10. Tout's personal communication on the same subject in March 2013 confirmed the same.

71. Chris Beer, A. Rose, and K. Tout, "AIDS: The Grandmother's Burden," in *The Global Impact of AIDS*, Proceedings of the First International Conference on the Global Impact of AIDS, cosponsored by the World Health Organization and the London School of Hygiene and Tropical Medicine, held in London, March 8–10, 1988, ed. Alan F. Fleming, Manuel Carballo, David W. FitzSimons, Michael R. Bailey, and Jonathan Mann (New York: Alan R. Liss, 1988), 164–71. See more at www.popline.org/node/360936#sthash.DWlANJoy.dpuf.

See also *Missing Voices: Views of Older Persons on Elder Abuse: A Study from Eight Countries: Argentina, Austria, Brazil, Canada, India, Kenya, Lebanon and Sweden* (Geneva: WHO, 2002), http://www.who.int/ageing/publications /missing_voices/en/.

72. James Ferguson, *Expectations of Modernity: Myths and Meanings of Urban Life in the Zambian Copper Belt* (Berkeley: University of California Press, 1999), 1–37.

73. HelpAge International, "The Situation of Older Persons in Tanzania," in *The Aging and Development Report* (London: Earthscan, 1999), 138, 136–42.

74. Donald J. Adamchack and Adrian O. Wilson, "The Situation of Older People in Zimbabwe," in *The Aging and Development Report*, 145, 143–46.

75. HelpAge International, "The Situation of Older Persons in Tanzania," 138.

76. M. Chazan, "Seven 'Deadly' Assumptions: Unravelling the Implications of HIV/AIDS Among Grandmothers in South Africa and Beyond," *Aging and Society* 28 (2008): 935–58; S. Madhavan, "Fosterage Patterns in the Age of AIDS: Continuity and Change," *Social Science and Medicine* 58, no. 7 (2004): 1443–54; J. May, "Chronic Poverty and Older People in South Africa," CPRC Working Paper Number 25 (Manchester, UK: University of Manchester, Chronic Poverty Research Center, 2003); HelpAge International, *Age and Security: Summary Report—How Social Pensions Can Deliver Effective Aid to Poor Older People and Their Families* (London: HelpAge International, 2004); A. R. Moore and D. Henry, "Experiences of Older Informal Caregivers to People Living With HIV/AIDS in Lome, Togo," *Ageing International* 30, no. 2 (2005): 147–66; Tawega Nhongo, *The Changing Role of Older People in African Households and the Impact of Ageing on African Family Structures* (Johannesburg, South Africa: HelpAge International, 2004). I am thankful to Tawega Nhongo and Monica Ferreira for their insights about these years, when their own work and engagements intersected closely with these debates in South Africa in particular and at a regional level.

77. "A Success Story from Belize," *Ageing International* 13, no. 1 (Spring 1986): 15–16.

78. Interview with the late Professor Nana Apt, sociologist and founder of ties with HelpAge International (HAI) in Ghana in the 1980s, following the Vienna Assembly, June 12, 2015. She was of the opinion that all the gerontological knowledge and experience of aging programs that a first cohort of aging activists received was from HAI.

79. "Taking Account of Older People in Development Cooperation: A Review of the Status of Ageing in Major Bilateral and Multilateral Agencies," in *The Aging and Development Report*, 174–78. The report added that the World Bank, after producing its report *Averting the Old Age Crisis* (1994), was mostly looking at the costs of insurance and pensions, and the economic impacts of

aging on healthcare systems in states such as Chile, Mexico, Brazil, Vietnam, and Indonesia, but had little interest in other countries.

80. Ibid., 178. The Australian government also offered some aid to countries in the Pacific region to train and sensitize policymakers about aging.

81. HelpAge India, "History," www.helpageindia.org/aboutus/history.html.

82. Hudson, *Help the Aged*, 151–52.

83. Cecil Jackson, who had been associated with the early success of Oxfam, was also known as "Mr. Charity." Hudson, *Help the Aged*, 156–57, 180–81.

   Meetings and correspondence with Mark Gorman (June 2014 and September 2015), Strategic Relations Officer, HelpAge International and interviews with Mathew Cherian, HelpAge India (August 2015) in New Delhi.

84. Hudson, *Help the Aged*, 66.

85. Ibid. At an eye hospital in Aligarh, where cataract surgeries were performed.

86. "First National Symposium on Aging in India," 34.

87. Ibid., 35.

88. Ibid.

89. Ibid., 34.

90. South Africa was a significant exception to this in Sub-Saharan Africa, as it provided universal pensions.

91. Among the surveyed countries, Chile, Cuba, Jamaica, Singapore, and Sri Lanka had developed and implemented national aging policies. See "National Policies on Ageing and Older People," 155–78.

92. Statement by the chief executive of HelpAge International, in *United Nations: Difficult Situation of Africa and Countries in Conflict in Support of Older People Highlighted at Ageing Assembly in Madrid*; and "Taking Account of Older People in Development Cooperation: A Review of the Status of Ageing in Major Bilateral and Multilateral Agencies," 174.

93. Kate Forrester Kibuga and Alex Dianga, "Older People in Tanzania: A Research Report from HelpAge International," HAI, Dar Es Salaam, September 1998, quoted in HelpAge International, "The Situation of Older Persons in Tanzania," in *The Aging and Development Report*, 139.

94. Charlotte Nusberg, "Aging China: Policies in Transition," Conference Reports, *Ageing International* (Winter 1987): 19–20.

95. Megan L. Dolbin-Macnab, Shannon E. Jarrott, Lyn E. Moore, and Kendra A. O'Hora, "Dumela Mma: An Examination of Resilience among South African Grandmothers raising Children," *Ageing and Society*, September 2015, 1–31. There is a huge literature in this field stressing challenges, coping mechanisms, and social support over the past years.

96. B. Hayslip and G. C. Smith, eds., *Resilient Grandparent Caregivers: A Strengths-based Perspective* (New York: Routledge, 2013). Hayslip's work flags its approach right at the beginning: "this book speaks to the other side of grand-

parent caregiving with the glass being half full rather than falling victim to the established half-empty pessimistic view."

97. For a searching critique of these generalizations and an effort to move beyond debates on reforming formal social security for those who have no retirement or to rescuing those who are "left behind" and try to address rapid and complex social changes, see Peter Lloyd-Sherlock, *Old Age and Poverty in the Developing World: The Shanty Towns of Buenos Aires* (London: Macmillan, 1997). Sherlock contests the World Bank's views in its report (1994) that extending formal pension programs in sub-Saharan Africa could undermine informal sources of support. Lloyd-Sherlock, "Older People's Strategies in Times of Social and Economic Transformation"; HelpAge International, "The Situation of Older Persons in Tanzania," in *The Aging and Development Report: Poverty, Independence and the World's Older People*, ed. Judith Randel, Tony German, and Deborah Ewing (London: Earthscan Publications, 1999), 71–81.

98. Esther Duflo, "Grandmothers and Granddaughters: Old Age Pension and Intra-household Allocation in South Africa," NBER paper, 8061, January 14, 2003. See obssr.od.nih.gov/pdf/wberduflofinal.pdf.

99. Mark Gorman, "The Situation of Older People in the Transitional Economies of Eastern and Central Europe"; and HelpAge International, "The Situation of Older Persons in Tanzania," 148, 147–51.

100. United Nations Department of Economic and Social Affairs, *Regional Dimensions of the Ageing Situation* (New York: United Nations, 2009), https://www.un.org/development/desa/dspd/2010/10/22/regional-dimensions-of-the-ageing-situation/.

101. WHO, AFR/HEE/1, Coordinated Action on Aging, Report of the First NGO/WHO Roundtable, Brazzaville, January 27–29, 1988 (Brazzaville, Congo: Regional Office for Africa, 1988). This was hosted by the WHO's Programme for the Health of the Elderly, which was established after a WHA resolution targeted at the healthcare of the elderly in 1979. See "Taking Account of Older People in Development Cooperation," 178.

Epilogue

1. Rajya Sabha Proceedings (parliamentary session held on December 6, 2007), 395–96. These are uncorrected and unpublished proceedings available at the library of the Indian Parliament, New Delhi. The law pertains to those aged sixty years and above.

2. The law lays down that if a senior citizen (aged sixty years and above) or parent is unable to maintain themselves from their own earnings or out of their property, it is obligatory for the child to maintain his/her parents so that they may lead "a normal life." *Report of Standing Committee on Social Justice and*

Empowerment, 28th Report, Session of Fourteenth Lok Sabha, 2007–08, Lok Sabha Proceedings, Library of the Indian Parliament (New Delhi, August 2007), 4; *Maintenance and Welfare of Parents and Senior Citizens Bill,* December 5, 2007, Lok Sabha Proceedings, item 26, 495–500.

3. *Maintenance and Welfare of Parents and Senior Citizens Bill.* For later developments on this legislation and its debates, I am indebted to a discussion with Mathew Cherian for sharing the work done by HelpAge India under his initiative, which has provided valuable input to the government policy process on family support. See their Report of the Preliminary Study on Efficiency and Efficacy of the "Maintenance and Welfare of the Parents and Senior Citizens Act, 2007," March 2017.

4. For discussions in China on family support agreements, see Rita-Jing Ann Chou, "Filial Piety by Contract? The Emergence, Implementation, and Implications of the 'Family Support Agreement' in China," *Gerontologist* 51, no. 1 (2011): 3–16; Yuebin Xu, "Family Support for Old People in China," *Social Policy Administration* 35, no. 3 (July 2001): 307–20. The literature on this subject is dense, and current debates on long-term care in China continue to look at the crucial role of family in providing care to elders.

5. In the case of Singapore, Act 35, 1995, which has been amended several times since it was originally passed. See http://statutes.agc.gov.sg/aol/search/display/view.w3p;page=0;query=DocId%3A1ce29500-b64a-4000-b8ae; Charlotte Ikels, "Introduction," in *Filial Piety: Practice and Discourse in Contemporary East Asia* (Stanford, CA: Stanford University Press, 2004), 1–16; for a background, see Roger Goodman and Sarah Harper, *Ageing in Asia: Asia's Position in the New Global Demography* (London: Routledge, 2013). On debates related to intergenerational support and drivers of social change in Africa, see Isabella Aboderin, *Intergenerational Support and Old Age in Africa* (New Brunswick, NJ: Transaction, 2006). I am indebted to Isabella Aboderin for a discussion on issues relating to family and intergenerational politics in various parts of Africa, after our panel at the Age Boom Academy meeting, held in June 2015 at Columbia University, and another discussion following the meeting on global aging held in Shanghai, October 2016. All the views expressed are my own.

6. See "Our History" on the website of the South African Older Persons Forum, founded in 2005: www.saopf.org.za/history-vision-and-mission; "Mothers and Fathers of the Nation: The Forgotten People," Report of the Ministerial Committee on the Abuse, Neglect and Ill-Treatment of Older Persons, February 26, 2001, vol. 1: Main Report. See www.polity.org.za/polity/govdocs/reports/welfare/2001/elder.html. I am thankful to Jaco Hoffman, past President of the South African Gerontological Association (SAGA) and cofounder / coordinator, with Isabella Aboderin, of the African Research Network on Ageing

for providing background regarding recent developments in South Africa and in the region.

7. James Ferguson, *Expectations of Modernity: Myths and Meanings of Urban Life on the Zambian Copperbelt* (Berkeley: University of California Press, 1999), 6, 9–12.

8. Political Declaration and Madrid International Plan of Action on Ageing, www.un.org/en/events/pastevents/pdfs/Madrid_plan.pdf (2002).

9. Ibid. The second global review of the MIPAA document and its goals was undertaken in 2013 at the UN Commission for Social Development. See www .unescap.org/resources/madrid-international-plan-action-ageing.

10. See "Second World Assembly on Ageing (8–12 April 2002, Madrid, Spain)," www.un.org/en/events/pastevents/ageing_assembly2.shtml for a short overview of the Madrid Meeting, with links to meeting documents, such as the Political Declaration and Madrid International Plan of Action on Ageing (2002) and the Report of the Second World Assembly on Aging (May 23, 2002).

11. United Nations, Department of Social and Economic Affairs, *World Population Ageing*, ST/ESA/SER.A/260 (New York: United Nations, 2007); see also the UN report *World Population Ageing*, ST/SEA/SER.A/348 (New York: United Nations, 2013).

12. The SDGs were framed by the UN to replace the Millennium Development Goals. In September 2015, the United Nations adopted 17 SDGs and 169 targets as a global action plan, with indicators of progress. See *Transforming Our World: The 2030 Agenda for Sustainable Development*, https:// sustainabledevelopment.un.org/post2015/transformingourworld.

13. HelpAge International, "Post-2015 and Sustainable Development Goals," www.helpage.org/what-we-do/post2015-process/post2015-and-population -ageing/.

14. Final Stakeholder Group on Ageing, May 18, 2015, Follow and Review Intergovernmental Meeting, www.helpage.org/what-we-do/post2015-process/.

15. Ibid.

16. See Chapters 1 and 3.

17. See Chapter 1.

18. Statement by Bangladesh, "UN: Difficult Situation of Africa and Countries in Conflict in Support of Older People Highlighted at Ageing Assembly in Madrid," Reported by M2 Presswire (Coventry), April 11, 2002.

19. See discussion in Chapter 5 on Townsend's work, and Meredith Minkler and Coroll I. Estes, eds., *Critical Perspectives on Aging: The Political and Moral Economy of Growing Old* (New York: Baywood, 1991), 1–36.

20. National Consultation and Preparatory Workshop for the Second World Assembly on Aging, *Towards Secure Ageing: Proceedings of the National*

Preparation for the Second World Assembly on Ageing, February 20, 2002, Nepal Administrative Staff College.

21. The four-day meeting was held in Bombay and Pune, with support from the Economic and Social Commission for Asia. The same month, the president of the IFA was invited to address the UN General Assembly.

22. International Federation on Ageing, *The Report of First Global Conference on Ageing on New Century, New Hopes, New Thinking about Ageing Policies and Programmes and Select Papers*, August 30 to September 3, 1992, Bombay-Pune, India (Pune: n.p., 1992), 1–17. In the same book, Julia Tavars de Alvarez, in her "IFA Acceptance Speech," mentioned that Charlotte Nusberg of the IFA had asked her to help secure a UN Declaration on the Rights of the Aged at the 14th Congress on Gerontology held in Acapulco. They had anticipated that since the UN had taken 20 years to affirm the rights of the child, it might take even longer for those at the other end of life's chronology; therefore they decided not to follow the conventional path through the UN General Assembly and approached the Commission on Social Development. See pages 176–80.

23. Though this subject is often raised at global aging meetings, there is still very little concrete thinking on what these lessons and strategies could offer. Ibid., 17–18.

24. Some delegates had emphasized at the Madrid Assembly that the objective was also to see beyond international conferences, because "most old people" were unaware that Vienna had occurred and that Madrid was taking place, and planning development initiatives without involving older persons as "responsible agents" was a challenge. Intervention by H. E. Msgr. Renato R. Martino at the Third Committee of the 57th General Assembly of the United Nations on Ageing, Monday, October 7, 2002, www.vatican.va/roman_curia /secretariat_state/documents/rc_seg-st_doc_20021007_martino-ageing_en .html.

25. Author's interview with officials in Department of Social Welfare, New Delhi in 2012, followed by discussion with Mathew Cherian, HelpAge, India.

26. The same meeting also discussed the neglect of older widows in particular, and a scheme of financial assistance for the needy and old was enacted (2008), led by the Human Rights Minister Ansar Burney. Burney's language in introducing this policy was reminiscent of Meira Kumar's in India; he said, "We as a society lack in extending respect to parents and elders, are morally bound to acknowledge the services of the aged group of the society who spent their lives for our better future." See the SHARP, Islamabad, January 24, 2008 meeting to discuss "Aging Issues in Pakistan and Older People's Rights in the Spirit of the MIPAA, 2002," online seminar report, 18, 10, 19, sharp-pakistan .org/reports/u.pdf.

27. Interview with Jaco Hoffman, who assisted with the SALGA project.

28. For an introduction of the current framework of the UN's seventeen Sustainable Development Goals, https://sustainabledevelopment.un.org/index.php?page=view&type=400&nr=2116&menu=35.

29. Peter Lloyd-Sherlock et al., "A Premature Mortality Target for the SDG for Health ISs Ageist," *Lancet* 385 (May 30, 2015): 2147–48.

30. On non-contributory pensions for older persons in Lesotho, Namibia, and South Africa, see N. Kakawani and K. Subbarao, "Ageing and Poverty in Africa and the Role of Social Pensions," Working Paper no. 8, International Poverty Centre (Brazil: United Nations Development Programme, 2005); Stephen Devereux, "Social Pensions in Namibia and South Africa," IDS Discussion Paper 379 (2001); Laura Pelham and Andrew Nyanguru "The Old Age Pension in Lesotho: A Case Study for 'Making Cash Count'—A Study of Cash Transfers in Eastern and Southern Africa" (Sussex: IDS, 2005). For an overview, see Peter Lloyd-Sherlock, ed., *Living Longer: Ageing, Development and Social Protection* (London: Zed Books, 2013). I am grateful to Professor Kefasi Nyikahadzoi at the University of Zimbabwe for guiding me to Professor Andrew Nyanguru's work.

31. *Himachal Pradesh Maintenance of Parents and Dependents Act, 2001* and interview with Ms. Anuradha Thakur, Joint Secretary, Social Welfare Department, Simla, Government of Himachal Pradesh, September 2009; see also http://indiatogether.org/seniors-laws for details on this early legislation.

32. John B. Willamson and Fred C. Pampel, "Ethnic Politics, Colonial Legacy and Old Age Security Policy: The Nigerian Case in Historical and Comparative Perspective," *Journal of Aging Studies* 5, no. 1 (1991): 19–44.

33. Ibid.

34. *African Conference on Gerontology*, Dakar, December 10–14, 1984 (under the patronage of H. E. Mr. Abdou Diouf, President of the Republic of Senegal, organized by the Government of Senegal with the International Center for Social Gerontology, in collaboration with the UN, UNESCO and UNFPA), 9.

35. Interviews with Dr. Monica Ferreira, pioneering gerontologist, president of the International Longevity Center, South Africa until 2015. Dr. Ferreira closely engaged with drafting this framework at an initial meeting in Uganda in 2002, and I am grateful to her for guiding me to speak with Terezinha da Silva, long-time spokesperson for aging in Mozambique. Dr. Isabella Aboderin, senior research scientist and head of the program on aging and development at the African Population and Health Research Center, Nairobi and Mark Gorman from HelpAge International were also valuable informants regarding recent development in aging-related policies and programs in Africa; Professor Nana Apt offered further insight into these efforts as a representative from Ghana. I am also thankful to Tawega Nhongo, regional representative of HelpAge International in Africa, for sparing time to speak with me. See

"Organization of African Unity Framework and Plan of Action on Ageing" (Nairobi, Kenya, HelpAge International Africa Regional Development Center and the African Union, n.d.); Nana Apt, "30 Years of African Research on Ageing: History, Achievements and Challenges for the Future," *Generations Review* 15 (2005): 4–6; Monica Ferreira, *The State of Older People in Africa—2007 Regional Review and Appraisal of the Madrid International Plan of Action on Ageing* (Addis Ababa: UNECA, African Union, 2007); HelpAge International, *Expert Group Meeting on Ageing in Africa*, November 19–20, 2007, Addis Adaba, Ethiopia; HelpAge International, *AU Policy Framework and Plan of Action on Ageing*, Africa Regional Development Centre, Nairobi, Kenya, 2003; HelpAge International, *Report of the Africa Regional Workshop*, Accra, Ghana, September 27–29, 2004; Tawenga M. Nhongo, "Advocacy, Awareness Creation and Evolution of Policies and Programmes on Ageing in Africa," in *HelpAge International Expert Group Meeting on Ageing in Africa*, 19–20 November 2007, Addis Adaba, Ethiopia (Addis Ababa: UNECA, African Union, 2007).

36. W. P. Amarabandu, "Elderly Population and Social Security in Sri Lanka, in Population Association of Sri Lanka and UNFPA," in *Ageing Trends in Sri Lankan Population Problems and Prospects* (Colombo: PASL and UNFPA, 2004); G. R. Andrews and M. M. Hennink, "The Circumstances and Contributions of Older Persons in Three Asian Countries: Preliminary Results of a Cross-National Study," *Asia-Pacific Population Journal* 7, no. 3 (1992): 127–46; Phillip Kreager, *Ageing in Indonesia: A Comparative Study in Social Demography*, Final Report for the Welcome Trust Project 052626, Oxford, 2001.

37. Alexandre Sidorenko, *Progress in Implementing the MIPAA at the Global Level*, n.d., www.cepal.org/celade/noticias/paginas/4/23004/asidorenko1_p.pdf.

38. Ibid.

39. UNDESA, *Review of MIPAA Goals, Asia and Asia Pacific Region, June 2013, Bangkok* (Bangkok, 2013).

40. Professor N. K. Ganguly, Director, Indian Council of Medical Research, in World Health Organization, "Development of Health and Welfare Systems: Adjusting to Ageing," *Proceedings of Valencia Forum*, Spain, April 1–4, 2002, WHO/WKC/SYM 02.8: 18.

41. WHO, "Development of Health and Welfare Systems: Adjusting to Ageing," statements from Dr. Narimah Awin, Director of Family Health Development, Malaysia, 56–57, and from Dr. Agus Suwandono, National Institute of Health Research and Development, Indonesia, 85–86.

42. I am deeply grateful for two interviews conducted with the late Professor Nana Araba Apt at Ashesi University, Ghana who passed away recently. Her knowledge of the history of aging networks in Africa and her insights on how aging-related advocacy was pioneered in Ghana and other parts of Africa were invaluable.

43. Christian NGOs, for instance Hogar De Christo (Christ's Home) in Chile, have had a remarkably effective and enduring presence in addressing the needs of older persons in Latin America; see Javier Perriera, Ronald G. Angel, and Jacqueline J. Angel, "A Case Study of the Elder Care Functions of a Chilean Non-Government Organization," *Social Science and Medicine* 64, no. 10 (May 2007): 2096–106. See also Richard A. Settersten, Jr. and Jacqueline L. Angel eds., *Handbook of Sociology of Aging* (New York: Springer, 2011), 554.

44. Interview with Monsignor Charles J. Fahey, Roman Catholic Diocese of Syracuse, representative of the Holy See Delegation to the WAA, Vienna (1982), October 2015.

45. Walter Fernandes, "Aging in South Asia as Marginalization in a Neo-Colonial Economy: An Introduction," in Alfred de Souza and Walter Fernandes, *Ageing in South Asia Theoretical Issues and Policy Implications*, papers presented at the Asian Regional Conference on Active Aging, Manila, 1982, sponsored by the UNFPA and Opera Pia International (New Delhi: Indian Social Institute, 1982), title page. Yes, fine.

46. Interview with Monsignor Charles J. Fahey, Roman Catholic Diocese of Syracuse, representative of the Holy See Delegation to the WAA, Vienna (1982), October 2015.

47. Interview with Professor Du Peng, Director, Institute of Gerontology, Renmin University, November 2015.

48. See Katrien Pype, "Caring for 'Worthless' People: Kinshasa's Retirement Homes between the Family, the Church and the State," draft, work-in-progress (2015), and K. Pype, S. Van Wolputte, and A. Melice, eds., "Religion and Transformation within and beyond Africa," *Canadian Journal of African Studies* 46, no. 3 (2012): 355–65.

49. See the office website of the conference at http://ifa2014.in/about_hyderabad.php.

50. In a BRICS and global-aging session, speakers compared lessons from Brazil, China, South Africa, and India regarding recent policy changes for aging populations, http://ifa2014.in/about_hyderabad.php is the official website of the conference.

51. Bhagirath Singh Bijarnia, "Whither Economic Governance? The Emerging Role of BRICS, an Alternative," *Indian Journal of Asian Affairs*, 26, nos. 1/2 (January 6, 2013): 75–92; Francis A. Kornegay and Narnia Bohler-Muller, *Laying the BRICS of a New Global Order: From Yekaterinburg 2009 to Ethekwini 2013* (Pretoria: African Books Collective, Africa Institute of South Africa, 2013), 2–7.

52. Global Alliance, International Longevity Center meeting in May 2012 in Prague. Report of minutes from ILC, GA from its secretariat at the Mailman School of Public Health, Columbia University.

53. Vegaard Skirbekk, M. Stonawski, E. Bonsang, and U. M. Staudinger, "The Flynn Effect and Population Aging," *Intelligence* 41 (2013): 169–77.

54. X. Y. Shang and X. M. Wu, "The Care Regime in China: Elder and Child Care," *Journal of Comparative Social Welfare* 27, no. 2 (2011): 123–31; R. M. Marsh and C. K. Hsu, "Changes in Behaviour Concerning Extended Kin in Taipei, Taiwan, 1963–1991," *Journal of Comparative Family Studies* 26, no. 3 (1995): 349–69; Jieyu Liu, "Ageing, Migration and Familial Support in Rural China," *Geoforum* 51 (January 2014): 305–12.

55. UN Resolution 65/182 in December 2010, the UN General Assembly established an Open-Ended Working Group on Ageing for the purpose of strengthening the protection of the human rights for older persons. The task of the group was to evaluate the current international human rights framework for older persons, to identify gaps and how best to address them, and to consider the possibility of additional instruments and measures (United Nations Open-Ended Working Group on Ageing, 2011). For an analysis of the discussions for and against a Convention on the Rights of Older Persons, see Martha Fredvang and Simon Biggs, "The Rights of Older Persons: Protection and Gaps Under Human Rights Law," Social Policy Paper no. 16, The Centre for Public Policy, University of Melbourne, Brotherhood of St. Laurence (August 2012), 1–21. I am thankful to Helen Hamlin (representative of the IFA at the UN and chair of the Non-Governmental Committee on Ageing from 1997 until 2003) and Erika Dhar (AARP, International) for discussions and insights on the workings of this group and related developments.

56. Frederick Cooper, *Colonialism in Question: Theory, Knowledge, History* (Berkeley: University of California Press, 2005).

Acknowledgments

Many people and institutions have contributed to this book in profound ways. My initial interest in age and aging stemmed from my time as a David E. Bell Fellow at the Harvard Center for Population and Development Studies (HCPDS). My work with the group, pretesting the Longitudinal Aging Study in India (LASI) among older persons in the villages bordering Delhi, inspired me to ask questions about the historical and contextual politics of aging and how it has evolved as a public issue in India and, more broadly, in the Global South. I am grateful to Lisa Berkman and David Bloom for being stellar mentors during those years and afterward, and also to Allan Brandt at Harvard University, who has been a real inspiration, for allowing my training in South Asian history and my interest in global health politics and policies to take shape along their own pathways.

I have many debts to my colleagues at Columbia University that are hard to repay. At the Mailman School of Public Health, I thank the dean of the Mailman School, Linda Fried, for her indispensable mentorship and special kindness in supporting this book from its inception. This work has been shaped by our mutual interest in global aging. In the Department of Sociomedical Sciences, I found crucial support from my department chair, Lisa Metsch, especially as the book entered the long production process. Several other senior colleagues reputed for their work on aging and global health have also been invested in this research. I would like to thank Ursula

Staudinger and the Robert N. Butler Columbia Aging Center at the Mailman School for their support, and Richard Parker for his intellectual generosity in our discussions on global health politics.

Most of all, at the Center for History and Ethics of Public Health at the Mailman School, I have found my closest intellectual solidarities, inspiration, and a wonderful space to think about and debate my work. For their careful reading and guidance, I want to thank my closest friends and colleagues: Ronald Bayer, Merlin Chowkwanyun, James Colgrove, Amy Fairchild, Dave Johns, Gerry Oppenheimer, and David Rosner, who read through each of my rough drafts and were insightful and rigorous critics and, to my surprise, asked for more. To Connie Nathanson (honorary member of our center), I owe special thanks for close friendship and razor-sharp insights on messy first drafts and article outlines; for federal grant ideas; and for unfailingly egging me on at every turn. All of their input pushed me toward shaping my final manuscript. Elisa Gonzalez was a trusted anchor who assisted with years of searches, discussions, and exchanges during her time at Mailman, as was Laura Sutter, whose research and analytical skills were immensely valuable. I thank others at SMS for generously exchanging ideas, including Jennifer Hirsch, Kim Hopper, Ana Abraido Lanza, Helen-Maria Lekas, Rachel Shelton, and Karolynn Siegel; and yet others who stimulated thoughtful discussions: Lisa Bates, John Santelli, Bhaven Sampat, and Ezra Susser.

In the Department of History and the Department of Middle Eastern, South Asian, and African Studies (MESAAS) at Columbia University, and also at Barnard College, a number of colleagues and close friends read chapter drafts, foraged for references from their own work, introduced me to essential contacts, and responded to my queries with unfailing generosity and shared interests. I would like to especially thank Matt Connelly and Pamela Smith for taking interest in this book. Rhiannon Stephens has been an understanding friend and colleague, offering both critique and encouragement during the various ups and downs of writing. For referring me to further reading and framings in African history and for conversations around age, gerontocracies, and the lifecourse in history writing and literature, I especially want to thank Greg Mann, Mamadou Diouf, and Abosede George; and I owe a special intellectual debt to Sudipta and Nilanjana Kaviraj for long evenings of discussions on changing generational ties and social lives in India.

Several scholars have offered invaluable help in locating sources, have assisted with translations, and have shared their local contacts on my visits during conferences and field work. Helen Tilley and Karl Ittman offered advice at crucial moments regarding demographic surveys and sources, as did Pat Thane during my work in London; Alison Bashford introduced me to the life and times of key demographers and directed me to sources; Arunabh Ghosh, Sumit Guha, and Projit Mukharji offered vital leads relating to my demographic and disease searches in India and China; Anne-Emmanuelle Birn and Laurence Monnais helped me identify the main questions, especially the moral, political, and geographical concerns and gaps, that underlie this project; and Julie Livingston and Cathy Burns gave me feedback on vital parts of this work when I was attempting comparative arguments between India and South Africa. Sarah Lamb visited my class and pointed me toward people and intellectual resources, and Lawrence Cohen was vital in mentoring this project through many of its stages as I grappled with being a historian examining anthropological research in South Asia and Africa. Megan Vaughan has been a good friend and a thoughtful reader of my work and provided significant input when I sought to ground this work in local field voices rather than telling it from a more distant Western perspective. Sunil Amrith encouraged me to write this book, even as I was still mulling over its relevance, and he offered comments on it from its most primitive form, when he was visiting Cambridge, to its final form, when he returned to settle there. Sana Aiyar has always been there as adopted family and fellow historian, offering perceptive and spot-on advice on my drafts and always making time for me.

Others have offered critical insights, clarified my queries, and shared ideas: Andrew Achenbaum, Jeremy Greene, Susan Greenhalgh, Paul Greenough, Mark Harrison, Randall Packard, Scott Podolsky, K. Sivaramakrishnan, Jay Sokolovsky, David Troyansky, and, at the Columbia Aging Center, Ruth Finkelstein, Vegard Skibekk, and David Weiss. David Jones has been a good friend and terrific collaborator over the past few years, working on a proximate research project, and contributing to discussions on aging even as we tried to trace histories of heart disease and its risks in India. Thibault Moulaert provided insights on debates in critical gerontology in Europe, including critiques and discussions of active aging and of Elise Feller's work. At the Harvard Pop Center, those who helped me understand debates at the intersections of aging, health disparities, and global health include Mauricio Avendano, David Canning, Guenther Fink, Maria Glymour, Santosh Kumar, S. V. Subramanian (Subu), and Rohini Pande at the Kennedy School for her social policy insights.

In Delhi, Mumbai, and Chennai, I owe a string of debts dating back many years to overlapping ties of close friendship, illuminating conversations, and shared historical and public health projects that have allowed me to develop ideas and to mine interviews, private archives, and leads for this book. Conversations with Rama Baru, my longtime friend and colleague from the Center for Social Medicine at the Jawaharlal Nehru University, are reflected in many parts of this book, as are discussions on health governance, law, and the politics of social and welfare policies with Keshav Desiraju, Ramachandra Guha, Prateek Jalan, S. Krishnan, Debashree Mukherjee, Smitha Nagaraj, Mahesh Rangarajan, and Tejveer Singh. Many others have shaped the themes and questions raised in this work: Seema Alavi, Mohan Rao, Radhika Singha; and also Neeladri Bhattacharya, Burton Cleetus, and Indivar Kamtekar, especially through their intellectual hospitality during my time as a visiting scholar in the UGC-supported CAS program (2016). The influence of Majid Siddiqi, my graduate supervisor at the Center for Historical Studies at JNU, and of Anil Seal at Trinity College remains enduring over the years. Colleagues and scholars from the Public Health Foundation of India—Dr. Srinath Reddy, Dr. Prabhakar, and several others from the Delhi office—worked together in sustaining an abiding interest in health inequalities and public health ethics that is anchored in Indian resources and context.

I have had the good fortune to be in contact with the eminent policymakers, researchers, and advocates who form part of the global alliance of the International Longevity Centers, and I am grateful for their generosity in sharing their experiences of international meetings and transnational aging issues. In particular, I thank Du Peng for support in Beijing, for interviews and input, and for inviting me to join meetings around BRICS and aging issues; and Baroness Sally Greengross, Alex Kalache, Sebastiana Kalula, Jaco Hoffman, Rosy Peryra, Louise Plouffe, Mary Ann Tsao, and others; and among the WHO leadership, John Beard, for insights on current global aging and health policy framings. Warm thanks to Srinivas Tata for showing interest in this research during his stint at the UN Division for Social Policy and Development at New York, and also to others associated with the UN Divisions (past and present): Rosemary Lane, Tarek Shuman, Robert Venne, and Bridget Sleap at HelpAge International, and Rajiv Chandran at the UN office in New Delhi. For his generosity in sharing insights relating to his early career and the workings of international NGOs and campaigns to protect and promote the rights of older persons, I am truly grateful to Mark Gorman, who also introduced me to a pioneer in aging and international development programs, Ken Tout. I am indebted to friends and contacts in Kenya, India, South Africa, New York, and Ghana: Isabella Aboderin, Mathew Cherian, Monica Ferriera, Helen Hamlin, Tavengwa Nhongo, and the late Nana Araba Apt.

The work on this book and access to primary sources were made much easier due to the interest taken by librarians and archivists at the United Nations High Commission for Refugees library; the World Health Organization and International Labour Organization archives in Geneva; and the United Nations archive in Long Island, New York, of the Economic and Social Council; as well as the United Nations Population Fund and records of the UNESCO archives in Paris. In South Africa, I am grateful to the University of Witwatersrand library collections, and in India, to the library of the Tata Memorial Institute and the Tata archives. In Delhi, I worked at the libraries of the Ministry of Health and of Social Welfare, Central Secretariat Library at the Nehru Memorial Museum and Library, and the Planning Commission Library on material relating to international development projects, national correspondence regarding international population conferences, and private papers of key welfare and population actors. Material from smaller libraries and NGO holdings with documentation on social work and welfare, urban sociological surveys, and studies and reports published by activists and field-workers have been critical in piecing together the accounts in this book.

Private papers and recorded interviews of gerontologists, chronic disease pathologists, and demographers located at libraries and oral history collections in the universities of Michigan, Chicago, Missouri, and Princeton have also been consulted, as well as the holdings of the Rockefeller Archive Center in Sleepy Hollow. Stephen Logsdon at the Bernard Becker Library and Lee Hiltzik at the Rockefeller archives were of great help. The White Fathers Records were consulted at the Charles E. Young Research Library, UCLA Library, Department of Special Collections. I am also grateful to the National Library of Medicine for granting me access to the Leroy Stewart Papers and gerontological publications, and to Columbia University, which has preserved interviews with Leroy Stewart in its Oral History Collections. The Lamont and Law Libraries and the

South Asia Collections at Harvard University were consulted for rare issues of social work and gerontology journals and reports, and the Countway Medical Library for rare books relating to the Gillman's, Paul Dudley White, and South African medical research. Papers relating to cancer and gerontological research at the Wellcome Library for the History of Medicine, London, were invaluable; also Christian Aid records at the library of the School of Oriental and African Studies. For late colonial and development-related debates, I consulted the Indian Office Collections at the British Library and the National Archives at Kew, London. I also conducted interviews and meetings with retired and serving UN experts, gerontologists, social workers, and functionaries of various international NGOs located in Beijing, Ghana, India, Malta, South Africa, the United Kingdom, Zimbabwe, and other sites in Asia and Africa, and I am immensely grateful to them for the time they spent with me. Most of all, I owe a huge debt to Eugene F. Robinson, librarian at the Health Sciences Library at Columbia University, for unwavering and patient support in procuring documents and microfilms.

This work has relied greatly on ideas and questions raised by many students, and on the research forays they undertook in archives and holdings across the United States, the United Kingdom, Asia, and Africa, and on their assistance with interviews. I thank Camilla Burkot, Sohini Chattopdhyay, Purbasha Das, Alice Sophie Duquesnoy, Devon Golaszewski, Radhika Gore, Preeti Gulati, Ganesh Gupta, Joshua Leifer, Zachary Makowski, Vaibhav Ramani, Sarah Cook Runcie, Aparajita Sarkar, Shilpa Sharma, Pranjali Srivastava, Nick Tackes, Renee Van der Wiel, Faridah Zaman, and Dongxin Zhu for their enthusiasm, insights, and help with data collection.

A book that required searches and travel on this scale simply would not have been possible without wide-ranging institutional support and grants. A Scholar's Award from the National Science Foundation Scholars (Award 1230534: *The Coming of Age: The Formation of the Global Science and Policy of Aging*) was crucial in helping to execute most of the research toward writing this book. In addition, I was also supported by the Center for History and Ethics of Public Health (and give special thanks to the directors, Ronald Bayer and David Rosner, for their generosity); the Robert N. Butler Aging Center; the Dorothy Borg Fund at the Weatherhead East Asia Institute (thanks especially to Eugenia Lean for her support); the Presidential Scholars Grant in Neuroscience and Society (based at the Center for Science and Society); the Leonard Hastings Publication Fund; and the Society of Fellows at Columbia University. My deep thanks to my editor, Andrew Kinney, for his critical support in making this book materialize. Special thanks to Rimli Borooah and Shyama Warner in Delhi for their editorial inputs and lasting friendship, and also to Kerry Higgins Wendt.

Many others have provided warmth, friendship, and advice as the writing on this book raced and stalled. A heartfelt thank you to Anuradha Roy and Rukun Advani for being there always throughout the past, present, and future lives of my books; to Latha Venkataraman and Gita Johar for providing space to think and write, and for sharing their views at vital moments; and to Kathy Conway for generously discussing her writing and reflections on the politics of health and caregiving in the United States.

I thank Amrit Singh and Kavita Issar for true and lasting understanding, friendship, and humor as this book has progressed. Many other close friends from St. Stephens College—Romonika and Vibhu, Manika and Sanjay, Renu and Hitendra, and so many others in Delhi—connected me with news archives and reports, policy interviews, and wider debates that have contextualized this work.

Within my family, my parents and in-laws and their love and boundless faith in this book have sustained me. Radha and Sivaramakrishnan, my parents, have helped in more ways than I can express here. They encouraged this research enterprise, from its tentative and risky start as I sailed to Cambridge, Massachussetts, to its last stages, when they listened and cared about deadlines for chapter drafts, revisions, and reviews, were undaunted by my gloom, and always saw a happy end in sight. Nandita has been a critical anchor in the New York household while I dashed around presenting various stages of this work at conferences; and in India, Ashok stepped in at a vital point in Delhi, ensuring that the book progressed seamlessly. Many other family members—my extended Jamshedpur clan, but most notably my formidably articulate and wise older aunts across north and south India—are thanked warmly for their lively interest in age and aging, and their grasp of its social and cultural significance.

Finally, to Karuna and Krishna, I owe everything for their endurance, laughter, and love over the challenging journey of seeing this book come to fruition. My writing and world would not be the same without both of them.

Index

AARP (American Association for Retired Persons), 176, 200

Abandonment, 18, 52, 129, 203; of aged refugees, 180–182; Christian charities and, 188; concerns about, 52–53; of grandmothers, 187; in India, 197, 199; missionaries and, 180, 181; of refugees, 178–180; transnational migration and, 197; urbanization and, 187

Abuse, elder, 186–188, 195, 213

Activists, 171. *See also* Charities; NGOs

Adaptation, 56, 57, 89–90, 98

Adjustment, 89–90, 92, 98, 104

Africa: aging of, 1; anthropologists' study of, 39; Association for Social Work Education in Africa (ASWEA), 123; cancer research in, 73–74; colonial legacies and, 208 (*see also* Africa, Anglophone; Africa, Francophone); communication in, 208–209; contrast with West, 96; Dakar Recommendations for Action on Aging, 164; data on, 27, 28, 29, 33–34, 137–138; demographic forecasts for, 133–136; demographic transition in, 138; family in, 40, 163; family support in, 197–198; fertility in, 138; focus on, 20, 21; HIV crisis (*see* Grandparents; HIV/AIDS); humanitarian relief in, 127; ICSG meetings in, 106; industrialization in, 40, 161–162; Institute for Medical Research, 79; intergenerational relations in, 40; internal displacement in, 172 (*see also* Refugees); life expectancy in, 77; migration in, 42–43, 162; old age threshold and, 179; Population Conference, 137–138; regional consultations for WAA, 150–151; social change in, 40, 42–45; social gerontology research and, 104; social security in, 45–46, 163; social work schools in, 122–125; speed of aging in, 3; stereotypes about aging in, 114; studies of, 28; traditional societies in, 164; urbanization in, 40, 161–162; viewed by insiders, 41–45. *See also individual countries*

Africa, Anglophone, 162, 208–209

Africa, British, 39

Africa, Francophone, 105, 162, 208–209, 212

African Americans: cancer and, 75; as medical subjects, 20; migration of, 24; rise in aging in, 58; vulnerability of, 58

African Conference on Gerontology, 1–2, 5, 6, 7, 161–164, 165, 171, 208–209

African identity, 164

African Survey of 1938, 27–28

Age, 111; in Bantu society, 42; criterion of, 45; determining, 23, 31–36, 37–38, 129; invisibility of, 24; misstatements about, 32

Age classes, in colonial censuses, 30

Aged in Rural Society, The (Smith), 57–58
Aged persons: change in status, 55; defined by conditions, 167; marginalization of, 1, 6; overlooked in population assessments, 26; pagan beliefs and, 50–51; responsibility for dependence, 44; responsibility of, 126; UN's definition of, 150. *See also* Elderly; Old age; Older populations
Age grades, in primitive tribes, 39
Ageing and Society (journal), 193
Ageism, 172
Age regiment, 45
Age thresholds, 6, 202
AGHE (Association for Gerontology in Higher Education), 110, 112–113, 122
Aging: active, 119, 161, 191, 192–193; association with dependence, 43; assumptions about, 2, 5; beginning of, 108; as biological and medical challenge, 13–14; conflicting views on, 70; continuities and, 210–211; contradictions in, 198; as developmental issue, 2; domestic concerns about, 56; in England, 25; as global agenda, 4–5, 113, 215 (*see also* Global aging); international discourse on, 15–16; interpreting implications of, 157; invisibility of, 24; local contexts and, 10; as manageable process, 63; as mark of civilization, 91; as moral issue, 2; normative models of, 10; paradigms of, 192; as pervasive, 200; premature, 70–74; as problem, 87, 99; productive, 117; regulation of experience of, 8–9; resilient, 56; rise in, 57; social aspects of, 86–87 (*see also* Social aging); speed of, 3; as subject of interest, 8; Victorian notions of, 52; viewed beyond West, 60; as Western problem, 67–68. *See also* Aged persons; Old age; Older populations
Aging, rural, 203–204, 208
Aging in Primitive Cultures (Simmons), 56
Aging in Western Societies (Burgess), 91, 94, 96
Aging populations. *See* Aged persons; Elderly; Old age; Older populations
Aging programs, in China, 140–141
Agriculture, 137, 166
AIDS. *See* HIV/AIDS
Alma Ata declaration, 85
Alvarez, Julia Tavares de, 206

American Association for Retired Persons (AARP), 176, 200
American Cancer Society, 74, 77
American Gerontological Society, 100
Analysis of Social Change (Wilson and Wilson), 43–44
Anthropologists/anthropology, 22, 38–40; focus of, 38–40; Indian, 47; insiders, 41–45; leverage over demographers, 45; social, 47; social change and, 40–41; subversive use of, 44–45
Apt, Nana, 211
Arab world, 108
Argentina, 20
Armed conflict, 108. *See also* Refugees
Arteriosclerosis, 68–69
Asia, 136; cancer research in, 73–74; contrast with West, 96; demographic forecasts for, 133–136; family support in, 197; focus on, 20, 21; gerontology in, 112; policies in, 158–159; population growth in, 137; social gerontology research and, 104; stereotypes about aging in, 114; transition to aging in, 21. *See also* South Asia; *individual countries*
Asian, 137
Asian Population Conference, 136
Asian Regional Conference on Active Ageing, 161
Association for Gerontology in Higher Education (AGHE), 110, 112–113, 122
Association for Social Work Education in Africa (ASWEA), 123
Australia, 94
Autonomy, exerting, 146. *See also* Independence

Bantu, 42, 60, 75, 77, 78, 79
Bashford, Alison, 8, 134
Beattie, Walter, 102, 104, 106, 110, 113–114, 122, 154
Beer, Christopher, 173, 177, 178, 181
Belize, 188
Berman, Bruce, 45
Berman, Charles, 76, 77
Birth control, 84. *See also* Fertility; Population control
Birth planning programs. *See* Fertility; Population control

Births, registration of, 34

Blacker, C. P., 25

Bogomolets, A. A., 107

Booth, Charles, 97

Bose, Ashish, 120

Botswana, 194

Bourgeois-Pichat, Jean, 67–68

Brazil, 20

BRICS nations, 214

British Empire: health of army, 29; population assessment of, 28; population problems of, 27. *See also* Colonialism; Great Britain; India

British Indirect Rule, 39

British Society for Research on Ageing, 61

Bulletin on Aging (UN), 171

Burgess, Ernest, 55, 86, 88, 90, 91, 93, 95, 97, 98, 99, 119; *Aging in Western Societies*, 91, 94, 96

Butler, Robert, 214

Cairo Declaration on Population and Development, 140

Caldwell, John, 138

Canada, 94

Cancer: in Africa, 75–79; African Americans and, 75; among Bantu, 60, 77; civilization and, 83; environment and, 78–79, 81; in India, 79–83; modernity and, 80, 82, 83–84; race and, 73; research in Asia and Africa, 73–74; research on, 60; Union for International Cancer Control, 70, 74, 76, 79, 83. *See also* Diseases, chronic

Cancer Institute, 68

Cancer Research Commission, 80

Care, expectations for, 126

Caribbean, 148

Carnegie Corporation, 26, 27, 88

Carrel, Alexis, 61

Caste hierarchies, 47–49

Catholic Church, 212, 213. *See also* Christianity; Missionaries

Censuses, 26–27, 30–31, 33–37. *See also* Data

Centre de Gérontologie (ICSG), 100, 102–103, 162, 163

Centre for Social Development and Humanitarian Affairs (CSDHA), 142, 143

Chakrabarty, Dipesh, 7, 75

Chandrasekar, Sripati, 37

Change, social, 4, 15, 197; in Africa, 42–45; in colonies, 3; effects of, 104; marginalization of older persons and, 6; need for social security and, 45–46; observed by missionaries, 49–54; pace of in West, 11; speed of, 46; study of, 38; transnational, 197; in US, 91; viewed by insiders, 41–45; in Western culture, 95–96. *See also* Industrialization; Migration; Urbanization

Changes, sudden, 56

Charities, 175; Christian, 175, 177, 211–213; new approach to, 204; publicity, 181. *See also* NGOs

Charter for Older People, 159

Chebotarev, D. F., 106–107, 108, 154

Chicago, University of, 88, 90, 98, 102

Child marriage, 33

Child mortality, 82. *See also* Infant mortality

Children: during crises, 179–180; Declaration on the Rights of the Child, 180; emphasis on, 208; lack of protection of, 72; refugees, 185–186

Children, adult. *See* Family responsibility/support; Filial responsibility

Chile, 20

China, 21; active aging in, 119, 192–193; aging programs in, 140–141; community services in, 212; Confucianism, 115, 116, 118; development in, 141; family support in, 114–115, 197; Gerontological Society of China, 117; gerontology in, 116–119, 141; International Forum on Ageing, 192; life expectancy in, 118; political system, 159; population control in, 115, 117, 118–119, 134, 140, 192; retirement in, 115; rural aging in, 204; Sino-American Conference on Ageing, 117; studying aged in, 114–117; Wu Cangping, 117–119, 120, 141, 159. *See also* Asia

Chowkidars, 37

Christian Aid, 177, 180. *See also* Charities; NGOs

Christianity: African Christian morality and, 51; charity and, 175, 177, 211–213; colonial rule and, 45; old age and, 51

Church, Frank, 152, 154

CIBA Foundation, 59–60, 67, 75

Cities, 203. *See also* Urbanization

Civilization: aging as mark of, 91; cancer and, 83; race and, 83. *See also* Industrialization; Migration; Modernity; Urbanization

Clifford, William, 128–129

Club for Research on Aging (CRA), 61, 62, 63, 68, 70

Coale, Ansley J., 136

Cohen, Lawrence, 120, 121

Cold War, 14, 20, 71, 93–94, 106, 109, 115. *See also* Communist countries

Cole, Cecil Jackson, 175

Collectivism, 118

Colloquium on Aging (1954), 59–60, 75

Colombia, 20

Colonialism: funding for NGOs and, 175; investigation of old age during, 13; legacies, 208; officials, 22; population decline and, 25–26; poverty and, 54. *See also* British Empire; Censuses; Decolonization

Colonial Office, 23, 27

Colonial Populations, 26–27

Colonies: anxieties about, 27; data on, 29; elders in, 39–40; interpretation of age and aging in, 23; pensions in, 34; population in, 26. *See also* British Empire; Censuses

Coming of age, migration as, 43

Communist countries, 95, 106–109, 115, 159, 201. *See also* Cold War; *individual countries*

Community: responsibility of, 128; roles of, 127; in social work, 125

Community development, 148

Community services, 212–213

Compassion, politics of, 177

Conference on Gerontology (Dakar), 1, 5, 6, 7

Confucianism, 115, 116, 118

Connelly, Matt, 134

Continuities, 210–211

Cooper, Frederick, 164

Costa Rica, 150–151

Cowdry, E. V., 61–62, 63, 64–66, 68, 69, 72, 73, 74, 76, 81, 87, 102, 107, 113, 117

Cowgill, Donald, 110, 111–112, 113, 114–116, 117, 122

CRA (Club for Research on Aging), 61, 62, 63, 68, 70

Crises, 38, 170, 179. *See also* HIV/AIDS; Refugees

Critical inquiries, 4

Critical social gerontology, 20

Cross-cultural theory of aging, 111

CSDHA (Centre for Social Development and Humanitarian Affairs), 142, 143

Cumming, Elaine, 89

Dakar. *See* African Conference on Gerontology

Dakar Recommendations for Action on Aging, 164. *See also* African Conference on Gerontology

Daniel, Samson, 189, 190

Darfur, 177

Darfur Diaries, 178

Data: in Africa, 27, 28, 29, 33–34, 137–138; anthropologists and, 45; on colonies, 29; debates and, 137–138; efforts to improve, 30–31; from UN agencies, 133–134. *See also* Censuses

Davis, Kingsley, 56, 87, 93, 97, 98, 115–116, 119, 120, 136, 215

Death rates, 3, 137, 139. *See also* Child mortality; Infant mortality

Deaths, registration of, 34

Deccani Hindus, 81

Declaration on the Rights of the Child, 180

Decolonization, 3; aging narratives tied to, 2; assessment of old age during, 22–55; censuses and, 36–37; and Indian village hierarchies, 47–49; research on aging and, 14. *See also* Development; Industrialization

Delhi, conference in, 6–7

Democratic Republic of Congo, 212

Demographers, 22, 45, 134. *See also* Experts

Demographic dividend, 214

Demographic inertia, 139

Demographic models, linear, 11–12

Demographic patterns, in global South, 3

Demographic Survey of the British Colonial Empire (Kuczynski), 28, 30

Demographic transition, 134–135, 138, 150

Deng Xiaoping, 117, 119

Dependence, 21, 171, 197, 205; aging associated with, 43, 105; in anthropological studies,

40–41; criteria for, 35–36; on elders, 48–49; fracture of social relations and, 41; income/work and, 172; in Kikuyu community, 44–45; in Masai, 39; older persons' responsibility for, 44; in South Asia, 120. *See also* Family responsibility/support; Filial responsibility; Intergenerational ties

Dependency ratios, 93

De Souza, Alfred, 121

Developing countries, 14; demographic transition in, 138; in discussions on aging, 200; gerontology in, 111–113, 122; neoliberalism in, 191; participation in IAG, 110; research in, 201. *See also* Africa; Asia; India; South Asia; *individual countries*

Development, 3, 140, 157; aging-related policies linked with, 207–208; assumptions about, 2; in China, 141; critiques of, 127, 205; disenchantment with, 203; effects of, 104; failures of, 122, 132; focus on, 84; focus on youth in, 130; human aspect of, 169–170; importing Western models of, 163–164; models of, 10; in social work education, 124; Sustainable Development Goals, 200–201, 208. *See also* Industrialization; Migration; Urbanization

Developmental approach, 200

Disability, old age threshold and, 179

Disasters, 38, 179. *See also* Refugees

Disasters Emergency Committee (DEC), 185

Discourse, shifting, 215

Diseases: in British army, 29; childhood, 34; infectious, 12, 34, 71, 214; of poverty, 80; tropical, 80. *See also* Diseases, chronic; Diseases of aging

Diseases, chronic, 14, 202, 214; age and, 60–61, 84; assumptions about, 14; boundary with acute diseases, 12; effects on aging, 70–74; environment and, 60, 78–79, 81; manpower and, 72; in non-Western societies, 75–84; old age's similarity to, 64; plan to map, 74; race and, 72–73; sex and, 72–73; viewed beyond West, 60. *See also* Cancer

Diseases of aging: debate over, 62–63; focus on, 14; race and, 20. *See also* Cancer; Diseases, chronic

Diversity: of aging populations, 6, 200; of IAG, 103–104; in NGOs, 210

Donahue, Wilma, 11, 91, 102, 106, 110

Dorn, Harold, 69

Dorobo tribe, 41

Duara, Prasenjit, 83

Dying, Victorian notions of, 52

Economic and Social Council (ECOSOC), 17–18, 88, 142, 162

Economic Commission for Asia and the Far East (ECAFE) regions, 136. *See also* Asia; Developing countries; South Asia; *individual countries*

Economic crises, 145, 158, 169

Economic instabilities, 19

Economic survival, lack of means for, 7

Economy, effects on aged, 157–158

ECOSOC (United Nations Economic and Social Council), 17–18, 88, 142, 162

Education, gerontological, 102, 110–111, 122

Egypt, gerontology in, 112–113

Elder abuse, 186–188, 195, 213

Elderly, 92. *See also* Aged persons; Old age; Older populations

Elders: in Bantu society, 42; focus on, 38; fracture of social relations and, 41; in Indian villages, 48–49; role of, 39–40

Empathy, 171–172, 181, 216

Employment: adjustment and, 98; in colonial censuses, 36; focus on, 144–145. *See also* Productivity; Retirement

Encyclopaedia of Social Work in India, 126

Endogamy, 81

England. *See* British Empire; Great Britain

Environment: as agenda, 139, 206; cancer and, 60, 78–79, 81

Epidemiological transition model, linear, 12

Equity, 139

Eriksson, Lars-Gunnar, 185

Eritrea, 178

Escobar, Arturo, 140

Estes, Carol, 205

Ethiopia, 178

Ethnographic accounts, by missionaries, 49–54

"Ethnological" knowledge, 36

Eugenics Society, 25

EURAG (European Federation for the Welfare of the Elderly), 143–146, 149

Europe: Central, 194; compared to US, 96–97; Eastern, 95, 104, 194; exclusion of at WAA, 143–145; focus on, 95–96; as laboratory of aging, 92; provincializing, 12; relevance of to US, 109; as source of norms, 4; Western, 11, 94. *See also* West; *individual countries*

European Federation for the Welfare of the Elderly (EURAG), 143–146, 149

Evans Pritchard, E. E., 39, 47

Events, used to estimate age, 37–39

Ewing, Oscar R., 72

Expertise: emergence of, 16–19; objectivity and, 97; proliferation of, 26

Experts: American, 100–102, 109, 122; anthropologists, 38–40; desire to understand local society, 28; development, 16–17; gerontological, 2, 86–87; influence of, 202; local, 17; networks of, 162–163; role of, 16–19, 100, 215–216; WAA agenda and, 133. *See also* Demographers; Social workers

Fahey, Monsignor, 212

Faith-based networks, 211–213

Family: absence of, 92; in Africa, 163; decline in relations, 168, 198; in developing countries, 158; intergenerational, 48–49; migration and, 137; in social work, 125; urbanization and, 137

Family Care Council, 151

Family planning. *See* Fertility; Population control

Family responsibility/support, 126, 128, 146, 192, 194, 197–198; assumptions about aging and, 199; failures of, 18–19; mandated in India, 196–197, 208. *See also* Filial responsibility; Intergenerational ties

Fassin, Didier, 108, 161, 172

Federal Security Agency (FSA), 65

Ferguson, James, 187, 198

Fernandes, Walter, 120, 121, 161, 164

Fertility: in Africa, 138; decline in, 3, 25, 27, 96, 135; forecasts of, 134; reducing, 138. *See also* Demographic transition; Population control

Filial responsibility, 18, 114–116; in anthropological studies, 40–41; in China, 114–115, 197;

communism and, 115; mandated in India, 196–197. *See also* Family responsibility/ support; Intergenerational ties

Finkle, Jason, 140

First International Conference on the Global Impact of AIDS, 187

First Population Conference (Ibadan), 137–138

Flesch, Joseph, 105, 106, 113, 162

Forecasts, 7–8, 133–136

Fortunes of Primitive Tribes, The (Majumdar), 47

Foucault, Michel, 8

Foundations, private, 211

France: Centre de Gérontologie (ICSG), 100, 102–103, 162, 163; dependency ratios in, 93; expertise in, 26; gerontology in, 104–106; relevance of to US, 109; research in, 97; rural, 105

Francis, Sybil, 148

Frank, Lawrence, 70, 72

Frenk, Julio, 12

Funding: lack of, 17, 18, 211; for NGOs, 188–189; private partnerships, 213; of state-level initiatives, 210; for Vienna Plan, 170–171

Fundraising, 204

Gates Foundation, 211

Gelinek, Ingrid, 147, 148–149

Geriatric services, 107

Gerontocracies, 39

Gerontological associations, 14. *See also individual associations*

Gerontological education, 102, 110–111, 122

Gerontological knowledge: disseminating, 113–114; influence of research in colonies on, 54–57

Gerontological Society, 62

Gerontological Society of China, 117

Gerontologists, 20; American, 109; differences among, 92. *See also* Experts

Gerontology: in Asia, 112; assumptions in, 60; biological aspects of, 89; in China, 116–119, 141; collaboration with other sciences, 65; communist countries and, 106–109; comparative, 107; course on, 103; critical, 20; described, 99; disseminating, 99–100;

Europe as laboratory of, 92; expansion of networks, 104; in France, 104–106; in IAG, 100–101; interest in, 87; international, 58; as international social science, 86; mission of, 98, 99; networks, 65 (*see also* Networks); prestige of, 101; race and, 58, 74–75; relevance of, 104, 202; research in, 63, 64 (*see also* Research); scientific legitimacy of, 63; support for research in, 101–102; tied to human welfare, 64; values of, 102; views of, 67; welfare policies and, 104. *See also* Experts; *individual associations*

Ghana, 79, 207, 211

Gillman, Joseph, 72, 75–76, 78, 79, 83, 84

Gillman, Theodore, 59–60, 73, 75–76, 77, 79

Glass, D. V., 25

Global Age-Friendly Cities, 203

Global agenda, 204

Global aging, 131, 139–140, 160–161, 198–199. *See also* Madrid International Plan of Action on Ageing (MIPAA); World Assembly on Aging (WAA), second

Global Alliance of International Longevity Centers, 214

Global Program on Aging, 17–18

Global South: demographic patterns in, 3; WAA and, 150–151. *See also* Developing countries; *individual countries*

Gluckman, Max, 42

Godfrey, Nancy, 178, 179, 184

Gokhale, Sharad, 205, 206

Goldhamer, Herbert, 88

Gorman, Mark, 176

Gourou, Pierre, 26

Grandmothers, abandoned, 187. *See also* Grandparents

Grandparents: custodial, 193; HIV/AIDS and, 193, 197–198; urbanization and, 187

Granville Edge, Percy, 30–31

Gray Panthers, 172, 200

Great Britain: aging in, 25; army, 29; declining fertility in, 25; Disasters Emergency Committee (DEC), 185; expertise in, 26; Population Investigation Committee (PIC), 25–27; population shift in, 25; research in, 97. *See also* British Empire

Habitat, 203

Hailey, Malcolm, 27, 28, 29, 30

Hampson, Joseph, 124, 162, 165, 167, 212

Handbook on Social Gerontology, 55

Hardy, Dorcas R., 153

Harris, Louis, 153

Hauser, Philip, 90, 93–94, 95

Havighurst, Robert, 55, 88, 89, 95, 97, 100, 118

Health: in British army, 29; in British India, 29–30; crises, 170 (*see also* HIV/AIDS); emphasis on children/youth, 208; global, 4, 9–10, 211 (*see also* Public health); neoliberalism and, 192; NGOs and, 194–195; privatization of, 192; social goals of, 85. *See also* Public health

Healthcare, in cities, 203

HelpAge India, 189–190

HelpAge International (HAI), 159, 165, 168, 173–174, 175, 179, 180, 181, 187, 188, 200, 207; collaboration with social workers, 182–184; impact of campaigns, 185–186; influence of, 209–210; motivating philosophy, 176; priorities, 190–191; work of, 216

Help the Aged, 159, 161, 173, 175, 178, 189

Henry, Warren Earl, 89

Higginson, J., 78–79, 84

Hindus, Deccani, 81

Historiography, 3–4

HIV/AIDS, 170, 206; children and, 180; elder abuse and, 186–188, 195; First International Conference on the Global Impact of AIDS, 187; grandmothers and, 193, 197–198; intergenerational ties and, 187

Hollis, Alfred, 39

Holmes, Lowell, 111–112, 117

Hong Chang Ping, 140, 141

Huet, Jean Auguste, 105

Human development, 124

Human Development Services, 153

Humanitarian campaigns, 182–184, 206

Humanitarian interventions, 127, 174–175, 177. *See also* Refugees

Humanitarian issue, aging as, 122, 170, 185

Humanitarian reason, 161, 172

Human Relations Area Files (HRAF), 55

Human rights, 185, 215, 216

Hungary, 194

IAG (International Association of Gerontology). *See* International Association of
    Gerontology (IAG)
IASW (International Association for Social
    Work), 147
Ibo, 41
ICSG (International Center for Social
    Gerontology), 102–103, 105–106, 113, 162, 163
ICSW (International Council on Social
    Welfare), 147–148, 149, 205
Identity, African, 164
Identity, cultural, 44
Idleness, 57
IFA (International Federation on Aging).
    See International Federation on Aging (IFA)
Illife, John, 54
ILO (International Labor Organization), 67,
    105, 106, 162–163
Inbreeding, 81
Income, 172. *See also* Productivity
Independence, 97, 98, 192
India: abandonment in, 197, 199; aging in,
    79–83; anthropologists in, 38, 47; assessment
    of population in, 27; cancer in, 79–83; caste
    hierarchies in, 47; census operations in, 31;
    determining age in, 32; *Encyclopaedia of
    Social Work in India*, 126; family in, 168;
    family responsibility in, 196–197, 208;
    forecasts regarding, 136; generalizations
    about elderly in, 191; gerontological views in,
    121–122; independence of, 37; intergenerational families in, 48–49; lack of accurate
    data on, 29–30; life expectancy in, 82;
    national initiatives in, 207; National
    Population Conference, 139; as neutral, 94;
    NGOs in, 189–191; Partition of, 126; pensions
    in, 35; population control policies, 134;
    private partnerships in, 213; purposes of
    age-related statistics in, 32–33; retirement in,
    120–121, 168; rural aging in, 204; social work
    in, 122–125, 130, 211; state-level initiatives,
    209; studies in, 10; Vienna Plan of Action
    and, 168; village hierarchies in, 47–49; vital
    statistics in, 37; women in, 209
Indian Association of Gerontology, 213
Indian Science Congress, 80
Indian Social Institute (ISI), 168, 211

Industrialization: in Africa, 40, 161–162; aging
    and, 95, 96; assumptions about, 1–2; creation
    of elderly by, 92; effects of, 18; risks to bodies
    and, 90; US's lag in, 91. *See also* Change,
    social; Migration; Urbanization
Inequalities, 4, 6, 10, 58, 203, 205
Infant mortality, 34, 82, 120
Institute for Medical Research (Ghana), 79
Institute for Social Gerontology (ISG), 165
Institute of Economic Growth, 213
Interchurch Aid, 177
Intergenerational ties, 24, 40, 187; anxieties
    about, 24; in China, 115; in India, 48–49.
    See also Family; Family responsibility/
    support; Filial responsibility
Internal displacement. *See* Refugees
International African Institute, 27, 41
International Association for Gerontology
    and Geriatrics (IAGG), 209–210. *See also*
    International Association of Gerontology
    (IAG)
International Association for Social Work
    (IASW), 147
International Association of Gerontology
    (IAG), 62, 66, 71, 86, 88, 113, 154, 209–210;
    developing countries' participation in, 110;
    diversity of, 103–104; geostrategic tensions
    and, 108; international representation in, 65;
    scientific character of, 105; social gerontology
    in, 100–101; social scientists and, 87; support
    for, 68–70. *See also* International Gerontological Congress (IGC)
International Center for Social Gerontology
    (ICSG), 102–103, 105–106, 113, 162, 163
International Council on Social Welfare
    (ICSW), 147–148, 149, 205
International Demographic Congress, 26
International Federation on Aging (IFA), 142,
    148, 181, 186, 188, 200, 205; conference in
    India, 213; influence of, 209–210; president
    of, 205; work of, 216
International Forum on Ageing, 192
International Association of Gerontology
    (IAG), 154
International Gerontological Committee, 88
International Gerontological Congress (IGC),
    62, 63, 64, 67, 69, 71, 91, 134, 176; agenda of,

69; influence of Americans at, 101; international representation at, 65; in Kiev, 107; representation at, 104; social gerontology at, 88; social research committee, 100. *See also* International Association of Gerontology (IAG)

International Labor Organization (ILO), 67, 105, 106, 162–163

International Refugee Year, 176

International Social Science Journal, 86, 99–100

International Social Security Association, 163

International Union Against Cancer, 70, 76. *See also* Union for International Cancer Control (UICC)

Interventions, local/regional, 204

Ireland, 38

ISG (Institute for Social Gerontology), 165

Isolation, 7, 92

Israel, 107, 123

Jackson, Cecil, 189

Jamaica, 148

Japan, 112, 135

Jensen, Howard, 98

Jesuit missions, 51. *See also* Hampson, Joseph; Missionaries

Kalache, Alexandre, 184

Kaplan, Oscar, 87–88

Karve, Iravati, 49

Kaunda, Kenneth, 167

Kenya, 148, 157–158

Kenyatta, Jomo, 44–45

Kerrigan, William, 155–156

Khanolkar, V. R., 59, 60, 76, 79–83, 84

Kiev Institute of Gerontology, 108

Kikuyu community, 43–44

Kinship: decreasing value of, 43; dependence and, 44–45. *See also* Family; Intergenerational ties

Kirkley, Leslie, 175, 176–177, 181

Knowledge, "ethnological", 36

Knowledge, politics of, 4

Korea, 72, 158–159

Korenchevsky, Vladimir, 61, 62, 63, 64, 66, 71, 88, 102

Kosovo, 194

Kuczynski, Robert, 23, 25, 26–27, 28, 30, 33–34, 36

Kuhn, Maggie, 200

Kumar, Meira, 196

Kuplan, Robert, 100

Kuwait, 112, 122

Labor force, 78, 79, 82–83, 97–98. *See also* Productivity; Retirement

Lambert, Georges, 162

Laroque report, 105

Latin America, 20; demographic transition in, 150; regional consultations for WAA, 150–151. *See also individual countries*

League of Arab States, 108

League of Nations, 29

Lerner, Baron, 73

Leroy Stewart, Harold, 70, 74, 75, 78

Life cycle, in White Fathers' inquiry, 50–52

Life expectancy, 3, 71, 96; in Africa, 77; in China, 118; in India, 82; in South Asia, 18–19, 120

Life insurance, 35

Lifespan approach, 146–147, 155

Life stages, in social work education, 124

Liver cancer, 60, 77, 78. *See also* Cancer

London School of Economics, 28, 100

London School of Hygiene, 23, 30

Loneliness, 158–159

Longevity. *See* Life expectancy

Lonsdale, John, 45

MacNider, William, 70

Josiah Macy Jr. Foundation, 61, 68, 72, 175

Madras School of Social Work, 126

Madrid. *See* Madrid International Plan of Action on Ageing (MIPAA); World Assembly on Aging (WAA), second

Madrid International Plan of Action on Ageing (MIPAA), 162, 200, 203, 206–207

Majumdar, Dina Nath, 47–48

Maladjustment, 43, 47, 90, 202

Malawi, 158

Malinowski, Bronislaw, 41, 44, 47

Malnutrition, 78, 79

Manpower, 72, 78, 79. *See also* Labor force; Productivity

Mao Zedong, 117

Marks, Shula, 28

Marxism, 118

Masai, 39

McCay, Clive, 70

Medalia, Leon, 71

Medical subjects, 20

Medvedev, Zhores, 107

Memories, 38

Men, research and, 72–73

Mexico, 20

Migrant labor, caste structure and, 49

Migrant Labour and Tribal Life (Schapera),
    42–43

Migration, 18, 19, 214; abandonment and, 197;
    adaptation of aged and, 56; in Africa, 42–43,
    162; of African Americans, 24; in China, 116;
    as coming of age, 43; concerns about, 15;
    controlling, 26; effects of, 7, 104; family and,
    137; in India, 197; interdependence and, 24;
    intergenerational relations and, 40; and roles
    of older people, 179; in United States, 57.
    See also Change, social; Industrialization;
    Urbanization

Military: aging and, 71–72; British army, 29

Minkler, Meredith, 205

MIPAA (Madrid International Plan of Action
    on Ageing), 162, 200, 203, 206–207

Missionaries, 22, 50–54, 165, 180, 181. *See also*
    Hampson, Joseph

Models: challenging, 12–13; normative, 10–12.
    See also Norms

Modernity: assumptions about, 14; cancer and,
    80, 82, 83–84

Modernization: in Africa, 40; concerns about,
    14–15; critiques of, 205; effects of, 120;
    failures of, 132; family relations and, 198;
    knowledge of age and, 34; linear stages of,
    94–95; marginalization of older persons and,
    6; views of, 21; in Western culture, 95–96.
    See also Change, social; Industrialization;
    Migration; Urbanization

Moffat, Robert, 52, 180

Montreal Protocol, 139

Morality, African Christian, 51

Mortality, 137, 179. *See also* Child mortality;
    Infant mortality

Mugabe, R. G., 165, 166, 167

Mupedziswa, R., 183, 184

Murdock, George Peter, 55

Narasimhan, M. C., 168

National Cancer Institute, 74

National Conference on Aging, 65, 66, 69, 72

National Council on Aging, 153

National initiatives, 207

National Institute for Mental Health, 88

National Institute of Child Health and Human
    Development, 89

National Institute of Mental Health, 89

National Institute on Aging, 154, 172, 214

National Institutes of Health (NIH), 62, 78, 87

National Plan for the Elderly, 167

National Population Conference, 139

Need, 216

Neoliberalism, 4, 16, 133, 145, 152, 153, 191, 192,
    199, 203, 205

Networks, 162–163; development of, 60–64,
    66–70; expansion of, 104; NGOs and, 176,
    177, 189; relief projects and, 170. *See also*
    Experts

New International Economic Order
    (NIEO), 152

New Zealand, 94

NGOs, 17, 54, 142, 159, 161, 170, 175, 188, 192;
    afterlives of WAA and, 160; appeals of,
    180–181; campaigns by, 171; diversity in, 210;
    focus of, 191; funding for, 188–189; fund-
    raising techniques, 189–190; goals of, 210;
    humanitarian crises and, 176–177; impact of
    campaigns, 185–186; in India, 189–191;
    mainstreaming aging and, 194; networks
    and, 177, 189; Open-Ended Working Group
    on Ageing, 215; participatory action networks
    and, 205; rights of older persons and, 186;
    rise of, 160; roles of, 190–191, 194–195,
    209–210, 215–216; SDGs and, 200; support for
    old by, 51; work with national governments,
    188. *See also* HelpAge International

Nigeria, 158; census in, 36; gerontology in, 112;
    regional consultations for WAA, 150–151

NIH (National Institutes of Health), 62, 78, 87

Non-governmental organizations (NGOs).
    See NGOs

Norms: challenging, 12–13, 14; sources of, 4.
    See also Models
Notestein, Frank, 93, 135
Nuers, 39
Nuffield Foundation, 67, 100, 175
Nyakyusa, 51
Nyerere, Julius, 186

Objectivity, 97
Odio, Rodrigo Carazo, 151
Oettle, A. G., 78, 79, 84
Office of Aging, 86
Office of Population Research, 134, 135, 138
Officers, British, 34
Old age: Christianity and, 51; criteria for,
    35–36; during decolonization, 22–55;
    defining through memories, 38; interpreta-
    tions of, 54–58; as social category, 128;
    threshold of, 6, 179. See also Aged persons;
    Aging; Elderly; Older populations
Old Age Pensions Act, 38
Older persons. See Aged persons; Elderly; Old
    age; Older populations
Older Persons Forum, 198
Older populations: in Africa, 1; changing
    perspectives on, 2–3; global health histories
    and, 9; growth of, 8; linked with future and
    promise, 2–3. See also Aged persons; Aging;
    Elderly; Old age; Older persons
Old People in Three Industrial Societies
    (Shanas), 92
Open-Ended Working Group on Ageing, 215
Oppenheimer College, 129
Organization for Economic Co-operation and
    Development, 189
Organization of African Unity, 3, 197, 209, 215
Orphans, AIDS. See HIV/AIDS
Oxfam (Oxford Committee for Famine Relief),
    174, 175, 180
Oxford, University of, 27
Oxford Committee for Famine Relief (Oxfam),
    174, 175, 180
Ozone discourse, 139

Packard, Randall, 78
"Pagan" beliefs, preservation of, 50–51
Paillat, Paul, 105, 154

Pakistan, 207
Pan-American Congress of Gerontology,
    First, 64
PanAmerican Health Organization, 189
Paradigms, 4. See also Models; Norms
Parental Maintenance and Senior Citizens
    Act, 196
Parsis, 81, 82
Past, sense of, 38
Patriarchy, 205
Peace Corps volunteers, 17
Peggs, Reverend, 53
Pension disease, 108. See also Retirement
Pensioners, 121. See also Retirement
Pensions, 145; availability of, 7; in colonies, 34;
    criteria for, 35–36; determining eligibility for,
    38; French, 106; for informal workers, 209.
    See also Retirement
Pepper, Claude, 153, 154
Pères Blancs, 50–52, 53
Petersen, Todd, 185
PIC (Population Investigation Committee),
    25–27
Policies, 7–8, 192, 208. See also Population
    control
Politics: aging and, 14, 92–94; refashioning,
    214; in social work education, 124; of
    suffering, 108
Pollock, Ann, 72
Population changes, interest in, 8
Population control, 132; in Asia, 136; in China,
    115, 117, 118–119, 134, 140, 192; confrontations
    over, 212; focus on, 84; funding for, 175;
    policies, 134, 135, 140, 159, 192
Population decline, 24–27
Population growth, 67, 137
Population Investigation Committee (PIC),
    25–27
Poverty, 7, 15, 203; of age, 19; assumptions about
    chronic disease and, 14; colonial rule and,
    53; diseases of poverty, 80; UN and, 192;
    urban, 19; white, 45
Poverty Reduction Strategy Papers, 207
Predictions, aging populations and, 7–8
Preventive approaches, 125, 148, 155
Primer of Social Case Work in Africa,
    A (Clifford), 128–129

Principles for Older Persons, 186, 205–206

Private sector, 213–214

Problems of Ageing, The (Cowdry), 62, 70

Productivity, 82–83, 97–98, 195; chronic diseases and, 72; in colonial censuses, 36; developmental goals and, 191–192; focus on, 97, 144–145; lack of adjustment and, 89–90; older refugees and, 172. *See also* Aging, active; Retirement

Progress, linear stages of, 94–95

Psychological aspects of aging, 14, 88. *See also* Social aging

Public health, 96, 159; infectious disease and, 12; life expectancy and, 18–19

Pumpernig, Eduard, 143, 145

Qian Xuesen, 119

Race: assumptions about chronic disease and, 14; civilization and, 83; gerontology and, 58, 74–75; malnutrition and, 78; science and, 72–73; in social security, 128

Recession, 15. *See also* Economic crises

Refugee camps, 127, 178, 179, 183

Refugees, 170, 171, 172–174, 175, 177–180, 193–194; abandonment of, 178–182; awareness of, 189; Christian charities and, 188; developmental approach to, 182–183, 184; European, 194; human rights of, 185; impact of NGO campaigns, 185–186; social status of, 183, 184; social workers and, 182–184; women, 183. *See also* NGOs

Relief projects, 170. *See also* NGOs; Refugees

Remembered Village, The (Srinivas), 48

Report on Aging in Slums (UN), 126–127

Report on Improvement of Slums and Uncontrolled Settlements (UN), 127

Research: in Africa, 73–74, 104; agenda of, 60; on aging and cancer, 60; applicability of to Asia and Africa, 104; in Asia, 73–74; in developing countries, 201; diseases of old age and, 63; on environmental causes, 78–79; in Europe, 97; focus of, 97–98; generalizability of, 60; in non-Western societies, 75–84; priorities of, 201; silos in, 84–85; support for, 64, 77–78, 80, 81–82, 101; in United States, 100

Researchers, tensions between, 20

Resilience, 193

Respect, forms of, 52–53

Responsibility, for care of aged, 126, 128. *See also* Family responsibility/support; Filial responsibility; Intergenerational ties

Retirement, 87, 103, 104, 108, 153; adaptation to, 98; in China, 115; in India, 120–121, 168; mandatory, 172. *See also* Pensions; Productivity

Rhodesia, 167

Rhodes-Livingston Institute (RLI), 10, 42, 46, 47, 162, 187

Rights, of older persons, 186

Rockefeller Foundation, 27, 66, 88

Rockefeller Institute for Medical Research, 61, 66

Rockefeller Medical University, 62

Role of the Aged in Primitive Societies, The (Simmons), 55

Rosenmayr, Leopold, 146

Rural aging, 203–204, 208

Rural decline, 19. *See also* Urbanization

Russia, 95, 104, 201. *See also* USSR

Sagner, Andreas, 52

Samiti, Kalyan, 190

Saunders, Carr, 25

Sauvy, Alfred, 93, 103

Schapera, Isaac, 42–43, 45, 46, 48, 187

Scholarship, focus of, 9

School of Social Work (Harare), 165, 167

Science, race and, 72–73

SDGs (Sustainable Development Goals), 200–201, 208

Security, threats to, 93

Security analysts, 7–8

Self-help, exerting, 146

Self-reliance, 153, 192, 195

Senegal, 163

Senility, 61, 63

Serampore mission, 53

Shanas, Ethel, 88, 92, 102, 107, 118, 147, 154, 155

Shock, Nathan, 62, 63, 73, 88, 104, 107, 108

Shuman, Tarek, 142–143, 146

Sickness insurance, 35

Simmons, Leo, 55, 56
Sino-American Conference on Ageing, 117
Skweyiya, Zola, 198
Slums, 126–127
Smith, T. Lynn, 57–58
Social aging, 87, 88–89
Social benefits, 90. *See also* Social security; Welfare
Social category, old age as, 128
Social change. *See* Change, social
Social Contours of an Industrial City (Majumdar), 48
Social control, age and, 33
Social harmony, 117–118
Socialism, 159, 166
Social Policy for Old Age, A, 105
Social problems of aging, 14. *See also* Social aging
Social relations, 38, 41
Social science, 55, 87. *See also* Anthropologists/ anthropology; Gerontology
Social Science Research Council (SSRC), 88, 89
Social scientists, ties with UN, 18
Social security, 90; in Africa, 45–46, 163; for African Americans, 58; availability of, 7; colonial legacies and, 208; expectations for, 126; idleness and, 57; in poor countries, 120; pressure for, 45–46; race in, 128; in United States, 154. *See also* Pensions; Welfare
Social security reform, 87
Social work, 126; biases in, 129; stress on nation building, 130
Social work education, 128–130, 147, 211; Association for Social Work Education in Africa (ASWEA), 123; course development in Africa, 125; in India and Africa, 122–125; School of Social Work, 165, 167
Social workers, 17; afterlives of WAA and, 160; collaboration with HelpAge International, 182; critiques of development, 127; in developing nations, 122–125; in India, 130; International Association for Social Work (IASW), 147; preventive approaches, 125; refugees and, 182–184; urbanization and, 125. *See also* Experts; Hampson, Joseph
Society, local, 28–31

Society for Human Rights and Prisoner Aid (SHARP), 207
Sociologists, 24, 111, 203
Sociology, 57
Somalia, 173
Soodan, Kirpal Singh, 121
South Africa, 76; cancer and aging in, 77–79; custodial grandmothers in, 193; elder abuse in, 187–188, 195; HIV/AIDS in, 193, 197–198; liver cancer in, 75; malnutrition in, 78; Older Persons Forum, 197; pensions, 208. *See also* Gillman, Theodore
South African Local Government Association (SALGA), 207
South Asia, 6–7; conferences on aging in, 121; dependence in, 120; life expectancy in, 18–19, 120; problems for aged in, 120–121; retirement in, 120–121. *See also individual countries*
Sri Lanka, 209
Srinivas, M. N., 48
SSRC (Social Science Research Council), 88, 89
Standing Committee on Relief of Distress Among the Aged, 148
Standing Conference of Refugees, 181
State, responsibility for care of aged and, 145. *See also* Social security; Welfare
State-level initiatives, 209, 210
Statistics, age-related, 32–33. *See also* Data
Status, change in, 55, 183, 184
Steiner study, 73
Struggle for Population, The (Glass), 25
Sudan, 178, 179
Suffering, discourse of, 216
Surveys, imputing age in, 31–36
Sustainable Development Goals (SDGs), 200–201, 208
Szreter, Simon, 134

Taeuber, Irene, 135, 136
Tanzania, 192, 194
Tata (family), 82
Tata, Naval, 80
Tata Institute of Social Sciences, 213
Technology, 6, 96
Thailand, 112, 122

Thematic frames, 13

Third World: framing of, 140; meaning of, 103. *See also* Developing countries

Tibbits, Clark, 55

Tibbitts, Clark, 11, 86, 87, 88, 89, 90, 91, 99–100, 101, 102, 106, 110, 117

Tiers monde, 103

Titmuss, Richard, 93

Tobacco, 81

Tout, Kenneth, 159–160, 165, 173–174, 179, 181, 186

Townsend, Peter, 92, 205

Traditional societies, 55–56, 114–115, 164

Traditions, in Africa, 129

Tropical diseases, 80

Truman, Harry, 65

Tswana, 42

UICC (Union for International Cancer Control), 70, 74, 76, 79, 83

UK. *See* Great Britain

UNDP (United Nations Development Programme), 166

UNESCO, 67, 68, 86, 99–100, 102, 104

UNFPA (United Nations Population Fund), 6, 212

UNHCR (United Nations High Commissioner for Refugees), 172, 174–175, 184

UNICEF, 67, 68, 180

Union for International Cancer Control (UICC), 70, 74, 76, 79, 83

United Nations (UN), 20; approach to aging, 166; *Bulletin on Aging*, 171; Declaration on the Rights of the Child, 180; distrust of, 152; in field of aging, 17–18; humanitarian interventions, 174–175; lack of support for gerontological research, 66–68; mainstreaming aging and, 194–195; Population Branch, 67; poverty and, 192; Principles for Older Persons, 186, 205; *Report on Aging in Slums*, 126–127; *Report on Improvement of Slums and Uncontrolled Settlements*, 127; reports, 8; Social Affairs division, 152; Social Development division, 152; ties with social scientists, 18; World Population Conferences, 132, 133–134. *See also*

Sustainable Development Goals (SDGs); World Assembly on Aging (WAA); World Assembly on Aging (WAA), second

United Nations Development Programme (UNDP), 166

United Nations Educational, Scientific and Cultural Organization (UNESCO), 67, 68, 86, 99–100, 102, 104

United Nations High Commissioner for Refugees (UNHCR), 172, 174–175, 184

United Nations Population Fund (UNFPA), 6, 212

United Nations Trust Fund, 171

United States: aging in, 57; compared to Europe, 94, 96–97; as demographic laggard, 90–91; dependency ratios in, 93; discomfort with welfare, 97; elderly in, compared to traditional societies, 55–56; Europe's relevance to, 109; inequalities in, 58; lag in industrialization, 91; as leader of free world, 94; migration of African Americans in, 24; models of aging in, 11; modernization in, 96; norms and, 18; Office of Aging, 86; research in, 97–98, 100, 101; self-reliance of aged in, 153; as source of norms, 4; support for WAA by, 152–154. *See also* West

United States Senate Committee on Aging, 106–107

Urbanization, 157–158; abandonment and, 187; in Africa, 40, 161–162; agriculture and, 166; concerns about, 14–15; effects of, 7; family and, 137; need for social security and, 46; and old age as social category, 128; in social work, 125; US's lag in, 91. *See also* Change, social; Industrialization; Migration

USSR, 94, 107. *See also* Communist countries; Russia

Values, European, 102

Vargas, Raul, 93–94

Vienna. *See* World Assembly on Aging (WAA)

Vienna Plan of Action, 140, 156, 160, 163; afterlives of, 160; funding for, 170–171, 175;

India and, 168; local adaptations of, 204–205; relevance of, 161

Vietnam, 181

Visibility, of aging, 19, 22

Vital statistics: collection of, 36; in context of decolonization, 36; in India, 37. *See also* Data

Vulnerability, 216; of aged, 7, 206; perceptions of, 187; translated into strength, 193

Vulnerable persons, exclusion of in international discourse, 16

WAA (World Assembly on Aging). *See* Vienna Plan of Action; World Assembly on Aging (WAA)

WAA (World Assembly on Aging), second. *See* Madrid International Plan of Action on Ageing (MIPAA); World Assembly on Aging (WAA), second

Wahi, Premnath, 84

Wailoo, Keith, 73

War, 108. *See also* Refugees

Weisz, George, 63

Welfare: in Africa, 45–46; American discomfort with, 97; availability of, 7; during economic crises, 133; in Korea, 159; from state, 96; in United States, 97, 152. *See also* Social security

Welfare policies, social gerontology and, 104

Welfare societies, exclusion of old within, 103

Welfare state, 68

West: confining age to, 94–96; linear models and, 12; models of aging and, 11; models of development and, 163–164; as reference point, 109; social distinctions in, 20. *See also* Europe; United States

Western culture, qualifications for, 95. *See also* Industrialization; Modernity; Urbanization

Western society, transformation of, 92. *See also* Industrialization; Social change; Urbanization

WFI (White Fathers' inquiry), 50–52, 53

White, Paul Dudley, 71

White Fathers, 50–52, 53

White House Conference on Aging, 153, 154

Whites, 20

WHO (World Health Organization). *See* World Health Organization (WHO)

Wilson, Godfrey, 43–44, 187

Wilson, Monica, 42, 43–44, 51

Witchcraft, 213

Women: during crises, 179; developmental approach to, 184; in EURAG's concerns, 145; in India, 82, 209; lack of research on, 73; old age threshold and, 179; refugees, 183, 185–186

Work, 172. *See also* Labor force; Productivity; Retirement

Workers, 144. *See also* Labor force; Productivity; Retirement

World aging. *See* Global aging

World Assembly on Aging (WAA), 5–6, 15, 17–18, 106, 108, 131, 143, 152, 203; agenda of, 133; as benchmark, 165; criticism of UN approach, 146; debates at, 133, 156–160; economic crisis and, 169; expectations of, 149; focus on West, 147–149; global South and, 150–151; Kerrigan at, 155–156; origins of, 132–133; pressures leading to, 152–155; recommendations of, 160; regional consultations for, 149–151; responses to agenda, 142–151; vision of, 142. *See also* Vienna Plan of Action

World Assembly on Aging (WAA), second, 15, 185, 199–200, 203, 205, 206–207, 215. *See also* Madrid International Plan of Action on Ageing (MIPAA)

World Bank, 203

World Congress of Gerontology, 117

World Health Organization (WHO), 17–18, 68, 83, 85, 106; "Ageing and Health" program, 189; cancer research and, 74; Global Age-Friendly Cities, 203; Global Program on Aging, 17–18; ICSG and, 106; integrated health services and, 210; interest in aging, 151; NGOs and, 194; support for gerontological research, 67; at Zimbabwe meeting, 165–166

World Population Conferences, 58, 114, 132, 133–134, 152, 212

World War II, 64

Wu Cangping, 117–119, 120, 141, 159
Wylie, Diana, 78

Xhosa, 52, 180, 181

Youth: anxieties about, 24; emphasis on, 130, 208, 214; migration of, 15 (*see also* Migration; Urbanization); in social work, 130
Yugoslavia, 194
Yu Guanghan, 159

Zambia, 10, 167
Zimbabwe, 19–20, 162, 165–167, 178; adaptation of Vienna Plan in, 204–205; collaboration of social workers and HelpAge International in, 182–184; National Plan for the Elderly, 167; National Plan on Aging, 193; social security in, 128; social work education in, 165, 167, 211. *See also* Hampson, Joseph
Zimbabwe African National Union (ZANU), 167